AF598662

RESEARCH PROGRESS IN ALZHEIMER'S DISEASE AND DEMENTIA (VOL. 4)

RESEARCH PROGRESS IN ALZHEIMER'S AND DEMENTIA SERIES

Research Progress in Alzheimer's Disease and Dementia, Vol. 1
Miao-Kun Sun
2007. ISBN: 1-59454-949-4

Research Progress in Alzheimer's Disease and Dementia, Vol. 3
Miao-Kun Sun
2008 ISBN: 1-60021-960-8

Research Progress In Alzheimer's Disease and Dementia, Vol. 4
Miao-Kun Sun
2009 ISBN: 978-1-60876-152-4

RESEARCH PROGRESS IN ALZHEIMER'S DISEASE AND DEMENTIA SERIES

RESEARCH PROGRESS IN ALZHEIMER'S DISEASE AND DEMENTIA (VOL. 4)

MIAO-KUN SUN
EDITOR

Nova Biomedical Books
New York

For permission to use material from this book please contact us:
Telephone 631-231-7269; Fax 631-231-8175
Web Site: http://www.novapublishers.com

Library of Congress Cataloging-in-Publication Data

Available upon request

ISBN 978-1-60876-152-4

Published by Nova Science Publishers, Inc. ✢ New York

Contents

Preface	*Miao-Kun Sun*	**vii**
Chapter I	**Emotional Memory in Alzheimer's Disease** *Jill D. Waring and Elizabeth A. Kensinger*	**9**
Chapter II	**Mechanisms of AMYLOID-β Clearence in Alzheimer's Disease** *Joseph El Khoury and Suzanne E. Hickman*	**37**
Chapter III	**Synaptic Transmission Regulates Amyloid-β Dynamics** *John R. Cirrito*	**67**
Chapter IV	**Anti-Aβ Antibodies for the Treatment of Alzheimer's Disease** *Bin Liu, Hongjun Fu, Jeffrey L. Frost and Cynthia A. Lemere*	**85**
Chapter V	**The Failure of the APP Transgenic Mouse Models to Predict Efficacy of Agents in Five Clinical Trials of Alzheimer's Disease Suggests that there is a Need for a New Paradigm for Drug Development** *Jordan L. Holtzman*	**113**
Chapter VI	**Apolipoprotein E and Alzheimer's Disease: An Update on Allele-Specific Effects of Disease Etiology** *Ann M. Saunders*	**145**
Chapter VII	**Chronic Inflammation and Alzheimer's Disease** *Douglas G. Walker, Jason Yuan and Lih-Fen Lue*	**161**
Chapter VIII	**Cathepsins in Alzheimer's Disease and Dementia: Cathepsin Inhibitors as Potential Anti-Dementic Therapeutics** *Azizul Haque, Naren L. Banik and Swapan K. Ray*	**185**
Chapter IX	**Role of Gelsolin in Alzheimer's Disease** *Lina Ji, Abha Chauhan and Ved Chauhan*	**199**

Chapter X **Declarative Memory Impairment and Hippocampal Atrophy in Parkinson's Disease** **219**
Carme Junque

Chapter XI **Fronto-Temporal Dementia** **243**
Alfredo Postiglione, Graziella Milan and Sabina Pappatà

Chapter XII **Cognitive Impairment in Schizophrenia** **263**
Verity C Leeson and Eileen M Joyce

Index **281**

In: Alzheimer's Disease and Dementia (Vol. 4) ISBN:978-1-60876-152-4
Editor: Miao-Kun Sun

Preface

Research Progress in Alzheimer's Disease and Dementia (Volume 4)

Miao-Kun Sun
Blanchette Rockefeller Neurosciences Institute, USA

Dementia, including Alzheimer's disease (AD), progressively robs the cognitive ability of those affected, i.e., the ability to learn, memorize, reason, communicate, judge, and carry out daily activities. AD is characterized pathologically by extracellular amyloid plaques containing amyloid β peptide (Aβ) in the brain and intracellular neurofibrillary tangles containing hyperphosphorylated microtubule protein tau, pathophysiologically by synaptic dysfunction/synaptic loss, and clinically by a progressive loss of memory.

The main focuses of research efforts in AD and dementia are to define the underlying pathogenic mechanisms and to develop methods that are reliable for the diagnosis of early AD and therapies that directly target the underlying causes of the disorders. In AD, the ability for emotion to influence memory is particularly disrupted. Accumulation of Aβ is still believed to play a critical role in the AD pathogenesis, including those patients with familial early-onset AD, a rare disease, and late-onset AD, the sporadic and common form of the disorder. Aβ clearance from the brain depends on three major pathways: uptake of Aβ by specific receptors expressed on microglia and astrocytes followed by intracellular degradation, extracellular degradation by surface bound or released Aβ-degrading enzymes, and transport across the blood brain barrier. The pathways linking synaptic activity and Aβ, on the other hand, may provide opportunities to interrupt relationship between synaptic activity and Aβ dynamics. Numerous efforts are also underway to develop refined, highly effective and possibly safer active and passive immunotherapeutic approaches. The failure of the APP transgenic mouse models to predict efficacy of agents in several clinical trials of AD, however, suggests that there is a need for a new paradigm for drug development.

Remarkable progress has been made in understanding the susceptibility genetics of *APOE* and AD and the influence of a common polymorphism on recovery from acute brain stresses and in understanding neuroinflammation and acidic cathepsins in AD pathogenesis. Gelsolin as an anti-amyloidogenic agent that can reduce amyloid load by acting as Aβ-sequestering agent and/or as an inhibitor of Aβ fibrillization. Memory impairments are not only observed in AD, but also in other neurodegenerative diseases and behavioral disorders, such as the Parkinson's disease, fronto-temporal dementia, and schizophrenia, all of which demand effective cognitive therapeutics.

All these new developments further indicate the multi-disciplinary nature of AD and dementia research. The emergence of an effective cure of AD and dementia depends on how well we understand the underlying pathogenic mechanisms. Our hope is that effective therapeutic agents that target memory-relevant AD pathogenesis and other dementic disorders are developed soon, through the intensive research efforts worldwide, as evidenced in this book volume.

In: Alzheimer's Disease and Dementia (Vol. 4)
Editor: Miao-Kun Sun

ISBN:978-1-60876-152-4

Chapter I

Emotional Memory in Alzheimer's Disease

Jill D. Waring and Elizabeth A. Kensinger
Department of Psychology, Boston College, Chestnut Hill, MA USA

Abstract

Events that elicit an emotional response usually are more likely to be retained in mind than more mundane experiences. This beneficial effect of emotion on memory has been proposed to arise from a combination of two types of processes: emotion can directly modulate memory processes, and it also can exert indirect influences on memory via its effects on attention and elaboration (see Talmi, Anderson, Riggs, Caplan, & Moscovitch, 2008). In this chapter, we describe the effects of healthy aging on emotional memory, and we discuss how the neurocognitive changes that occur with Alzheimer's disease (AD) may lead to a disruption in many of the effects of emotion on memory. We hypothesize that AD may particularly disrupt the ability for emotion to influence memory via indirect effects on attention and elaboration, and we consider directions for future research that would allow this hypothesis to be examined directly.

Abbreviation List

AD = Alzheimer's disease

aMCI = MCI amnestic variety;

md-MCI= MCI multiple domains;

BDS = Blessed Dementia Rating Scale (Blessed, Tomlinson, & Roth, 1968)

beh. = behavioral study; ERP = event-related potentials

fMRI = functional magnetic resonance imaging; MCI = Mild Cognitive Impairment,

MMSE= mini mental state examination (Folstein, Folstein, & McHugh, 1975); rcg. = recognition; y/n= yes/no forced choice recognition; wm = working memory;

n/a = not applicable;
nr = not reported;

Introduction

Strong emotions often punctuate our most significant life experiences, leaving a seemingly indelible mark in our memory. Instances of forgetting supposedly unimportant, everyday information - like what we had for lunch yesterday or the weather report from last month - are frequent and generally unremarkable events for most people. In sharp contrast, forgetting events with great emotional importance - like the birth of a grandchild or a natural disaster - seems more unusual and surprising. Emotional memory is a particularly interesting concept to examine across the adult lifespan because although there are declines in many skills and abilities arising with aging, the ability for emotional experiences to be preferentially processed and maintained in memory is largely preserved in healthy older adults (Hess, 2005; Mather & Carstensen, 2005). By contrast, for many people who develop dementias like Alzheimer's disease (AD) as they age, emotional information may not hold the same degree of salience or the same privileged status in memory.

In order to understand the effects of aging and AD on emotional memory, it is first necessary to consider the processes that support emotional memory in a healthy, young adult. A tremendous amount of research in this area has revealed that emotion can directly modulate memory processes. At a neural level, this modulation appears to occur via interactions between the amygdala and the hippocampus: the amygdala, when activated by a release of stress hormones, can modulate hippocampal function and thereby increase the likelihood that an emotional experience is consolidated, or solidified in memory (McGaugh, 2004; Phelps & LeDoux, 2005). Although much of the research examining interactions between emotion and memory has focused on these amygdala-hippocampal connections, it is becoming clear that emotion can also influence memory via other means as well. Emotion can influence the likelihood that attention is allocated to information, that sensory details are processed, or that the significance of information is considered and elaborated upon (reviewed by Kensinger, 2004; Vuilleumier & Driver, 2007). All of these influences are likely to have downstream consequences for memory (see Hamann, 2001). It is well known that information is remembered best when it is attended to and processed in a deep, meaningful fashion (Craik & Lockhart, 1972). Indeed, a number of neuroimaging studies have revealed that in addition to amygdala-hippocampal interactions, the amount of activity elicited within sensory regions, within attentional circuits, and within semantic elaboration regions can predict the likelihood that emotional information is remembered (Mickley & Kensinger, 2008; Kensinger, in press; Talmi et al., 2008).

When examining the effect of emotion on memory, it is therefore important to consider whether the effect of emotion is likely to result from a direct modulation of mnemonic processes or from indirect influences on other attentional, sensory, or conceptual processes (discussed by Talmi et al., 2007). Although many studies have assumed that disruptions in emotional memory – with AD or with other pathologies – are due to disruptions in the direct modulation of memory, it must be considered that the disruption could also arise from a reduced effect of emotion on attentional, sensory, or conceptual processes. We will return to this important issue later in the chapter, when we hypothesize about the core deficit underlying the changes in emotional memory that accompany AD. But first, we outline the neurocognitive changes that accompany healthy aging and AD, and we describe the behavioral effects of emotion on memory in these groups of older adults.

Neurocognitive Changes in Healthy Aging and Alzheimer's Disease: Links to Emotional Memory

The contrasting effects of healthy aging versus AD on emotional memory can be better understood by first considering the types of brain changes that occur with each trajectory. The normal aging process is marked by some reduction of the brain's grey and white matter volumes, as well as by alterations in the strength of the connections between brain regions. Importantly, aging has relatively little impact on the volume of structures within the limbic and paralimbic/sensory-integration circuits that are relevant for emotion processing, with structures including the amygdala, hippocampus, thalamus, and cingulate gyrus showing only modest volumetric and connectivity reductions with advancing age (Chow & Cummings, 2000; Salat, Kaye & Janowsky, 2001). The relative preservation of these regions contrasts with the more significant changes within the frontal and parietal lobes, regions that are responsible for more controlled cognitive processing and which are more vulnerable to age-related changes (Grieve, Clark, Williams, Peduto, & Gordon, 2005; Ziegler, Piguet, Salat, Prince, Connally, & Corkin, in press). It has been proposed that this pocket of preservation within the limbic system explains why older adults focus upon, and remember emotional information at least as readily as young adults (e.g., Cacioppo, Berntson, Bechara, Tranel, & Hawkley, in press).

It is well known that AD – the most common form of dementia - presents a number of challenges to the integrity of brain structure and function, with the pathological features that develop in AD (i.e., the extracellular accumulation of amyloid plaques and the intracellular deposition of neurofibrillary tangles) following a different pattern of distribution across the brain from the changes arising within the course of normal aging (Head, Snyder, Girton, Morris, & Buckner, 2004; Knopman et al., 2003). These pathological features interfere with normal neural connectivity and subcortico-cortical neural projections, which in turn lead to a breakdown in neural circuits and increase cognitive dysfunction. Of most importance for our discussion of emotional memory, in contrast to the relative preservation of limbic structures in healthy aging processes, limbic areas are the hardest hit in AD, pointing to the likely root of qualitative and quantitative differences in emotional memory content for those with AD pathology relative to those following a normal course of aging.

Structural brain images reveal severe volumetric loss in the hippocampus as one of the most obvious anatomical changes of the AD brain relative to the non-pathological aging brain (see Shi et al., in press, for meta-analysis). The left and right amygdalae also have significantly reduced volume in patients with AD as compared to healthy older adults (Horinek, Varjassyova, Hort, 2007; Wright, Dickerson, Feczko, Negeira, & Williams, 2007); compared with approximately 2% loss in amygdala volume in normal aging, there is approximately 26% loss in the amygdala volume of AD patients (for review see Chow & Cummings, 2000). The amygdala is also one of the brain regions most susceptible to plaques and tangles pathology, and it is among those regions affected earliest in the disease process, along with the entorhinal and hippocampal cortices (Mori, Ikeda, Hirono, Kitagaki, Imamura, & Shimomura, 1999; Scott, DeKosky, & Scheff, 1991).

Given the amygdala's vital role in proficient emotion processing and emotional memory (for review see Phelps & LeDoux, 2005), deficiencies in this region's structure and function would be likely to interfere with emotional memory. More specifically, given that amygdala-hippocampal connections are integral for creating emotional memories, the extensive involvement of both of these regions, even within mild cases of AD, leads to the prediction that AD should disrupt memory for emotional information more than should healthy aging. In general, this prediction seems to be upheld; impairment in emotional memory abilities is generally more dramatic in AD than what is evidenced in healthy aging adults. However, as will be discussed later in this chapter, results have been mixed regarding the extent to which emotional memory is affected in AD. The discrepant results may have arisen because a wide variety of methodologies have been employed in the published studies examining emotional memory in AD, and there has been little replication of specific methodologies. It is also likely that the models of emotional memory that are currently being used to examine changes in AD are too simplified to draw a solid distinction between the aspects of the memory system that are impaired and those that are preserved. As noted earlier in this chapter, recent research has emphasized that emotional memory is supported not only by direct effects of emotion on amygdala-hippocampal interactions but also by indirect effects of emotion yielded by influences on regions within sensory and frontal cortices (Dolcos, LaBar, & Cabeza, 2004; Kensinger & Schacter, 2006; Kensinger & Schacter, 2008b; Pourtois, Schwartz, Seghier, Lazeyras, & Vuilleumier, 2006). It remains untested to what extent these different types of processes are preserved in AD. For example, limbic structures beyond the amygdala and the hippocampus - including the thalamus, caudate, and basal ganglia - usually retain their normal volumes (Grieve et al., 2005). These findings leave open the possibility that some aspects of processing and memory for emotional information may be selectively impaired in AD while others may be better preserved.

Perception of Emotion in Healthy Aging and AD

Before considering the results of studies investigating emotional memory, it is important to first confirm that emotion is perceived in the same way by patients with AD and by healthy older adults. This first stage of emotion perception is necessary to equate because otherwise any differences or changes observed in AD may not be memory-specific; if AD patients did not perceive stimuli as emotional, or did not experience the same quality or magnitude of emotional response as a healthy individual, then it would neither be surprising, nor informative, to find that the AD patients did not retain that information in the same fashion as their healthy counterparts.

Results from the studies examining emotion labeling, identification, and priming in patients with AD have shown that these abilities often are well-preserved, at least in early disease stages (LaBar, Torpey, Cook, Johnson, Warren, Burke, & Welch-Bohmer, 2005; Koff, Zaitchik, Montepara, & Albert, 1999; Shimokawa, Yakomi, Anamizu, Ashikari, Kohno, Maki, et al., 2000; Bucks & Radford, 2004; but see Padovan, Versace, Thomas-Anterion, & Laurent, 2002; Spoletini, Marra, Iulio, Gianni, Sancesario, Giubilei, Trequattrini, Bria, Caltagirone, & Spalletta, 2008; Teng et al., 2007). The ability to correctly label emotional faces, voices, or body language (Burnham & Hogervorst, 2004; Koff et al., 1999), and to demonstrate normal skin conductance responses to emotional information (Hamann et al., 2000), is comparable in individuals with early AD and in healthy older adults. These findings have been essential for the study of emotional memory, because they indicate that any differences in emotional memory do not simply reflect differences in how AD patients initially perceive the emotional nature of a situation.

Emotional Memory in Older Adulthood

Because AD patients' ability to remember emotional experiences may be affected both by the pathology that is specific to AD and also by those changes that occur more generally because of advancing age, it is important to spend a bit of time outlining the way in which emotional memory is affected by nonpathological aging. Investigations of age-related changes in emotional memory have highlighted two important distinctions that must be made when discussing emotion processing. First, there is a need to appreciate the different dimensions that can describe an affective experience. Not all emotions need to be processed or remembered in the same way, and many of the models of age-related changes in memory have honed in on the need to consider separately the dimensions of *valence*, referring to the pleasantness or unpleasantness of an experience, and *arousal*, referring to the exciting/agitating or calming/subduing nature an experience (Burke, Heuer, & Reisburg, 1992; Libkuman, Stabler, & Otani, 2004; see Russell, 1980 for discussion of these dimensions). As will be elaborated below, age changes tend to be minimal if valence is ignored and only the dimension of arousal is considered; like young adults, older adults usually remember more arousing experiences than nonarousing ones (reviewed by Kensinger, 2009). However, when the valence of information is considered, age differences become more apparent (reviewed by Mather, 2006). Second, a distinction should be made between those processes that occur relatively automatically (i.e., without conscious effort) and those that occur because of the implementation of controlled strategies (see Satpute & Lieberman, 2006 discussion of for the importance of this distinction as it relates to emotion processing). Age-related changes seem to be most abundant when the controlled processing of emotional information is analyzed, whereas there seems to be little impact of aging on the more automatic processing of emotional information (e.g., Mather, 2006; Murphy & Isaacowitz, 2008).

Valence-Specific Effects on Memory: Age-Related Changes

Though consensus has not been reached as to the degree to which emotional memory changes as a function of age, when changes are noted, they have tended to reveal a "positivity effect" with age. As suggested by the name, the "positivity effect" denotes the fact that older adults will tend to remember proportionally more positive information than younger adults (Mather & Carstensen, 2005). In some instances, a *strong* positivity effect has been noted, revealing a valence-based reversal in the types of information retained by young and older adults; in these studies, young adults have remembered relatively more negative information while older adults have remembered relatively more positive information. More commonly, however, a *weak* positivity effect has been noted, with young adults remembering more negative than positive information, and older adults remembering an equivalent proportion of negative and positive information. The commonality across both of these instantiations (*weak* and *strong* ones) is that, as compared to young adults, proportionally more of what older adults remember is of positive emotional valence (see Kensinger, O'Brien, Swanberg, Garoff-Eaton, & Schacter, 2007 for further discussion).

Interestingly, the interaction between valence and age tends to occur most readily when memory for the "gist" or general theme of information is sufficient for task performance. In these instances – when all that is required is for participants to recall the general details of an event or to recognize global event features – older adults often show a positivity effect. By contrast, when it is necessary that participants recall the details of an event –how an event unfolded, or what a particular stimulus looked like – then both age groups show a benefit for remembering the details of negative experiences (e.g., Kensinger, O'Brien, et al. 2007; Kensinger, Garoff-Eaton, & Schacter, 2007). These results suggest that positive valence may benefit older adults' abilities to remember the "gist," but it does not allow them to retain the details. Corroborating evidence for this proposal has come from neuroimaging studies revealing that the regions that correspond with older adults' abilities to remember positive information tend to be frontal regions that are also implicated in self-referential processing and with conceptual elaboration (e.g., Addis, Leclerc, Muscatell, & Kensinger, in press; Kensinger & Schacter, 2008b).

Age-Related Differences are Driven by Changes in Controlled Processes

Many of the mechanisms underlying the positivity effect remain a topic of active debate; for example, it is not clear whether the effect is best characterized as an age-related shift away from the negative (i.e., to avoid and forget bad things) or as a shift toward the positive (i.e., to seek and remember good things; Murphy & Isaacowitz, 2008 for recent discussion). What has been proposed, however, is that the positivity effect arises from age-related changes in motivational goals: As a consequence of viewing lifetime as more limited, older adults tend to put a greater emphasis on emotion-relevant goals. This motivational shift may drive them to focus more on the positive, or less on the negative, and thus to remember emotionally valenced information in a different fashion than younger adults.

An intriguing aspect of the positivity effect is that it appears to be engaged only when older adults are able to implement controlled strategies to process the emotional information. Thus, the positivity effect arises when older adults have sufficient cognitive resources to devote toward emotional processing and when they are given ample time to devote those resources toward the emotional items (Isaacowitz, Wadlinger, Goren, & Wilson, 2006; Mather & Knight, 2005). For example, the positivity effect is most robust in older adults with good cognitive control, and on tasks that allow older adults to devote their full attention toward the processing of emotional information (Mather & Knight, 2005). The effect also exists on tasks, and for stimuli, that rely on controlled processing, but not on those that rely on more automatic phases of processing (discussed by Kensinger & Leclerc, in press; Mather, 2006). For example, older adults are just as likely to rapidly detect negative items in a spatial array as they are to detect positive items, and older adults do not show a facilitated ability to see positive words briefly presented within a series of distractor words (e.g., Leclerc & Kensinger, 2008; Mickley, Muscatell, & Kensinger, submitted). Yet the positivity effect is pervasive on tasks of sustained attention, with older adults focusing more on positive information than on negative information, and processing positive information more deeply and for a longer period of time than young adults (e.g., Isaacowitz et al., 2006; Mather & Knight, 2005). These lines of evidence converge to suggest that the positivity effect has more to do with age-related changes in how older adults sustain attention and elaborate upon emotional information than with changes in how older adults initially detect emotional information (see Mather, 2006 for further discussion). Though it is still not clear exactly how sustained attention and elaborative processing change with aging, it is possible that the changes are related to older adults' attempts to interpret and regulate their emotional responses (e.g., to make negative events seem less bad; Mather, 2006) and to process information in a self-relevant fashion (e.g., to think about a positive event's relation to one's life or self concept; Kensinger & Leclerc, in press).

Although there has not been much neuroimaging data gathered yet to examine how aging affects emotional memory, the extant data suggest that the age-related changes may not be tied to a failure of the amygdala to modulate hippocampal activity. Amygdala and hippocampal activity are predictors of subsequent-memory for emotional information in older adults just as they are in young adults (Kensinger & Schacter, 2008b), and connectivity between these regions can be strong for both positive and negative information (Addis et al., submitted). It therefore seems plausible that age-related changes in emotional memory have more to do with emotion's indirect influences on attentional, sensory, or elaborative processes than with emotion's direct modulation of mnemonic processes, and this conclusion would be generally consistent with the behavioral evidence outlined above. There is still a dearth of data speaking directly to this hypothesis, and so future research will be needed to examine its validity.

Emotional Memory in Alzheimer's Disease

When considering how Alzheimer's disease affects the interactions between emotion and memory, there are a number of factors that must be taken into consideration. First, as noted above, it is essential to consider the valence of the emotion that is elicited; positive and negative information are not always remembered in the same fashion, and the influence of valence on memory may change as older adults age (see Kensinger, 2009; Mather, 2006 for further discussion). Second, the type of stimulus must be considered; stimuli that evoke stronger or more sustained emotion (e.g., real-life experiences or video clips) may have different effects on memory from stimuli that evoke short-lived or weaker emotions (e.g., single words). Third, careful consideration must be given to the memory demands required by the task, such as whether information is retained over short or long delays, or whether memory for "gist" is sufficient or a detailed memory is required. Fourth, it should be considered whether changes in emotional memory reflect differences in how emotion modulates mnemonic processes directly or in how emotion exerts effects on memory indirectly via its influences on attentional, sensory, or elaborative processes. In the sections below, each of these factors is considered in turn.

Effects of Valence on Memory in Alzheimer's Disease

In contrast to the widespread interest in examining the effects of valence upon older adults' emotional memories, less attention has been paid to the valence dimension when assessing the memories of patients with Alzheimer's disease. Of the studies to examine emotional memory in Alzheimer's disease, over half have restricted their analyses to negative materials (see Table 1). Of those that have examined effects of both valences, many have not equated the positive and negative stimuli for arousal level (a common problem when using facial expressions, since many negative expressions are higher in arousal than positive expressions), making it impossible to isolate the influence of valence. From the remaining handful of studies that have included positive and negative stimuli matched in arousal level, there appears to be little evidence of a "positivity effect" in the memories of the Alzheimer's disease patients, with only one study showing better recall of positive than negative stimuli in these patients (Hamann, et al., 2000). In the other studies, patients either have shown no memory enhancement for either valence (Abrisqueta-Gomez, Bueno, Oliviera, & Bertolucci, 2002; Kensinger et al., 2002) or they have shown better memory for the negative stimuli than for the positive ones (Fleming, Kim, Doo, Maguire, & Potkin, 2003). Although more research is clearly needed, the extant data do not support maintenance of a "positivity effect" in Alzheimer's disease. If true, it will be important for researchers to examine why the effect disappears--do these patients not have the same motivational goals as their healthy counterparts, or is there something about the disease process that destroys the neural processes that are required for a positivity effect to emerge? We will return to these important questions later in this chapter.

Table 1. Summary of laboratory studies testing emotional memory in Alzheimer's disease.

Study	Participants			Paradigm						Results		Conclusions
	# controls	#patients	disease severity	measures	material type	emotions tested	exposure duration	study-test	type of memory	EEM observed?	Other results	
Abrisqueta-Gomez et al., 2002	19	16	19.9	beh.	pix	pos/neg/neu	6sec	30-min	rcg. y/n	AD no EEM, and poorer rcg. overall	emotion identification retained	AD affects emo memory, but not identification
Boller et al., 2002	12	10	19.6	beh.	6 stories & narrative	happy/sad/neu	nr	none & 10+ min	immediate & delayed recall (if incorrect, then 4-choice rcg.)	AD immed EEM (sad & happy) > neu. After delay, a floor effect, rcg. emo>neu	no correlation between memory and P300.	EEM preserved, but attn impairment indicated by MMN & P300 components
Brueckner & Moritz, 2009	20	27 MCI, 36 AD	AD=24, MCI=nr	beh.	semantically associated word lists	neg/pos/neu	2sec	none	rcg. y/n	AD no EEM, YA & MCI yes	YA show incr false rcg for neg items; MCI and AD show incr false rcg for all emo items (pos or neg)	MCI and AD patients more likely than YA to falsely rcg emotional items; EEM for veridical rcg disrupted in AD but not

Table 1. (Continued)

Budson et al., 2006	19	19	23	beh.	semantically associated word lists	neg/non-emo	2600ms	5-min	rcg. y/n	AD no EEM, YA & OA yes	AD conservative bias for emotional words, YA & OA liberal	amy. pathology in early disease state may affect normal criterion shift for emo stimuli
Dohnel et al., 2007	10	10 MCI	nr	beh.	pix-IAPS	pos/neg/neu	2700ms	2-back wm task	working memory	OA no EEM. MCI yes, with a negativity bias. MCI overall performance comparable to OA.		neg info can enh. memory in MCI
Dohnel et al., 2008	16	16 MCI	(-0.81= patients' MMSE z-score)	fMRI	pix-IAPS	pos/neg/neu	2700ms	2-back wm task, 20-100sec.	working memory	OA no EEM, aMCI yes with negativity bias	MCI: R precuneus neg>neu =fail to deactivate	emo did not sig. affect OA WM, overall MCI < OA . Neg valence may help MCI pts. to compensate for disease related changes, but may be confounded with higher
Fleming et al., 2003	19	25	21	beh.	words	pos/neg/neu	nr	none	recall	AD neg>pos or neu		memory for (neg) emo preserved in

Table 1. (Continued)

Hamann et al., 2000	24	12	21.5	emo arousal rating, recall, & recognition	pix-IAPS	pos/neg/neu	6 sec	none	recall & y/n rcg.	Recall, AD EEM pos., not neg; OA-EEM pos & neg. Rcg., AD no EEM; OA neg		reactions normal, but EEM impaired for neg & normal for pos.
Kazui et al., 2000	10	34	22.6	beh.	narrated slide show	neg/neu	20sec/slide, 11 slides total	5-min	recall cued by photos	AD-EEM for neg v. neu portions		similar enhancement for pts & controls, although pts lower memory overall
Kazui et al., 2003	n/a	56	23.3	beh.	narrated slide show	neg/neu	20sec/slide, 11 slides total	5-min	recall cued by photos	AD EEM spared to some extent	Emotional memory related to general visual, but not verbal	
Kensinger et al., 2002; Expt. 1	20	13	BDS m=4.8	beh.	pix	pos/ neg/ neu	5 sec, 2x each	none?	recall	AD no EEM		mild AD affects emo mem, but ratings/perception intact.

Table 1. (Continued)

Kensinger et al., 2002; Expt. 2	20	13	BDS m=4.8	beh.	word list	pos, neg, neu	3 sec, 2x each	none?	recall	AD no EEM for words, but trend toward pos>neg. Pos recall in AD n/s diff from OA.		mild AD affects emotional memory, but ratings & perception intact.□
Kensinger et al., 2004	51	80	23.2	beh.	NYU stories	neg/neu	~30sec to read	none, & delay (10-min in AD/ 24-h in OA)	recall, 4-choice rcg.	AD no EEM for any condition		AD disrupts EEM for verbal info.
Koff et al., 1999	19	23	20.3	beh. emotion identification	audio, video, pix	happy/sad/ angry/neu	nr	n/a	emo rcg. matching	variable results, in AD: audio identification mainly preserved, more impaired in identifying drawing and video		AD not an emotion processing problem
Moayeri et al., 2000	16	28	19.6	beh.	narrated slide show	neg/neu	time taken to read	5-min., after narrative heard	y/n rcg. of photos, and questions	AD EEM neg > neu; OA no EEM (ceiling effects?)		influence of emotion spared in AD

Table 1. (Continued)

Rosenbaum et al., in press	21	11	24	PET, connectivity	emotional facial expession identification	happy/neu	4 sec	variable, 1-16 sec.	2-alternative forced choice	AD performance declined with inc. delay length	effective connections to amygdala stronger in AD than OA, left lateralized	possibly compensatory recruitment of emotion network to compensate for frontal loss
Satler et al., 2007	10	10	nr	beh.	narrated slide show	neg/neu	time taken to read	5-min	recall cued by photos	AD EEM, controls no EEM (ceiling effects?)		
Spoletini et al., 2008	50	50 aMCI, 50 AD	MCI≥23, AD≥18	beh. emotion identification	emotional faces	high intensity/ low intensity/ neu	nr	n/a	emotion identification	AD more impaired identifying almost all emotional faces than MCI or OA		increased progression in global facial emotion rcg. deficit from OA to MCI to AD
Teng et al., 2007	68	9 aMCI, 14 md-MCI	aMCI= 26.9, md-MCI=	beh. emotion identification	emotional faces	happy, sad, angry, frightened, neutral	nr	n/a	5 tests to identify emotion	Intact in aMCI, impaired in md-MCI.	performance in md-MCI correlated with	facial affect processing impaired early in MCI
Wright et al., 2007	12	12	24.6	fMRI	emotional faces	novel fearful & familiar neutral	200ms	variable	passive viewing	exaggerated, non-specific amygdala response in AD		amygdala dysfunction present in early AD

Notes: # of patients = # with AD, unless otherwise specified; n/a = not applicable; nr = not reported;
OA = healthy older adult; YA = young adult; MCI = Mild Cognitive Impairment, aMCI = MCI amnestic variety; md-MCI= MCI multiple domains;
MMSE= mini mental state examination (Folstein, Folstein, & McHugh, 1975); BDS = Blessed Dementia Rating Scale (Blessed, Tomlinson, & Roth, 1968)
beh. = behavioral study; fMRI = functional MRI; rcg. = recognition; y/n= yes/no forced choice; wm = working memory

Effects of Stimulus Type on Emotional Memory in Alzheimer's Disease

Although the unique contribution of emotional valence is likely to be a very important factor, the influence of the stimulus type – and the way in which participants are asked to process the stimuli – are factors that should not be ignored. Depending upon the type of stimulus used, and the task required of participants, the resulting affective responses can either be minimal and very short-lived (e.g., when using facial expressions or single words) or longer-lasting and more intense (e.g., when assessing memory for autobiographical experiences or video clips). From the generally mixed findings, dividing the literature by whether the study investigators employed faces, word lists, pictures, or narrative stories as stimuli may reveal patterns in how AD may differentially enhance or impair memory for emotional information relative to the healthy aging process. These factors may have their own unique influences on emotional memory in AD, and they may also modulate the effect of valence.

The simplest level of task demands are studies assessing AD patients' ability to identify and remember emotional facial expressions. These studies usually require either passive viewing of facial expressions or very simple identification of facial expressions, so the encoding task is a basic and straightforward one. Often these studies evoke only minimal emotional responses from the participants – usually facial expressions are presented briefly, and it is well known that facial expressions rarely elicit any stress response in a participant (e.g., Anderson, Wais & Gabrieli, 2006). Although the range of facial emotional expressions examined has varied a great deal across studies, many of these studies have revealed a greater degree of impairment in correct identification and recognition memory of emotional faces by AD patients than healthy older adults. Interestingly, many of these studies have found that these abilities were generally preserved in those with mild cognitive impairment (MCI) (Spoletini et al., 2008; Teng, Lu, & Cummings, 2007), suggesting that the deficits may be related to changes in amygdala activation or connectivity that arise during the progression of AD (Rosenbaum, Furey, Horowitz, & Grady, in press; Wright et al., 2007).

Sequential lists of emotional words are another type of stimulus that is likely to elicit at most a low-intensity, short-lived emotional response. The limited number of studies currently available permit few conclusions about the presence or absence of an emotional memory enhancement for words in AD, and these studies also leave open questions about the specific contribution of the varied study methodologies upon the results observed. Across studies, it seems that there are instances where emotional words can have a beneficial effect upon AD patients' memory relative to neutral words; however this is not a reliable effect across studies (see Table 1). For example, one group of researchers found that the emotional enhancement in memory was preserved in AD for negative words more so than for than positive ones, yet the arousal level of the positive and negative emotional words may not have been equivalently matched (Fleming et al., 2003), complicating the interpretation of their results. However, in another study where the arousal level of the words was matched, there was no significant enhancement in AD patients' memory for positive or negative words, although there was a trend toward better memory for positive words (Kensinger et al., 2002, expt 2). Two other studies sought to probe several possible effects of emotion upon true and false recognition memory for semantically related emotional and neutral word lists (Brueckner & Moritz, 2009; Budson, Todman, Chong, Adams, Kensinger, Krangel, & Wright, 2006). Budson and colleagues' (2006) results demonstrated that in contrast to healthy older adults' memory, AD patients did not retain a memory benefit for negative words (positive words were not included), nor did they show an improvement in item-specific recollection (memory for a specific item) nor in gist memory (memory for the general theme of presented information). As compared to older adults, AD patients also showed the opposite effect of emotion upon their response bias (tendency toward endorsing recognition memory test items as 'old' or 'new'); AD patients evidenced a more conservative response bias to negative words than to neutral words (more like to say that negative words were novel or 'new'), whereas healthy older adults showed a more liberal response bias to negative words (more likely to say they had been studied previously, or 'old'). Brueckner & Moritz (2009) also observed that AD and MCI patients had higher false recognition of semantically-related emotional words. The emotional enhancement in memory was disrupted in AD patients but not in MCI. The lack of agreement among results of these three studies leaves remaining questions about distinctions between the effects of valence and arousal of emotional words on memory in AD, and the effect of study design on the observed results.

There is somewhat more consistency in results across studies assessing memory for emotional pictures, although results are still somewhat mixed and scant. Most previous studies drew their stimuli from the International Affective Picture System (IAPS; Lang, Bradley & Cuthbert, 1997), thereby providing continuity between studies at least for the stimuli selected. Across studies, the pictures chosen were drawn from a range of positively, negatively, and neutrally valenced images, however the mean arousal level between groups of positive and negative pictures was not always matched. Further, despite the similarity in stimuli used across studies, particular study methodologies varied quite a bit in terms of their task demands (see Table 1). The studies are divided among those assessing recall, recognition, and working memory for emotional pictures, with only a handful of studies assessing memory in each of those ways. Results have shown that patients with AD frequently have an impaired emotional enhancement in recognition memory for positive and negative pictures relative to healthy older adults (Abrisqueta-Gomez, et al., 2002; Hamann, et al., 2000). There has been extensive variability between studies in the effects of positive or negative pictures upon memory recall. One study reported a positivity bias in AD patients' memory for emotional pictures (Hamann et al., 2000), while another concluded there was no memory benefit for either negative or positive information in those with AD (Kensinger et al., 2002, expt. 1). Although limited in number, the studies of working memory revealed a negativity bias in the memories of MCI patients (but the negative items were also more arousing than positive items, making it impossible to attribute these differences to valence alone; Dohnel, Sommer, Ibach, Rothmayr, Meinhardt, & Hajak, 2008; Dohnel, Sommer, Reindl, Muller, Hajak, & Ibach, 2007). Further investigations carefully manipulating study methodologies would likely add greater consensus to the question of the impact of MCI and AD on memory for emotional words or pictures.

The research studies employing the most complex type of emotional stimuli, narrative stories, were also those that most often revealed the preservation of the emotional enhancement in memory in AD patients. Several studies have employed similar methodology, asking participants to view a narrated story accompanying a series of slides (methods adapted from Cahill & McGaugh, 1995). In this paradigm, there are two versions of the story, which differ only in the narration of the middle portion of the story; the beginning and end of the narrative story, and all of the slides that are shown to participants, are identical in the two versions. In the critical middle portion of the narrative, the 'neutral' version describes a boy visiting his father who works in a hospital, while the 'negative' version describes the boy being seriously injured and taken to the hospital for treatment. Results of these studies have revealed a preservation of the emotional enhancement in memory for the negative segment of the story in AD patients, suggesting that the addition of context or the continuity provided by a narrative structure may be an important factor influencing whether AD patients are able to demonstrate an emotional enhancement in recall or recognition memory, at least for negative information (Kazui, Mori, Hashimoto, et al., 2000, Kazui, Mori, Hashimoto, & Hirono, 2003; Moayeri, Cahill, Jin, & Potkin, 2000; Satler, Garrido, Sarmiento, Leme, Conde, & Tomaz, 2007). Two other studies examined memory for brief narratives without accompanying slides. These studies differed greatly from one another in their methodologies and results, in one case reporting that AD patients showed a benefit in recall and recognition memory for positive and negative short stories, with greater enhancement in memory revealed for the positive than negative stories (Boller, Massioui, Devouche, Traykov, Pomati, & Starkstein, 2002). The other study examined the effects of only negative compared to neutral narratives upon recall and recognition memory, finding no emotion-related enhancement in AD patients' memory (Kensinger, Anderson, Growdon, & Corkin, 2004).

As a whole, the studies examining emotional memory in AD using narrative stories have largely left unexplored the impact of positively valenced stories, with or without a visual component. A more inclusive approach to stimulus selection may lead to interesting revelations about the characteristics of an emotional bias in AD patients' memory and how it may differ from that observed in healthy older adults. Nevertheless, the existing data suggest that AD patients' memories may be most likely to benefit from the presence of emotion when there is more contextual information provided, and when the emotion elicited is longer lasting or more intense.

Effects of Memory Demands on Emotional Memory in Alzheimer's Disease

So far, our discussion has focused on the types of stimuli used and on the encoding task employed. But the retrieval tasks also can vary in the demands that they place on memory. Sometimes we are required to generate our own retrieval cues that will allow us to freely recall information. Other times we are given recognition prompts that will aide our mental search process. Sometimes we must retrieve the specific details of an event, whereas other times memory for "gist" is sufficient. Sometimes we must maintain information in mind for only a short period of time, while in other instances we must access information that we have not thought about for a while. In healthy adults, the effects of emotional arousal on memory tend to increase as memory demands intensify. The effects of emotional arousal are most noticeable after a delay (LaBar & Phelps, 1998; Payne, Stickgold, Swanberg, & Kensinger,

2008; Sharot & Phelps, 2004; Sharot & Yonelinas, 2008) and on tasks of recall rather than recognition (discussed by Kensinger & Schacter, 2008a).

In order to examine whether this pattern exists in AD, it would be prudent for a single study to assess the memory of AD patients after multiple delay intervals and to examine whether the enhancement in memory is more apparent after longer delays. In the absence of this type of within-subject design, it is impossible to draw strong conclusions, particularly because the methodologies of each study differ from one another in critical ways aside from retention interval (as noted earlier). Nevertheless, there is some evidence to suggest that delay can intensify the effects of emotion on AD patients' memories. The vast majority of laboratory studies have assessed recall performance after either no delay or a very short retention interval, and as noted earlier, the findings have not been consistent. In turn, AD patients have demonstrated no significant effects of emotion on memory (Kensinger et al., 2002, 2004; Budson et al., 2006), some benefit in memory for negative information (Boller et al., 2002; Kazui et al., 2000, 2003; Moayeri et al., 2000), or some benefit in memory for positive information (Hamann et al., 2000). Yet AD patients often show mnemonic benefits from emotion in studies that include much longer intervals (e.g., studies of "flashbulb memories"; Budson, Simons, Sullivan, Beier, Solomon, Scinto, Daffner, & Schacter, 2004; Ikeda, Mori, Hirono, Imamura, Shimomura, Ikejiri, & Yamashita, 1998). Although there are other differences, aside from the increased retention interval, which may contribute to this effect (such as the enhanced arousal associated with "flashbulb memories" as well as the increased event duration and the increased rehearsal likely to accompany such events), the extant data are at least consistent with the proposal that as the delay length increases, so does the probability of finding an effect of emotion.

There also is some evidence to suggest that the way in which retrieval is assessed can further influence the likelihood that emotion affects memory in AD. The studies that have used recognition have not found significant effects of emotion on AD patients' memories (Abrisqueta-Gomez et al., 2002; Budson et al., 2006; Hamann et al., 2000; Kensinger et al., 2002; Kensinger et al., 2004); by contrast, at least some of the studies that have assessed recall have noted an effect (Boller et al., 2002; Hamann et al., 2000; Kazui et al., 2000, 2003; Moayeri et al., 2000). Once again, a within-subjects design is necessary in order to give direct support to the claim (see Hamann et al., 2000 for the only such study), but the data seem to be compatible with the idea that as the retrieval demands increase, so does the likelihood of detecting an effect of emotion on AD patients' memories.

Interestingly, Budson, Simons, Waring, Sullivan, Hussion, & Schacter (2007) have proposed that many of the emotional memory deficits in AD may be related to initial encoding or storage problems, whereas AD patients may have less impairment maintaining or retrieving emotional memories. In their study, although AD patients initially remembered less about an emotional event than did control participants, over time, the slope of forgetting was no different for the AD patients than it was for the controls. These data suggest that the primary deficit in AD may be linked to the encoding phase, and the existing data from studies of emotional memory seem to be consistent with that proposal. AD patients show the least benefits from emotion when the ability to encode the information at the outset is assessed (e.g., by assessing memory after a short delay), whereas they show a greater benefit from emotion on tasks that assess the ability to retain information over time (e.g., by assessing the ability to maintain information across a long delay). Although no study has compared the decay of emotional *and* of neutral information across long delays in AD patients and in controls, if emotional information were to be better maintained by AD patients than neutral information, such a finding could suggest an important intersection between the effects of emotion on encoding and consolidation processes.

Direct Modulation of Memory Vs. Indirect Effects on Attention or Elaboration: What is the Core Deficit Underlying Emotional Memory Changes in AD?

Many of the initial investigations into the fate of emotional memory in Alzheimer's disease patients assumed that any deficits that arose would reflect reductions in emotion's direct modulation of memory, perhaps due to changes in amygdala function or in amygdala-hippocampal connectivity. This is a reasonable assumption, given the evidence for amygdala dysfunction and degeneration in AD discussed earlier, and we concur that part of the reason why AD patients often do not receive a mnemonic boost for emotional information is probably linked to declines in amygdala-based modulation of memory processes. However, we also propose that the changes in emotional memory with Alzheimer's disease may have a lot do with deficits in the indirect effects of emotion on attention, sensation, and elaboration. We believe that this proposal is consistent with the general findings that we outlined above regarding the effects of valence, modality, and delay on AD patients' memories for emotional events.

When considering the effects of valence, there is little evidence to suggest that AD patients show any positivity effect in memory. A preference for the positive was noted in only one study (Hamann et al., 2000), and a few other studies have noted a preference for the negative (Dohnel et al., 2007, 2008; Fleming et al., 2003). This pattern is in striking contrast to the pattern revealed by older adults, who often remember positive information better than negative information (Mather & Carstensen, 2005). Because older adults' positivity effect is believed to result from changes in how older adults' sustain their attention on emotional information and elaborate upon that information (Kensinger & Leclerc, in press; Mather, 2006), the absence of this effect in AD patients may indicate that these patients do not process emotional information in the same, controlled fashion as their healthy counterparts.

Further evidence - to support the conclusion that AD patients' deficits in emotional memory may reflect changes in how emotion guides attention, sensory processing, and elaboration in these patients - stems from the fact that AD patients show a blunted emotional memory enhancement effect even when information is not highly arousing and even when memory is assessed immediately after learning. It has been proposed (e.g., Kensinger, 2004; Talmi, et al., 2008) that when information is low in arousal, and when memory is tested after a short delay, emotional memory enhancement effects have more to do with attentional, elaborative and controlled processing effects than they have to do with direct modulatory effects of emotion on memory processes. The fact that AD patients do not show mnemonic enhancement for emotional information when memory is tested after these short delays may therefore suggest that they do not benefit much from these indirect effects of emotion on attention or elaboration. By contrast, AD patients seem more likely to show emotional memory enhancements when stimuli are higher in arousal (e.g., with narrated slide shows or "flashbulb" events), or when memory is tested after somewhat longer delays, perhaps because under these circumstances, they can rely on emotion's direct modulation of memory via more automatic linkages between the amygdala and the hippocampus. Taken together, these findings suggest that AD patients may benefit from direct modulation of memory processes but may not benefit from more indirect mediation effects that require emotion's effects to act via attentional or sensory means (Talmi et al., 2007, 2008).

Future Directions

There is little consensus or replication of results within the existing studies examining the presence (or absence) of an emotional enhancement in AD patients' memory, leaving much room in the future for careful and thorough manipulation of stimuli characteristics and task demands. There are still many open questions about the impact of these factors upon emotional memory in AD, and in the sections below, we outline some of those areas that we believe are most likely to yield important insights.

Understanding how MCI Affects Emotional Memory

The condition of mild cognitive impairment likely represents an intermediary stage between healthy aging and AD. Minor cognitive problems begin to arise in this stage, including increased difficulty with memory or attention processes, however the extent of these impairments is mild enough that they don't interfere with social interactions or with the normal completion of activities of daily living (Petersen, 2004). These changes are likely the result of initial disturbances in the integrity of limbic structures including the hippocampus, and amygdala, as well as in the frontal and parietal lobes (Chow & Cummings, 2000; Grieve, et al., 2005; Salat, et al., 2001; Ziegler, et al., in press).

It is unclear how emotional memory is impacted in MCI as compared to AD; it is possible that any impairment in processing or retaining emotional information follows in a graded fashion with increasing disease severity. This type of graded progression could lead to a gradual decline in functioning bridging to formal diagnosis of AD. By contrast, there may instead be a threshold effect, with most abilities retained upto a point, with a severe drop-off observed then. Research examining emotion processing and memory in MCI is even more scant than in AD, but a better understanding of these abilities in MCI would likely contribute beneficial information about the correspondence between emotional memory changes and the distribution of AD pathology during the course of the disease progression.

Investigating how Valence Affects Emotional Memory in AD

The vast majority of studies to date examining emotional memory in AD have only contrasted the effects of negative compared to neutral stimuli, yet given the literature suggesting a positivity bias in healthy older adults' memories (Mather, 2006), additional comparisons examining the effects of positive stimuli upon AD patients' memory may yield interesting results. There could be some circumstances under which a positivity bias is evident, and such a preservation of the effect could yield important insights into the types of motivation factors, or neurobiological factors, that underlie the effect, perhaps suggesting that AD leaves relatively intact the prefrontal processes that have been linked to the positivity effect (Leclerc & Kensinger, in press). Moreover, if further examination of valence effects reveals little difference between groups, yet there are noticeable group differences in response to stimulus arousal level, then that pattern of results could lead researchers to focus on how AD impacts brain regions responsible for processing stimulus arousal (e.g., amygdala and dorsomedial prefrontal cortex; Dolcos, LaBar, & Cabeza, 2004; Kensinger & Schacter, 2006). It is also possible that AD patients do not express a positivity bias. This would be an important finding as well, and would then lead to follow-up questions about what types of changes would lead to the dissipation of the positivity effect. For example, it could be indicative of the extent of damage to frontal brain regions, which are associated with controlled and self-referential mental processing, and goal-oriented behaviors. Alternatively, the motivational goals hypothesized to be driving the positivity effect in healthy older adults may not be comparable in AD patients due to generally reduced self-awareness and self-monitoring (Kaszniak & Zak, 1996; McGlynn & Kaszniak, 1991). Further exploration of the variations in memory impairment and preservation across a range of stimulus valence and arousal levels may lead to better understanding of the functional brain changes in emotion processing that develop during the progression from MCI to AD.

Examining how Sensory Integration Contributes to Emotional Memory Benefits in AD

In several instances, past research has shown that although the beneficial effects of simple, acontextual emotional stimuli upon memory are limited, more robust effects are observed with more complex or dynamic stimuli, which engage multiple sensory systems (e.g., auditory as well as visual). Although at first blush it might seem that adding information would create added burden for AD memory, paradoxically, the greater stimulus complexity may be beneficial to enhancing AD patients' memory because there is more information available to aid the construction of persisting mental representations. Subsequently, remembering any of several stimulus features could cue memory for more complex stimuli, and emotional information may grant these features additional saliency. The more reliable effects of complex stimuli upon emotional enhancements in memory also could be attributable to higher perceived stimulus arousal level arising from greater ecological relevance, or to the reduced attentional demands of maintaining one thematically coherent and continuous narrative context in mind rather than numerous discrete items. There are many candidate mechanisms responsible for these results, and future research that manipulates stimulus complexity may grant more information about the role of attentional processes and stimulus context in emotional memory in the neurodegenerative disease process. These investigations may also reveal how patients can best draw from abilities and skills that are preserved into later disease stages in order to help their ability to encode and retain information.

The Benefits of a Neuroimaging Approach to Studying Emotional Memory in AD

Neuroimaging studies employing fMRI or ERP technologies are likely to yield valuable information regarding the extent to which AD affects the neural systems recruited for processing and remembering emotional stimuli, and these results may in turn inform questions about how stimulus valence, arousal, or complexity influences the magnitude of emotional enhancements in memory. These methods may be particularly informative when behavioral patterns between AD patients and healthy individuals are similar, such as when both groups show an emotional enhancement in memory. In these instances, neuroimaging technology can reveal whether patients are recruiting the same processes as controls, whether the patients are recruiting differing brain regions in order to complete the task, or whether their neural activity occurs along a differing timecourse from healthy older adults. It is quite possible that when AD or MCI patients exhibit an emotional memory enhancement, it is because compensatory neural mechanisms are engaged or because there is intensified connectivity among involved regions, enabling comparable memory benefits amidst the increasing neuropathology and general memory decline in AD (Smith, Pankratz, Negash, Machulda, Petersen, Boeve, et al., 2007).

Acknowledgments

Preparation of this chapter was supported by grants from the Dana Foundation and the Searle Scholars program.

References

Addis, D.R., Leclerc, C.M., Muscatell, K., & Kensinger, E.A. (in press). There are age-related changes in neural connectivity during the successful encoding of positive, but not negative, information. *Cortex.*

Abrisqueta-Gomez, J., Bueno, O.F.A., Oliviera, M.G.M., & Bertolucci, P.H.F. (2002). Recognition memory for emotional pictures in Alzheimer's disease. *Acta Neurologica Scandinavia, 105,* 51-54.

Anderson, A.K., Wais, P.E., & Gabrieli, J.D.E. (2006). Emotion enhances remembrance of neutral events past. *Proceedings of the National Academy of Sciences, 103,* 1599-1604.

Blessed, G., Tomlinson, B. E., & Roth, M. (1968). The association between quantitative measures of dementia and of senile change in the cerebral grey matter of elderly subjects. *British Journal of Psychiatry, 114*, 797–811.

Boller, F., El Massioui, F., Devouche, E., Traykov, L., Pomati, S., & Starkstein, S.E. (2002). Processing emotional information in Alzheimer's disease: Effects on memory performance and neurophysiological correlates. *Dementia and Geriatric Cognitive Disorders, 14,* 104-112.

Brueckner, K. & Moritz, S. (2009). Emotional valence and semantic relatedness differentially influence false recognition in mild cognitive impairment, Alzheimer's disease, and healthy elderly. *Journal of the International Neuropsychological Society, 15*, 268-276.

Bucks, R. S., & Radford, S. A. (2004). Emotion processing in Alzheimer's disease. *Aging and Mental Health, 8,* 222-232.

Budson, A.E., Simons, J.S., Sullivan, A.L., Beier, J.S., Soloman, P.R., Scinto, L.F., et al. (2004). Memory and emotions for the September 11, 2001, terrorist attacks in patients with Alzheimer's disease, patients with mild cognitive impairment, and healthy older adults. *Neuropsychology, 18,* 315-327.

Budson A.E., Todman, R.W., Chong, H., Adams, E.H., Kensinger, E.A., Krandel, T.S., et al. (2006). False recognition of emotional word lists in aging and Alzheimer's disease. *Cognitive and Behavioral Neurology, 19,* 71-78.

Budson A.E., Simons J.S., Waring J.D., Sullivan A.L., Hussion T., & Schacter D.L. (2007). Memory for the September 11, 2001, terrorist attacks one year later in patients with Alzheimer's disease, patients with mild cognitive impairment, and healthy older adults. *Cortex, 43,* 875-888.

Burke, A., Heuer, F., & Reisberg, D. (1992). Remembering emotional events. *Memory and Cognition, 20,* 277-290.

Burnham, H., & Hogervorst, E. (2004). Recognition of facial expressions of emotion by patients with dementia of the Alzheimer type. *Dementia and Geriatric Cognitive Disorders, 18,* 75-79.

Cacioppo, J.T., Berntson, G.G., Bechara, A., Tranel, D., & Hawkley, L.C. (in press). Could an aging brain contribute to subjective well being?: The value added by a social neuroscience perspective. In A. Tadorov, S.T. Fiske, & D. Prentice (Eds), Social Neuroscience: Toward Understanding the Underpinnings of the Social Mind. New York: Oxford University Press.

Cahill, L., & McGaugh, J.L. (1995). A novel demonstration of enhanced memory associated with emotional arousal. *Conscious Cognition, 4,* 410-421.

Chow, T.W. & Cummings, J.L. (2000). The amygdala and Alzheimer's disease. In J.P. Aggleton (Ed), *The amygdala: A functional analysis.* pp. 656-680. Oxford, England: Oxford University Press.

Craik, F.I.M., & Lockhart, R.S. (1972). Levels of processing: A framework for memory research. *Journal of Verbal Learning and Verbal Behavior, 11*, 671-684.

Dohnel, K., Sommer, M., Ibach, B., Rothmayr, C., Meinhardt, J., & Hajak, G. (2008). Neural correlates of emotional working memory in patients with Mild Cognitive Impairment, *Neuropsychologia, 46,* 37-48.

Dohnel, K., Sommer, M., Reindl, G., Muller, J., Hajak, G., & Ibach, B. (2007). Information processing in patients with Mild Cognitive Impairment (MCI). *Psychiatric Praxis, 34, Supplement 1,* S117-S118.

Dolcos, F., LaBar, K. S., & Cabeza, R. (2004). Interaction between the amygdala and the medial temporal lobe memory system predicts better memory for emotional events. *Neuron, 42,* 855–863.

Fleming, K., Kim, S.H., Doo, M., Maguire, G., & Potkin, S.G. (2003). Memory for emotional stimuli in patients with Alzheimer's disease. *American Journal of Alzheimer's Disease and Other Dementias, 18,* 340-342.

Folstein, M.F., Folstein, S.E., & McHugh, P.R. (1975). A practical method for grading the cognitive state of patients for the clinician. *Journal of Psychiatric Research, 12,* 189-198.

Grieve, S.M., Clark, C.R., Williams, L.M., Peduto, A.J., & Gordon, E. (2005). Preservation of limbic and paralimbic structures in aging. *Human Brain Mapping, 25,* 391-401.

Hamann, S. (2001). Cognitive and neural mechanisms of emotional memory. *Trends in Cognitive Sciences, 5,* 394-400.

Hamann, S.B., Monarch, E.S., & Goldstein, F.C. (2000). Memory enhancement for emotional stimuli is impaired in early Alzheimer's disease. *Neuropsychology, 14,* 82-92.

Head, D., Snyder, A.Z., Girton, L.E., Morris, J.C., & Buckner, R.L. (2004). Frontal-hippocampal double dissociation between normal aging and Alzheimer's disease. *Cerebral Cortex, 15*, 732-739.

Hess, T.M. (2005). Memory and aging in context. *Psychological Bulletin, 131*, 383-406.

Horinek, D., Varjassyova, A., & Hort, J. (2007). Magnetic resonance analysis of amygdalar volume in Alzheimer's disease. *Current Opinion in Psychiatry, 20*, 273-277.

Ikeda, M., Mori, E., Hirono, N., Imamura, T., Shimomura, T., Ikejiri, Y., et al. (1998). Amnestic people with Alzheimer's disease who remembered the Kobe earthquake. *British Journal of Psychiatry, 172,* 425-428.

Isaacowitz, D.M., Wadlinger, H.A., Goren, D., & Wilson, H.R. (2006). Is there an age-related positivity effect in visual attention? A comparison of two methodologies. Emotion, 6, 511-516.

Kaszniak, A. W. & Zak, M. G. (1996). On the neuropsychology of metamemory: Contributions from the study of amnesia and dementia. *Learning and Individual Differences, 8,* 355-381.

Kazui, H., Mori, E., Hashimoto, M., Hirono, N., Imamura, T., Tanimukai, S., et al. (2000). Impact of emotion on memory: Controlled study of the influence of emotionally charged material on declarative memory in Alzheimer's disease. *British Journal of Psychiatry, 177,* 343-347.

Kazui, H., Mori, E., Hashimoto, M., & Hirono, N. (2003). Enhancement of declarative memory by emotional arousal and visual memory function in Alzheimer's disease. *Journal of Neuropsychiatry and Clinical Neuroscience, 15*, 221-226.

Kensinger E.A. (2004). Remembering emotional experiences: The contribution of valence and arousal. *Reviews in the Neurosciences,15,* 241-251.

Kensinger E.A. (2009). How emotion affects older adults' memories for event details. *Memory, 17,* 208-219.

Kensinger E.A. (2009). Remembering the details: Effects of emotion. *Emotion Review, 1, 99-113.*

Kensinger E.A., Anderson A., Growdon J.H., & Corkin S. (2004). Effects of Alzheimer disease on memory for verbal emotional information. *Neuropsychologia, 42,* 791-800.

Kensinger E.A., Brierley B., Medford N, Growdon J.H, & Corkin S. (2002). Effects of normal aging and Alzheimer's disease on emotional memory. *Emotion, 2,* 118-134.

Kensinger E.A., Garoff-Eaton R.J., & Schacter D.L. (2007). Effects of emotion on memory specificity in young and older adults. *Journal of Gerontology: Psychological Sciences, 62,* 208-215.

Kensinger E.A. & Leclerc C.M. (in press). Age-related changes in the neural mechanisms supporting emotion processing and emotional memory. *European Journal of Cognitive Psychology.*

Kensinger E.A., O'Brien J, Swanberg K, Garoff-Eaton R.J., & Schacter D.L. (2007). The effects of emotional content on reality-monitoring performance in young and older adults. *Psychology and Aging, 22,* 752-764.

Kensinger, E.A., & Schacter, D.L. (2006). Processing emotional pictures and words: Effects of valence and arousal. *Cognitive, Affective, and Behavioral Neuroscience, 6,* 110-126.

Kensinger E.A. & Schacter D.L. (2008a). Memory and Emotion. In M. Lewis, J. M. Haviland-Jones and L. F. Barrett (Eds.), *The Handbook of Emotion*, 3rd Edition. New York: Guilford.

Kensinger, E.A. & Schacter, D.L. (2008b). Neural processes supporting young and older adults' emotional memories. *Journal of Cognitive Neuroscience, 20,* 1161-1173.

Knopman D.S., Parisi J.E., Salviati A., Floriach-Robert M., Boeve B.F., Ivnik R.J., et al. (2003). Neuropathology of cognitively normal elderly. *Journal of Neuropathology and Experimental Neurology, 62,* 1087-1095.

Koff, E., Zaitchik, D., Montepare, J., & Albert, M.S. (1999). Emotion processing in the visual and auditory domains by patients with Alzheimer's disease. *Journal of the International Neuropsychological Society, 5,* 32-40.

LaBar, K.S., & Phelps, E.A. (1998). Arousal-mediated memory consolidation: Role of the medial temporal lobe in humans. *Psychological Science, 9,* 490-493.

LaBar, K.S., Torpey, D.C., Cook, C.A., Johnson, S.R., Warren, L.H., Burke, J.R., & Welsh-Bohmer, K.A. (2005). Emotional enhancement of perceptual priming is preserved in aging and early-stage Alzheimer's disease. *Neuropsychologia, 43,* 1824-1837.

Lang, P.J., Bradley, M.M., & Cuthbert, B.N. (1997). *International affective picture system (IAPS): Technical manual and affective ratings*. Gainesville: University of Florida, Center for Research in Psychophysiology.

Leclerc, C.M. & Kensinger, E.A. (2008). Effects of age on detection of emotional information. *Psychology and Aging. 23,* 209-215.

Libkuman, T.M., Stabler, C.L., & Otani, H. (2004). Arousal, valence, and memory for detail. *Memory, 12,* 237-247.

Mather, M. (2006). Why memories may become more positive as people age. In B. Uttl, N. Ohta, & A.L. Siegenthaler (Eds.), *Memory and emotion*. Malden, MA: Blackwell Press.

Mather M. & Carstensen, L.L. (2005). Aging and motivated cognition: the positivity effect in attention and memory. *Trends in Cognitive Sciences, 9,* 496-501.

Mather, M. & Knight, M. (2005). Goal-directed memory: The role of cognitive control in older adults' emotional memory. *Psychology and Aging,* 20, 554-570.

McGaugh, J.L. (2004). The amygdala modulates the consolidation of memories of emotionally arousing experiences. *Annual Review of Neuroscience, 27,* 1-28.

McGlynn, S. M. & Kaszniak, A. W. (1991). Unawareness of deficits in dementia and schizophrenia. In G. P. Priatano & D. L. Schacter (Eds.), *Awareness of deficit after brain injury: Theoretical and clinical aspects* (pp. 84-110). New York: Oxford University Press.

Mickley K.R. & Kensinger E.A. (2008). Emotional valence influences the neural correlates associated with remembering and knowing. *Cognitive, Affective, and Behavioral Neuroscience, 8,* 143-152.

Mickley, K.R., Muscatell, K.A., & Kensinger, E.A. (submitted). The effect of valence on young and older adults' attention: *More similarities than differences.*

Moayeri, S.E., Cahill, L., Jin, Y., & Potkin, S.G. (2000). Relative sparing of emotionally influenced memory in Alzheimer's disease. *NeuroReport, 11*, 653-655.

Mori, E., Ikeda, M., Hirono, N., Kitagaki, H., Imamura, T., & Shimomura, T. (1999). Amygdalar volume and emotional memory in Alzheimer's disease. *American Journal of Psychiatry, 156*, 216-222.

Murphy, N.A. & Isaacowitz, D.M. (2008). Preferences for emotional information in older and younger adults: A meta-analysis of memory and attention tasks. *Psychology and Aging, 23,* 263-286.

Padovan, C., Versace, R., Thomas-Anterion, C., & Laurent, D. (2002). Evidence for a selective deficit in automatic activation of positive information in patients with Alzheimer's disease in an affective priming paradigm. *Neuropsychologia, 40,* 335-339.

Payne, J.D., Stickgold, R., Swanberg, K., & Kensinger, E.A. (2008). Sleep and memory consolidation for complex emotional scenes. *Psychological Science, 19,* 781-788.

Petersen, R.C. (2004). Mild cognitive impairment as a diagnostic entity. *Journal of Internal Medicine, 256,* 183-94.

Phelps, E.A., & LeDoux, J.E. (2005). Contributions of the amygdala to emotion processing: From animal models to human behavior. *Neuron, 48,* 175-187.

Pourtois G, Schwartz S, Seghier ML, Lazeyras F, Vuilleumier P. (2006) Neural systems for orienting attention to the location of threat signals: an event-related fMRI study. *Neuroimage*, 31, 920-33.

Rosenbaum, R.S., Furey, M.L., Horowitz, B. & Grady, C.L. (in press). Altered connectivity among emotion-related brain regions during short-term memory in Alzheimer's disease. Neurobiology of Aging.

Russell, J. (1980). Russell, J.A. (1980). A circumplex model of affect. *Journal of Personality and Social Psychology, 39,* 1161-1178.

Satpute, A.B., & Lieberman, M.D. (2006). Integrating automatic and controlled processes into neurocognitive models of social cognition. *Brain Research, 1079*, 86–97.

Salat, D.H., Kaye, J.A., Janowsky, J.S. (2001). Selective preservation and degeneration within the prefrontal cortex in aging and Alzheimer disease. *Archives of Neurology, 58,* 1403-1408.

Satler, C., Garrido, L.M., Sarmiento, E.P., Leme, S., Conde, C., & Tomaz, C. (2007). Emotional arousal enhances declarative memory in patients with Alzheimer's disease. *Acta Neurologica Scandinavia, 116*, 355-360.

Scott SA, DeKosky ST, Scheff SW. (1991). Volumetric atrophy of the amygdala in Alzheimer's disease: quantitative serial reconstruction. *Neurology, 41,* 351-356.

Sharot, T., & Phelps, E.A. (2004). How arousal modulates memory: Disentangling the effects of attention and retention. *Cognitive, Affective, and Behavioral Neuroscience, 4,* 294-306.

Sharot, T. & Yonelinas, A.P. (2008). Differential time-dependent effects of emotion on recollective experience and memory for contextual information. *Cognition, 106,* 538-547.

Shi F, Liu B, Zhou Y, Yu C, Jiang T. (in press). Hippocampal volume and asymmetry in mild cognitive impairment and Alzheimer's disease: Meta-analyses of MRI studies. *Hippocampus.*

Shimokawa, A., Yatomi, N., Anamizu, S., Ashikari, I., Kohno, M., Maki, Y., et al. (2000). Comprehension of emotions: Comparison between Alzheimer type and vascular type dementias. *Dementia and Geriatric Cognitive Disorders, 11,* 268-274.

Smith, G. E., Pankratz, V.S., Negash, S., Machulda, M.M., Petersen, R.C., Boeve, B.F., et al. (2007). A plateau in pre-Alzheimer memory decline; Evidence for compensatory mechanisms? *Neurology, 69,* 133-139.

Spoletini, I., Marra, C., Di Iulio, F Gianni, W., Sancesario, G., Giubilei, F., et al. (2008). Facial emotion recognition deficit in amnestic mild cognitive impairment and Alzheimer's disease. *Journal of Geriatric Psychiatry, 16,* 389-398.

Talmi, D., Anderson, A.K., Riggs, L., Caplan, J.B., & Moscovitch, M. (2008). Immediate memory consequences of the effect of emotion on attention to pictures. *Learning & Memory, 15,* 172-182.

Talmi, D., Schimmack, U., Paterson, T., and Moscovitch, M. (2007). The role of attention and relatedness in emotionally enhanced memory. *Emotion* 7: 89–102.

Teng, E., Lu, P.H. & Cummings, J.L. (2004). Deficits in facial emotion processing in mild cognitive impairment. *Dementia and Geriatric Cognitive Disorders, 23*, 271-279.

Vuilleumier P, & Driver J. (2007). Modulation of visual processing by attention and emotion: windows on causal interactions between human brain regions. *Philosophical Trans of the Royal Society London B Biological Sciences,* 362, 837-55.

Wright, C.I., Dickerson, B.C., Feczko, E., Negeira, A. & Williams, D. (2007). A functional magnetic resonance imaging study of amygdala responses to human faces in aging and mild Alzheimer's disease. *Biological Psychiatry*, 62, 1388-1395.

Ziegler DA, Piguet O, Salat DH, Prince K, Connally E, & Corkin S. (in press). Cognition in healthy aging is related to regional white matter integrity, but not cortical thickness. *Neurobiology of Aging.*

In: Alzheimer's Disease and Dementia (Vol. 4)
Editor: Miao-Kun Sun ISBN:978-1-60876-152-4

Chapter II

Mechanisms of Amyloid -β Clearance in Alzheimer's Disease

Joseph El Khoury [*1, 2,] ***and Suzanne E. Hickman*** [1]
Center for Immunology and Inflammatory Diseases, Division of Rheumatology, Allergy, and Immunology[1]
Division of Infectious Diseases, Massachusetts General Hospital, Harvard Medical School, CNY 149, Room 8301, 149 13th Street, Charlestown, Massachusetts 02129, USA[2]

Abstract

Amyloid-β accumulation in the brain is regulated by equilibrium between Aβ production and clearance. Three major pathways regulate Aβ clearance from the brain. The first pathway involves uptake of Aβ by specific receptors expressed on microglia and astrocytes followed by intracellular degradation. The second pathway for Aβ clearance occurs via extracellular degradation by surface bound or released Aβ-degrading enzymes. The third pathway that regulates Aβ clearance is transport across the blood brain barrier (BBB) and the balance between Aβ efflux and influx into the brain. In this chapter we will review these three pathways relevant to Aβ clearance and discuss several recent advances in the field. We will also review the potential therapeutic applications of each of these pathways.

Abbreviations

Aβ	Amyloid β peptide
AD	Alzheimer's Disease
APP	Amyloid Precursor Protein

[*]Correspondence should be addressed to JEK (jelkhoury@partners.org or SEH (shickman@partners.org)

BBB	Blood Brain Barrier
PSEN1	Presenilin 1
MMP	Matrix Metalloproteinase
ACE	Angiotensin Converting Enzyme
ECE	Endothelin Converting Enzyme
CCR2	Chemokine Receptor 2
MCP-1/CCL2	Monocyte Chemotactic Protein-1
TGFβ	Transforming Growth Factor β
ApoE	Apolipoprotein E
GFAP	Gilal Fibrillary Acidic Protein
SR	Scavenger Receptors
CR3	Complement Receptor 3
FPRL1/FPR2	Formyl Peptide Receptor-Like 1
AGE	Advanced Glycation Endproducts
MARCO	MAcrophage Receptor with a COllagenous Domain
LPS	Lipopolysaccharide
NEP	Neprilysin
IDE	Insulin Degrading Enzyme

Introduction

Deposition of amyloid-β (Aβ) peptides in the brain is a pathological hallmark of Alzheimer's disease (AD) and plays a key role in the pathogenesis of this devastating disorder (Selkoe, 2000). Aβ accumulation in the brain is regulated by equilibrium between Aβ production and Aβ clearance. Aβ production has been fairly well characterized and involves the cleavage of the amyloid precursor protein (APP) by β- and γ-secretases (Thinakaran and Koo, 2008). Aβ clearance from the brain involves three distinct pathways. The first pathway involves intracellular Aβ degradation after phagocytosis and endocytosis, processes mainly mediated by microglia and astrocytes (Wyss-Coray et al., 2003; El Khoury et al., 2007). The second major pathway for Aβ clearance occurs via extracellular degradation by surface bound or released Aβ-degrading enzymes (Leissring, 2008; Miners et al., 2008a). The third pathway that regulates Aβ clearance is Aβ transport across the blood brain barrier (BBB) and the balance between Aβ exit and re-entry into the brain (Zlokovic, 2008). In this chapter we will discuss the three pathways that are relevant to Aβ clearance. We will review recent data on the role of microglia and blood-derived monocytes and astrocytes in phagocytosis and uptake of Aβ and the cellular receptors involved in this process. We will also discuss the role of the Aβ-degrading enzymes expressed by microglia, astrocytes and neurons in Aβ degradation. These enzymes include insulysin, neprilysin, matrix metalloproteases, plasmin, plasminogen activator, angiotensin converting enzyme, and endothelin converting enzyme. Finally we will discuss the role of Aβ transport across the BBB (efflux vs. influx) in regulating Aβ clearance from the brain.

Mouse Models of AD

Before we delve into the various pathways that regulate Aβ clearance, it is important to note that much of what we know about these pathways comes from work done in transgenic mouse models of AD. While some of this knowledge has been corroborated in human cells, much remains to be confirmed. Nonetheless, these mouse models of amyloidosis have proven to be invaluable tools in understanding the mechanisms of Aβ generation and clearance. Several mouse models of cerebral amyloidosis have been generated. Tg2576 mice and APP23 mice express the human APP with the Swedish mutation (APP695sw) associated with familial AD, and slowly develop AD-like pathology as they age (El Khoury et al., 2007; Lefterov et al., 2007). These mice develop senile-like plaques and diffuse Aβ deposits and have significant microgliosis and astrocytosis (Figure 1). Presenilin 1 (PSEN1) is a member of the γ secretase complex, an important Aβ generating enzyme. Mutations in the PSEN1 gene are also associated with early onset familial AD. Bigenic mice co-expressing the APP695sw transgene and a mutant exon-9-deleted variant of the human PSEN1 (PSEN1/dE9) transgene have also been generated (PS1-APP). In these mice, the APP and PSEN1 transgenes are integrated into a single locus, and are independently under the control of separate mouse prion protein promoter elements, which direct expression of the transgenes predominantly to central nervous system neurons. As a result, these mice develop accelerated AD-like pathology beginning at the age of six months. Studies with these transgenic mice confirmed earlier human immunohistochemical data (Hickman et al., 2008).

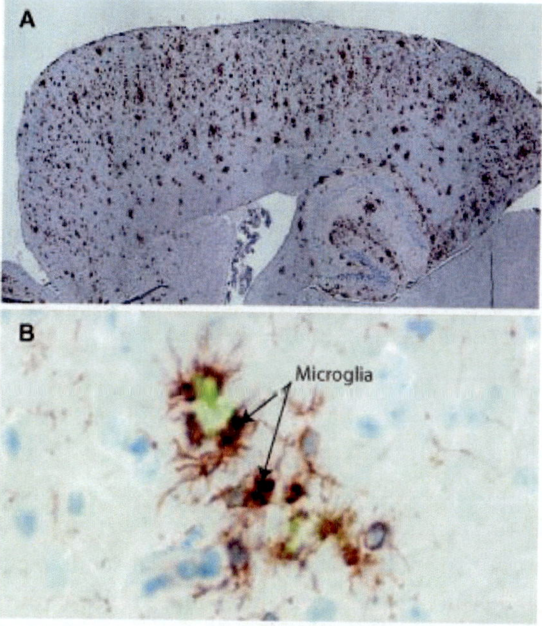

Figure 1. A. Brain section from a 522 day-old PS1-APP mouse stained with anti-AB antibodies showing florid plaques (40x original magnification). B. Co-staining of a PS1-APP mouse brain section with Thioflavin S for fibrillar AB (green) and anti-CD11b antibodies (red brown) shows intimate association between the AB deposit and microglia (200x original magnification).

Clearance of Aβ by Microglia and Astrocytes

Brain cells implicated in Aβ uptake and degradation include microglia and astrocytes. Since the early description of microglial association with senile plaques and Aβ deposits, their role in the pathogenesis of AD has been debated (Vostrikov, 1985) (Rozemuller et al., 1986). More recently, an emerging paradigm indicates that these cells may play a dichotomous role in AD pathogenesis. Early microglial accumulation delays disease progression by promoting clearance of Aβ before formation of senile plaques (El Khoury et al., 2007). However, persistent Aβ accumulation in spite of increasing microglial numbers suggests that the ability of microglia to clear Aβ may decrease with age and progression of AD pathology. Indeed, as disease progresses, pro-inflammatory cytokines produced in response to Aβ deposition downregulate genes involved in Aβ clearance, and promote Aβ accumulation, therefore contributing to neurodegeneration (Hickman et al., 2008). Similar to microglia, the interest in the role of astrocytes in Aβ clearance began several decades ago (Duffy et al., 1980). More recently, work done by several groups has indicated that these cells, similar to microglia, play a role in Aβ clearance (Wyss-Coray et al., 2003; Nielsen et al., 2008).

Aβ Clearance by Microglia

Microglia are mononuclear phagocytes/macrophages and constitute the principal innate immune cells of the brain. Strong evidence indicates that microglia in AD have a myeloid lineage and are derived from the bone marrow (El Khoury and Luster, 2008). Evidence for the presence of microglia in senile plaques derives from immunohistochemical studies that examined the brains of AD patients (Vostrikov, 1985; Rozemuller et al., 1986; McGeer et al., 1987). In contrast to normal brains where microglia are distributed uniformly throughout the gray and white matter (McGeer et al., 1987), in AD brains microglia are clustered in and around Aβ deposits (Heneka and O'Banion, 2007; El Khoury and Luster, 2008). Microglia are closely associated with Aβ (Perlmutter et al., 1990) and at times contain intracellular deposits of Aβ, indicating a possible role in Aβ clearance (D'Andrea et al., 2004).

Mouse models of intracerebral amyloidosis confirmed the close association of microglia with sites of Aβ deposition. In APP23, PS1-APP and APPsw Tg2576 transgenic mice microglia cluster around Aβ deposits (Figure 1B) and (Frautschy et al., 1998a; Hickman et al., 2008). Quantitative analysis of microglia as a function of distance from the center of senile plaques in Tg2576 mice revealed a 2-5 fold increase in microglia numbers in areas with plaques compared with neighboring regions (Frautschy et al., 1998a). Therefore, studies in transgenic mice confirm that microglial accumulation in senile plaques is an integral part of the disease process in AD and that microglia may indeed play a role in the pathogenesis of AD. Because of the close association between microglia and Aβ in human AD brain and because microglia were found to have some intracellular Aβ, it was suggested that these cells are involved in the clearance of Aβ. Indeed, we have found that accumulation of blood-derived microglia/mononuclear phagocytes prior to formation of visible Aβ deposits promotes Aβ clearance. Abolishing such accumulation, as occurs in Tg2576 mice deficient in the chemokine receptor 2 (CCR2), leads to development of early visible Aβ deposits, specifically around blood vessels, and was associated with increased mortality in these mice (El Khoury et al., 2007). In support of this protective role for microglia/mononuclear phagocytes, it was also found that bone marrow-derived microglia play an important role in restricting plaque formation in irradiated transgenic AD mice by promoting phagocytosis and clearance of Aβ (Simard et al., 2006). This concept was further supported when IL-1β was over expressed in the brain of PS1-APP mice. These mice had dramatically induced Monocyte Chemotactic Protein-1 (MCP-1/CCL2) expression in their brains, increased microglia/mononuclear phagocyte accumulation and activation, and reduced AD-like pathology (Shaftel et al., 2007). Furthermore, transgenic AD mice that are deficient in peripheral transforming growth factor β (TGFβ-SMAD2/3) signaling, have increased microglia/mononuclear phagocytes recruitment and reduced AD-like pathology (Town et al., 2008). Apolipoprotein E (Apo E) appears to enhance microglia/macrophage degradation of Aβ following phagocytosis (Jiang et al., 2008; Zhao et al., 2009b). These data in transgenic AD mouse models indicate that microglia/mononuclear phagocytes play important roles in Aβ clearance *in vivo*. Interestingly, the first evidence in support of a role for microglia in Aβ clearance in AD patients came before these mouse studies. In clinical trials of patients who received Aβ immunization, a significant microglia/macrophage infiltration was found (Nicoll et al., 2003), and *in vitro* studies confirmed that microglia play a role in clearing Aβ following immunization.

The data supporting a role for microglia in Aβ clearance is compelling, but these data also raise an important question. Why does Aβ continue to accumulate, and why does AD pathology progress in spite of continued microglia recruitment? One possible explanation for the failure of microglia to stop AD progression would be that these cells become overwhelmed by the excess amount of Aβ produced and cannot keep up with the pace of Aβ generation. Another possibility would be that as AD progresses, the phenotype of accumulating microglia changes and these cells become more pro-inflammatory and lose their Aβ-clearing capabilities, resulting in reduced Aβ uptake and degradation, and increased Aβ accumulation. We investigated this hypothesis in PS1-APP mice (Hickman et al., 2008). Our data show that as PS1-APP mice age, their microglia become dysfunctional and exhibit a significant reduction in expression of their Aβ-binding receptors and Aβ-degrading enzymes, but maintain their ability to produce pro-inflammatory cytokines. These cytokines may in turn act in an autocrine fashion and further reduce expression of Aβ-binding receptors and Aβ-degrading enzymes leading to decreased Aβ clearance and increased accumulation. If any AD therapy using microglia to clear Aβ is contemplated, activation of microglia or recruitment of microglial precursors from the blood, as occurs with Aβ immunization or bone marrow transplantation, may be a necessary step to restore microglial ability to clear Aβ in advanced AD.

Aβ Clearance by Astrocytes

In addition to microglia, astrocytes have been implicated in the clearance of Aβ. An early pathological event in AD is the accumulation of astrocytes at sites of Aβ deposition (Duffy et al., 1980). Astrocytes can release inflammatory cytokines and chemokines in response to Aβ stimulation (Johnstone et al., 1999). Cultured mouse astrocytes can degrade Aβ *in vitro* and *in situ* in senile plaques in brain slices from transgenic AD mice (Wyss-Coray et al., 2003). Furthermore, cultured adult and fetal human astrocytes can bind and internalize Aβ 1-42 *in vitro* (Nielsen et al., 2008). However, fetal astrocytes are more efficient in uptake of Aβ 1-42 than adult astrocytes perhaps explaining why Aβ continues to accumulate in spite of significant astrogliosis in AD. No definitive experiment so far has shown that astrocytes mediate Aβ clearance *in vivo* in humans or in mouse models of AD, but several reports have proposed that astrocytes participate in Aβ uptake *in vivo*. Following infusion of Aβ 1-40 into the rat hippocampus, immunostaining for the infused peptide co-localized with staining for glial fibrillary acidic protein (GFAP), a major astrocyte marker (Malm et al., 2006). Similar to its clearance by microglia, Apo E expression is necessary for astrocyte degradation of amyloid deposit since the process is significantly impaired in $APOE^{-/-}$ astrocytes (Koistinaho et al., 2004).

Receptors Involved in Aβ Binding and Uptake by Microglia and Astrocytes

Several receptors have been implicated in Aβ binding and uptake by microglia and astrocytes (summarized in Table 1). These include several members of the scavenger receptor family, such as the class A scavenger receptors (SRA), the class B scavenger receptors (SRB), CD14, CD47, $\alpha_6\beta_1$ integrins, the formyl peptide receptor-like 1 (FPRL1/FPR2), and complement receptor 3 (CR3).

Class A Scavenger Receptors (SRA)

SRA are a family of multiligand receptors that bind to modified lipoproteins, lipopolysaccharide (LPS) and lipoteichoic acid (Krieger and Herz, 1994; Thomas et al., 2000). We and others have shown that SRAI/II also bind fibrillar Aβ and advanced glycation end products. SRA have a collagen-like domain that is thought to mediate ligand binding (AGEs) (El Khoury et al., 1994; El Khoury et al., 1996; El Khoury et al., 1998). MAcrophage Receptor with a COllagenous domain (MARCO), another member of the SRA family, is encoded by a distinct gene from SRAI/II and has been implicated in binding of Aβ by rodent astrocytes (Alarcon et al., 2005). While SRAI/II null microglia and macrophages have a 60% reduction in binding and uptake of fibrillar Aβ (Chung et al., 2001; Husemann et al., 2001), it is not known if MARCO deficiency affects Aβ uptake in astrocytes. Since SRAI/II null microglia are not completely deficient in their ability to bind and phagocytose Aβ, it is likely that redundant pathways /and receptors are involved in this process. Indeed, SRA deficiency in one transgenic AD mouse model did not seem to affect AD like pathology (Huang et al., 1999) possibly because additional receptors may compensate for SRA deficiency. Interestingly, however, SRA expression is downregulated in microglia from aging transgenic

AD mice compared to their age-matched wild type littermates, suggesting that deficiency in this receptor may contribute to Aβ accumulation by decreasing microglial ability to clear Aβ (Hickman et al., 2008).

Class B Scavenger Receptors (SRB)

Table 1. Aβ binding receptors, their putative functions in relation to Aβ clearance and their location in the brain.

RECEPTOR	FUNCTION	CELL TYPE WHERE EXPRESSED	REFERENCES
SRAI/II	UPTAKE	MICROGLIA & MACROPHAGES	El Khoury et al., 1996
MARCO	UPTAKE	ASTROCYTES	Alarcon et al., 2005
SRBI	UPTAKE	ASTROCYTES & MICROGLIA	(Husemann et al., 2001
SRBII/CD36	UPTAKE & ACTIVATION	MICROGLIA & ENDOTHELIAL CELLS	El Khoury et al., 2003
CD14	UPTAKE & ACTIVATION	MICROGLIA & MACROPHAGES	Liu et al., 2005
RAGE	INFLUX ACROSS BBB	MICROGLIA, ASTROCYTES, NEURONS & ENDOTHELIAL CELLS	Deane et al., 2003
CD47	CO-RECEPTOR WITH CD36	MICROGLIA & MACROPHAGES	Koenigsknecht and Landreth, 2004
$\alpha_6\beta_1$ INTEGRIN	CO-RECEPTOR WITH CD36	MICROGLIA & MACROPHAGES	Koenigsknecht and Landreth, 2004
MAC-1/CR3	UPTAKE	MICROGLIA & MACROPHAGES	Goodwin et al., 1997
FPRL1/FPR2	UPTAKE & ACTIVATION	MICROGLIA & MACROPHAGES	Iribarren et al., 2005
LRP1	EFLUX ACROSS BBB	MICROGLIA, ASTROCYTES, NEURONS & ENDOTHELIAL CELLS	Shibata et al., 2000
LRP2	INFLUX ACROSS BBB-BINDS Aβ-Apo J COMPLEXES	ENDOTHELIAL CELLS	Sagare et al., 2007

SRB have also been found to mediate the binding and uptake of Aβ by microglia and astrocytes (Table 1). Like SRA, SRB are important in the innate host response to bacterial and fungal pathogens (Means et al., 2009). SRB are characterized by the presence of 2 transmembrane spanning domains. CD36 (SRBII), the first classified SRB, was initially identified as a receptor for thrombospondin and for malaria-parasitized erythrocytes (Ockenhouse et al., 1989; Yesner et al., 1996). Endemann and colleagues subsequently identified CD36 as the "second" modified lipoprotein receptor (Endemann et al., 1993), the first receptor being SRAI/II. By virtue of their ability to bind HDL and act as a fatty acid transporters SRB play major roles in cholesterol metabolism (Abumrad et al., 1993; Acton et al., 1996). In addition to binding to lipoproteins and microbial ligands, CD36 binds several modified "self" antigens. CD36 plays a role in removal of apoptotic cells (Lucas et al., 2006).

We have found that CD36 mediates the innate immune response to Aβ and plays a key role in the pathogenesis of Alzheimer's disease (Coraci et al., 2002; El Khoury et al., 2003). CD36 deficient microglia and macrophages fail to get activated when stimulated with Aβ and produced significantly less reactive oxygen species, chemokines and pro-inflammatory cytokines (Coraci et al., 2002; El Khoury et al., 2003). Similar to SRA, expression of CD36 is downregulated in aging transgenic AD mice suggesting that deficiency in this receptor may contribute to Aβ accumulation by decreasing the ability of microglia to clear Aβ (Hickman et al., 2008). However, the role of CD36 in Aβ clearance remains far from being confirmed. It is not known if CD36-deficient microglia phagocytose less Aβ and it also not known if CD36 deficiency in AD mice leads to increased Aβ levels in their brains. In addition to CD36, another SRB, SRBI is expressed on adult mouse astrocytes and can mediate biding to Aβ-coated surfaces. Interestingly SRBI is also expressed on neonatal microglia (Husemann et al., 2001). Unlike CD36, however, SRBI expression is not decreased in microglia isolated from transgenic AD mice compared to their wild type littermates (Hickman et al., 2008). It is not clear what role SRBI plays in Aβ clearance *in vivo*.

CD14

The LPS receptor CD14, which can mediate phagocytosis of bacterial components, shows pronounced immunoreactivity on parenchymal microglia spatially correlated to senile plaques in AD patients, but not in control subjects (Liu et al., 2005). CD14 interacts with Aβ1-42 and can mediate phagocytosis of this peptide (Liu et al., 2005). Similar to other Aβ binding receptors, it is not clear whether CD14 plays a key role in clearing Aβ *in vivo* in AD patients or in transgenic mice with AD like pathology.

Additional Putative Aβ Receptors

In addition to the above mentioned receptors, interactions of microglia with Aβ may involve two additional receptors , $\alpha_6\beta_1$ integrin and CD47, that are believed to form a receptor complex with CD36 (Koenigsknecht and Landreth, 2004). Inhibitors of each of these receptors block Aβ-stimulated phagocytosis. This β_1 integrin-linked process appears to be morphologically and mechanistically distinct from the classical type I and type II phagocytic mechanisms (Koenigsknecht and Landreth, 2004).

Less well characterized Aβ binding receptors include the formyl peptide receptor-like 1 (FPRL1/FPR2), and complement receptor 3 (CR3). FPRL1 and its mouse homolog FPR2 have been shown to be expressed by activated microglial cells and mediate the chemotactic activity of Aβ 1-42. FPRL1 also participates in Aβ internalization in macrophages and microglia-mediated neurotoxicity (Iribarren et al., 2005). The relative contribution of FPRL1/FPR2 to Aβ clearance *in vivo* has not been determined. CR3, also known as Mac-1 is thought to bind Aβ and may play a role in microglia activation by Aβ (Goodwin et al., 1997). However, it is not known if CR3 can actually mediate Aβ phagocytosis.

In summary, several microglial and astrocyte receptors have been implicated in binding of these cells to Aβ, and their collective deficiency *in vivo* is associated with increased Aβ deposition in transgenic AD mice. The contribution of individual receptors to Aβ clearance *in vivo* in mouse models of AD or in AD patients is an active area of investigation. Increasing Aβ clearance by upregulating expression of these receptors is a potential therapeutic modality to delay progression of AD by increasing phagocytosis and clearance of Aβ.

Aβ-DEGRADING ENZYMES

A major pathway for Aβ clearance occurs by intracellular degradation in astrocytes and microglia following Aβ uptake and via extracellular degradation by surface bound or released proteolytic enzymes (Leissring, 2008; Miners et al., 2008a). Proteases that have been shown to cleave Aβ include neprilysin (NEP), insulin degrading enzyme (IDE), matrix metalloproteinases (MMPs), endothelin converting enzymes (ECEs), angiotensin converting enzymes (ACE), plasmin, and Cathepsin B (CatB). Here we will discuss each of these enzymes and their potential role(s) in Aβ degradation (summarized in Figure 2).

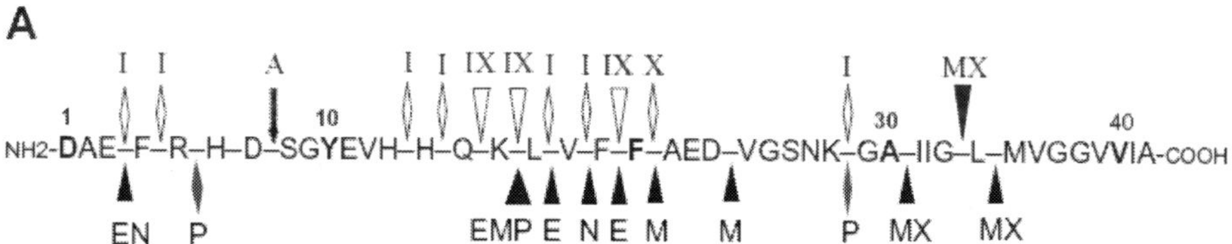

B

Protease	Cellular Location	Forms of Aβ cleaved
NEP	Extracellular , ER/Golgi	M, O(some)
ECE-1	Extracellular , ER/Golgi	M
ECE-2	Extracellular , ER/Golgi	M
MMP-2	Extracellular , ER/Golgi	M, O, F
MMP-9	Extracellular , ER/Golgi	M, O, F
IDE	Extracellular, cytosol, peroxisomes	M
Plasmin	Extracellular	M, O, F
CatB	Extracellular, lysosomes	M, O, F
ACE	Plasma membrane, perinuclear region	M
PreP	Mitochondria	M

Figure 2. A. Sites on human Aβ (1-42) cut by: ECE-1 (E), IDE (I), MMP-9 (M), NEP (N). The cleavage sites noted for these four enzymes are for human recombinant enzymes acting on human Aβ (Yan et al., 2006). Aβ-degrading enzymes derived from other animal sources have been shown to cleave at additional residues not shown in this figure. ACE (A) (Hu et al., 2001); Plasmin (P) (Van Nostrand et al., 1999; Tucker et al., 2000); PreP(X) (Falkevall et al., 2006). B. Cellular location and forms of Aβ cleaved by various enzymes. Abreviations: Endoplasmic reticulum (ER). Abreviations for Aβ forms: Monomeric (M); Oligomeric (O); Fibrillar (F) (Leissring MA, 2008; Miners et al., 2008).

Neprilysin

Neprilysin, also known as CD10, is a 90-110 kd plasma membrane glycoprotein of the neutral zinc-dependent metalloendopeptidase family (Turner and Tanzawa, 1997; Turner et al., 2001). Within the brain, neprilysin has been mainly detected on pre-synaptic membranes and axons of neurons in the hippocampus and neocortex (Barnes et al., 1992; Fukami et al., 2002; Iwata et al., 2002; Iwata et al., 2004). Neprilysin is also found on microglia (Hickman et al., 2008; Jiang et al., 2008; Shimizu et al., 2008). It is generally accepted that neprilysin preferentially degrades soluble monomeric Aβ but not oligomeric or fibrillar Aβ (Qiu et al., 1997; Leissring et al., 2003a). However, human neprilysin can cleave dimeric and trimeric forms of synthetic Aβ (1-42) (Kanemitsu et al., 2003).

Several lines of evidence suggested that neprilysin may be a major contributor of degradation of soluble Aβ in the brain. In post-mortem studies with AD patients, neprilysin mRNA and protein levels were significantly reduced in the hippocampus and temporal gyrus regions of AD brains compared with control subjects (Yasojima et al., 2001). In animal studies, injection of radiolabelled Aβ1-42 into rat hippocampal region resulted in degradation of Aβ that was inhibited by the neprilysin inhibitor thiorphan (Iwata et al., 2000). Further studies with neprilysin-knockout mice, showed that degradation of exogenously administered Aβ was decreased compared with wild type controls and that endogenous Aβ levels in these mice were significantly elevated compared with wild-type controls (Iwata et al., 2001). APPsw mice that were genetically modified to over-express neuronal neprilysin exhibited reduced Aβ levels and plaque formation compared with control animals and had improved survival when compared to regular APPsw mice (Leissring et al., 2003b). These data suggest that neprilysin upregulation may be beneficial in reducing AD pathology. This was confirmed recently in another AD mouse model that over-expresses neprilysin. In this model, soluble Aβ levels were reduced by 50%, effectively preventing early plaque formation in these mice. However, levels of neurotoxic Aβ oligomers and spatial and learning deficits were not improved in these mice suggesting that therapeutic upregulation of neprilysin may not be sufficient to prevent cognitive defects in AD (Meilandt et al., 2009).

Insulin Degrading Enzyme

Insulin degrading enzyme (IDE), also known as insulysin, is another protease that may play an important role in regulating Aβ levels in the brain. IDE is a 110 Kd zinc-dependent metalloprotease that is highly expressed in liver, testis, muscle and brain (Kuo et al., 1993). In the brain, IDE is expressed in neurons, microglia and astrocytes and is located primarily in the cytosol (with smaller amounts in peroxisomes, rough endoplasmic reticulum and plasma membranes (Authier et al., 1996; Morita et al., 2000; Zhao et al., 2009a). IDE is also secreted by a variety of cell types, including microglia and astrocytes (Dorfman et al., 2008; Jiang et al., 2008; Shimizu et al., 2008; Zhao et al., 2009a). IDE degrades a wide range of small peptides, including insulin (Vekrellis et al., 2000) and has been shown to preferentially degrade monomeric Aβ, but not oligomeric or fibrillar forms of Aβ (Leissring et al., 2003a).

Studies using IDE deficient mice showed increased cerebral accumulation of endogenous Aβ(Farris et al., 2003) compared with normal mice, suggesting that IDE may be involved in degradation of endogenous Aβ. Human postmortem AD brains, showed reduced levels and activity of IDE in hippocampal regions compared with non-AD control brains (Perez et al., 2000; Cook et al., 2003) suggesting that reduced IDE levels/activity may contribute to Aβ deposition in the brain. In support of these findings in AD patients, we found that mRNA levels of IDE and NEP were significantly decreased in freshly isolated microglia from old transgenic PS1-APP mice compared with their wild-type littermates (Hickman et al., 2008). In addition, APPsw mice that over-express neuronal IDE had improved survival, a dramatic decrease in Aβ brain levels, plaque formation and associated cytopathology compared to regular APPsw mice (Leissring et al., 2003b). Based on these animal and human studies, IDE appears to be a major Aβ-degrading enzyme that plays a key role in regulating Aβ deposition in AD.

Matrix Metalloproteinases

Matrix metalloproteinases (MMPs) are a family of zinc- dependent enodopeptidases that are involved in remodeling of the extracellular matrix (Rosenberg, 2002). They may play a role in influx of inflammatory cells into the brain and disruption of blood-brain barrier (Gurney et al., 2006; Yang et al., 2007). MMPs are expressed in an inactive pro-enzyme form that requires proteolytic modification before they become active (Ramos-DeSimone et al., 1999; Vartak and Gemeinhart, 2007). Some MMPs are secreted and others are found on the cell surface, but their proteolytic activity is probably confined to the cell surface and nearby extracellular space. At least 14 MMPs have been characterized (Chandler et al., 1997). MMP-2, -3, and -9 have been shown to degrade Aβ *in vitro* (Backstrom et al., 1996; Yin et al., 2006). Unlike neprilysin and insulysin, MMP-9 has been shown to degrade fibrillar Aβ in vitro and in compact plaques from brain slices of transgenic AD mice (Yan et al., 2006). Microglia, macrophages and astrocytes express a variety of MMPs (Chandler et al., 1997; Cross and Woodroofe, 1999; Crocker et al., 2008), but MMP-2 and MMP-9 are the most studied so far.

Several lines of evidence implicate MMP-2 and-9 in removal of Aβ in the brain. In PS1-APP transgenic mice, MMP-2 and -9 immunoreactivity was increased in astrocytes surrounding amyloid plaques (Yin et al., 2006). Laser capture and quantitative RT-PCR analysis of plaque-associated astrocytes and plaque-distal astrocytes from PS1-APP mice and astrocytes from normal mice showed a >20fold increase in both MMP-2 and MMP-9 RNAs in plaque-associated astrocytes (Yin et al., 2006). In astrocytes cultured from neonatal rats, soluble, but not fibrillar Aβ, induced MMP-9 expression (Deb et al., 2003). MMP-9 was also induced in response to Aβ in cultured rat microglia (Gottschall, 1996). Secretion of MMP-9 from adult rat microglia and human microglia cell line was enhanced by treatment with the chemokines MCP-1, MIP1β, and fractalkine (Cross and Woodroofe, 1999). MMP-9 expression was increased in response to LPS or tumor necrosis factor in microglia cultured from neonatal mice (Crocker et al., 2008). Collectively, these data suggest that MMP-2,

MMP-9 and possibly other MMPs can be up-regulated in response to chemokines and Aβ leading to enhanced clearance of Aβ.

Endothelin Converting Enzymes

Endothelin converting enzyme 1 and 2 (ECE-1/ECE-2) are type II membrane-associated zinc-dependent metallo-endopeptidases (Turner and Murphy, 1996). ECEs are localized in the endothelium throughout the human vasculature (Davenport et al., 1998). ECEs cleave endothelins to produce vasoconstrictors (Xu et al., 1994; Emoto and Yanagisawa, 1995). In human brain, ECE-1 is predominantly detected in the cerebrovascular endothelium (Miners et al., 2008a), with some expression seen in neurons of cerebral cortex (Schmidt-Ott et al., 1998). ECE-1 is localized predominantly in the plasma membrane (Schweizer et al., 1997) and in intracellular compartments (Azarani et al., 1998) and has optimum activity at neutral pH (Emoto and Yanagisawa, 1995). In human brain, ECE-2 is expressed predominantly in hippocampal pyramidal neurons (Miners et al., 2008a). ECE-2 is localized intracellularly and has optimum activity at acidic pH (Emoto and Yanagisawa, 1995).

ECE-1 cleaves synthetic Aβ at three sites (Eckman et al., 2001). Experimental models have provided *in vivo* evidence that ECE-1 and ECE-2 may be involved in degradation of Aβ (Eckman et al., 2001; Eckman et al., 2003; Eckman et al., 2006). Mice deficient in ECE-1 or ECE-2 showed significant increase in endogenous Aβ levels indicating that Aβ is a physiologically relevant substrate for these enzymes (Eckman et al., 2003; Eckman et al., 2006). Although there are few studies with human tissues, one study found significant decrease in ECE-2 mRNA expression in AD brains and immunostaining showed loss of ECE-2 from neurons (Weeraratna et al., 2007).

Plasmin

Plasmin is a serine protease involved in the degradation of fibrin generated during clot formation. Plasmin is generated from its inactive form, plasminogen, by proteolytic cleavage by two activators: tissue-type plasminogen activator (tPA) or urokinase-type plasminogen activator (uPA). Production of both tPA and uPA are induced by fibrin aggregates, which in turn, lead to generation of plasmin and degradation of the fibrin aggregates (Henkin et al., 1991). Recent data suggest that the plasmin pathway may be involved in degradation of Aβ in the brain. Brain tPA, uPA and plasminogen are produced by neurons and tPA is also produced by microglia (Tsirka et al., 1997). Plasmin has been shown to cleave Aβ at multiple sites (Tucker et al., 2000a; Tucker et al., 2000b) and prevent aggregation and formation of β-pleated sheets by Aβ1-42 ((Exley and Korchazhkina, 2001). Fibrillar Aβ binds to and enhances the proteolytic activity of tPA (Kingston et al., 1995; Wnendt et al., 1997). Furthermore, fibrillar Aβ (but not soluble) induces expression of tPA and uPA mRNA in cultured neurons (Tucker et al., 2000a).

In studies with mice deficient in plasmin, endogenous levels of Aβ were not found to be increased (Tucker et al., 2004) suggesting that plasmin may play only a small role in steady –

state maintenance of Aβ levels under non-pathological conditions in the brain. However, there is evidence that plasmin likely plays a role in clearance of pathogenic Aβ aggregates. Clearance of Aβ injected into the hippocampus of plasmin-deficient mice was much slower than in wild-type mice (Melchor et al., 2003). Furthermore, persistence of the injected Aβ in these mice resulted in activation of microglia and neuronal damage. In APP transgenic mice, mRNA levels of tPA and uPA were increased compared with non transgenic controls (Tucker et al., 2000b). However, in other studies with AD mice, the proteolytic activity of tPA was found to be reduced in transgenic mice compared with non-transgenic mice (Melchor et al., 2003; Cacquevel et al., 2007) and correlated with Aβ-accumulation. In summary, the tPA/plasmin system appears to favor Aβ clearance from the brain and impairment of tPA activity may decrease clearance and promote Aβ deposition.

Angiotensin-Converting Enzyme

Angiotensin-converting enzyme (ACE) is a membrane-anchored zinc metalloproteinase expressed throughout the vasculature where it plays an important role in regulation of blood pressure and fluid and sodium homeostasis (Skidgel and Erdos, 1987; Coates, 2003). In human brain tissue, ACE has been detected predominantly in pyramidal cortical neurons and cerebral vasculature (Savaskan et al., 2001; Miners et al., 2008a). Much of the evidence for an association between ACE and AD comes from human genetic studies assessing risk for AD development in patients with insertion or deletion polymorphisms in the ACE gene ((Kehoe et al., 1999; Elkins et al., 2004). The levels of ACE protein and activity were found to be elevated in AD postmortem brains compared with non-AD brains ((Savaskan et al., 2001; Miners et al., 2008b) raising the possibility for a role of ACE in Aβ clearance *in vivo.*

ACE can cleave synthetic Aβ and inhibit its aggregation and cytotoxicity *in vitro* (Hu et al., 2001; Oba et al., 2005). ACE can also degrade naturally produced Aβ in cell culture models and the degradation was blocked with an ACE inhibitor (Hemming and Selkoe, 2005). However, in vivo studies found that prolonged administration of ACE inhibitors to transgenic AD mice did not alter Aβ degradation (Hemming et al., 2007). Furthermore, mice genetically deficient in ACE did not have increased level of endogenous Aβ suggesting that ACE is not involved in steady-state regulation of Aβ (Eckman et al., 2006). Overall, these studies suggest that ACE does not appear to play a role maintaining Aβ balance in the normal brain, and that additional evidence is required to confirm that it may be involved in Aβ degradation in pathologic conditions.

Other Aβ-Degrading Enzymes

Two other enzymes, cathepsin B and PreP, have been found to degrade Aβ.

Cathepsin B (CatB) is a cysteine protease that has been found to degrade Aβ *in vitro* and *in vivo* (Frautschy et al., 1998b; Mueller-Steiner et al., 2006). CatB is located in the lysosomes where it degrades peptides/proteins that enter by endocytosis or phagocytosis (Chapman et al., 1997) and has been shown to be secreted in certain pathological conditions

(Buck et al., 1992; Mort and Buttle, 1997). In AD brains, extracellular CatB has been demonstrated in associated with amyloid plaques (Cataldo et al., 1997; Mueller-Steiner et al., 2006). Transgenic APP mice deficient in CAtB showed increased Aβ deposition and neuropathology (Mueller-Steiner et al., 2006), confirming a role for CAtB in Aβ clearance *in vivo.*

A novel mitochondrial peptidase, PreP, a functional analogue of IDE, has been shown to degrade Aβ *in vitro* (Falkevall et al., 2006). PreP shares some cleavage sites with IDE, but also cleaves in the hydrophobic carboxyl region of Aβ in sites also cut by MMP-9. Further studies are needed to assess the potential role of PreP in Aβ clearance.

Alpha Secretase

In addition to amyloidogenic processing of APP to generate Aβ, a non-amyloidogenic alternate pathway exists in which APP is cleaved within the Aβ peptide by α-secretase (Allinson et al., 2003; Deuss et al., 2008). As a result, a large non-pathogenic extracellular APP fragment is released. This cleavage prevents deposition of intact Aβ peptides, and therefore reduces Aβ accumulation in the brain (Allinson et al., 2003; Postina, 2008). Alpha-secretase is a zinc metalloproteinase, and several members of the adamalysin family of proteins, tumour necrosis factor convertase (TACE, ADAM17), ADAM10, and ADAM9, behave as α-secretases (Deuss et al., 2008; Postina, 2008). Interestingly, drugs such as muscarinic agonists, cholesterol-lowering drugs, steroid hormones, non-steroidal anti-inflammatory drugs, and metal ions increase α-secretase activity, which may explain some of the therapeutic actions of these agents in Alzheimer's disease (Allinson et al., 2003).

Efflux of Aβ Across the Blood Brain Barrier

Brain Endothelial Cells Regulate Influx of Aβ into the Brain

Specific influx and efflux transport of Aβ across the blood brain barrier (BBB) may play an important role in determining the concentration of Aβ in the brain (Deane and Zlokovic, 2007). The BBB regulates influx of plasma-derived Aβ into the brain parenchyma (Deane et al., 2003) and mediates efflux and clearance of brain-derived Aβ (Deane et al., 2004). While the exact pathways involved in Aβ transport across the BBB are not fully elucidated, the roles of at least two important receptors in this process have been well characterized. The endothelial receptor for advanced glycation endproducts (RAGE) mediates the transport of circulating Aβ across the BBB (blood→brain) leading to intracerebral accumulation of Aβ (Deane et al., 2003). In contrast, the LDL receptor-related protein-1 (LRP-1) is involved in the clearance pathway (brain→ blood) (Deane et al., 2004).

Aβ Influx Across the BBB

The blood appears to be a likely, continuous reservoir that supplies soluble Aβ to the brain (Clifford et al., 2007). Plasma-derived Aβ1-40 and Aβ1-42 can slowly cross the intact BBB via a common transport system (Martel et al., 1996). RAGE is expressed at relatively low levels in normal endothelial cells of the BBB. RAGE expression increases in cerebral vessels in AD patients and in transgenic mouse models of AD (Yan et al., 1996; Donahue et al., 2006), possibly as a result of endothelial activation by RAGE ligands (such as AGE proteins and Aβ) in the aging brain. In mouse AD models, Aβ-RAGE interactions at the luminal side of the BBB lead to transcytosis of circulating Aβ across the BBB into the brain parenchyma suggesting that RAGE may directly mediate influx of Aβ across the BBB in AD (Deane et al., 2003).

RAGE appears to be the only known receptor that mediates influx of free Aβ into the brain. However, other pathways for influx of Aβ into the brain have been described. Apolipoprotein J (Apo J), a circulating plasma Apolipoprotein, forms a complex with Aβ that binds to gp330 or low-density lipoprotein receptor related protein 2 (LRP2) and promotes the transport of Aβ-Apo J complexes across the BBB (Zlokovic et al., 1996). However, Apo J appears to play only a small role as a circulating binding protein for Aβ in human plasma (Sagare et al., 2007). While the data from animal models in support of a role for RAGE and Apo J/LRP2 in transport of Aβ from blood to brain is compelling, there is no definitive evidence that support the roles of RAGE or Apo J/LRP2-mediated transport of Aβ into the CNS in disease progression and development of CNS pathology in AD patients.

BBB Clearance of Aβ

While RAGE and Apo-J/LRP2 mediate influx of Aβ across the BBB and may promote accumulation of Aβ in the brain, a counter mechanism exists that mediates the clearance of Aβ from the brain, across the BBB, into the plasma. The low-density lipoprotein receptor related protein 1 (LRP1), a member of the LDL receptor family and a multifunctional scavenger and signaling receptor (Krieger and Herz, 1994), is expressed on the parenchymal side of the BBB. LRP1 binds Aβ and initiates Aβ efflux into the circulation, leading to Aβ clearance from brain→blood via transcytosis across the BBB (Shibata et al., 2000). In the liver, LRP1 also mediates systemic Aβ clearance and subsequent degradation (Tamaki et al., 2006).

In addition to its function in Aβ efflux, a soluble form of LRP1 (sLRP1) is generated as a result of β-secretase cleavage of the N terminus extracellular domain of LRP1. sLRP1 binds 70%–90% of Aβ in human plasma (Sagare et al., 2007) making it an effective peripheral "sink" that chelates Aβ in the plasma. Binding of Aβ to sLRP1 is compromised in AD, leading to increased "free" Aβ in the plasma and possibly contributing to elevated Aβ levels in the brain through influx via RAGE. In addition, LRP1 expression may be decreased during normal aging in nonhuman primates and in some AD patients, thereby reducing the Aβ efflux capabilities of the BBB, and possibly leading to increased Aβ accumulation around cerebral vessels (Shibata et al., 2000; Deane et al., 2004; Donahue et al., 2006). Recombinant LRP1 injected into APPsw mice, can effectively sequester Aβ in their plasma leading to decreased intracerebral Aβ deposits (Sagare et al., 2007). Thus recombinant LRP1 has been proposed as a novel therapeutic Aβ clearance agent that enhances the role of sLRP1 as a peripheral "sink" for Aβ.

In addition to LRP1, another protein that mediates efflux of Aβ from the brain has been identified. P-glycoprotein (Pgp) also known as ABCB1, is the 170-kD product of the multidrug resistance-1 (MDR1) gene. Pgp confers multidrug resistance to tumor cells by mediating efficient efflux of a variety of cytotoxic agents. Pgp is also highly expressed on the luminal surface of brain capillary endothelial cells, functionally limiting CNS accumulation of various chemotherapeutic agents, small peptides, antibiotics, HIV protease inhibitors, and antidepressant drugs by mediating their efflux (Zhou et al., 2008). Mice that lack Pgp at the BBB have reduced clearance of Aβ from the CNS, lower levels of LRP1 in brain capillaries and accelerated accumulation of Aβ deposition, raising a possibility that Pgp may influence Aβ clearance (Cirrito et al., 2005) .

While receptor-mediated transport appears to be the main mechanism for Aβ efflux from the brain it is not the only mechanism. Free diffusion has been estimated to account for up to 15% of Aβ removal from the brain in mice (Shibata et al., 2000).

Modulation of Aβ Clearance for Treatment of AD

Based on the above discussion, it appears very tempting to manipulate the various mechanisms of Aβ clearance in an attempt to delay or stop the progression of AD by enhancing clearance of Aβ and reducing its accumulation in the brain. Indeed several experimental models have been developed in mice that support the use of this approach as a therapeutic modality for AD. The first approach involves vaccination against Aβ to elicit an anti-Aβ humoral immune response. Such immune response promotes Aβ clearance either by phagocytosis of Aβ-anti-Aβ immune complexes or facilitating Aβ uptake via various Aβ receptors. The second approach includes the use of recombinant soluble Aβ binding receptors as a peripheral sink to promote efflux of Aβ across the BBB. The third approach uses umbilical cord cells or bone marrow transplant to enhance the accumulation of phagocytic cells in the brain and promote the cellular clearance of Aβ. Alternatively, agents that activate microglia/macrophages can be administered peripherally to upregulate these cells' abilities to clear Aβ. Finally, various vectors for gene therapy have been used to deliver high levels of Aβ degrading enzymes to the brain and enhance Aβ degradation.

Immunization

Perhaps the most successful experimental therapeutic approach to enhance Aβ clearance in AD in mice so far has been immunization against Aβ. In various mouse models of AD this approach successfully reduces levels of Aβ in the brain, prevents memory loss and improves spatial learning (Morgan et al., 2000; Arendash et al., 2001; Chen et al., 2007; Mouri et al., 2007). The mechanism by which vaccination with Aβ increases clearance of the peptides was believed to involve phagocytosis of Aβ-Anti-Aβ immune complexes via microglial Fc receptors. However, the ability of vaccination to clear Aβ appears to be equivalent in AD mice deficient in Fc receptors and AD mice with normal Fc receptor expression (Das et al., 2003). Furthermore, Fab fragments of the anti-Aβ antibodies applied directly to plaque-containing brain sections of transgenic AD mice also resulted in rapid clearance of Aβ, confirming that Fc receptors are not required for this process (Bacskai et al., 2002). Recently however, multiphoton *in vivo* imaging of events that follow passive immunization against Aβ showed that there was a marked increase in both the number of microglial cells and processes per cell and that these events required the Fc domain of the anti-Aβ antibodies. (Koenigsknecht-Talboo et al., 2008).

Alternate potential mechanisms of Aβ clearance following immunization include breakup of the Aβ aggregates followed by scavenging by other Aβ microglial or astrocyte receptors or anti-Aβ antibodies acting as a peripheral sink for Aβ in the circulation (Vasilevko et al., 2007).

Unfortunately, while immunization of mice is very effective in clearing Aβ deposits and appears to be safe, clinical trials with immunization against Aβ were halted in AD patients because of development of meningoencephalitis with T cell infiltrates in some enrolled patients, dramatically putting a stop, albeit temporary, to this therapeutic approach (Nicoll et al., 2003).

Recombinant Soluble Aβ Receptors as Peripheral Sinks

As discussed earlier, recombinant LRP1 injected into APPsw mice, can effectively sequester Aβ in their plasma leading to decreased intracerebral Aβ deposits (Sagare et al., 2007). Thus recombinant LRP1 has been proposed as a novel therapeutic Aβ clearance agent that enhances the role of sLRP1 as a peripheral "sink" for Aβ. It is not clear if additional receptors can be utilized in this manner.

Administration of Umbilical Cord Blood

Another experimental approach that harnesses the ability of immune cells to clear Aβ that has been proposed as a therapeutic modality for AD involves peripheral administration of human umbilical cord blood cells (HUCBCs). Such cells have unique immunomodulatory potential. Following multiple low-dose infusions of HUCBCs into PS1-APP mice, there was a marked reduction in Aβ levels/Aβ plaques and associated astrocytosis. HUCBC infusions also reduced cerebral vascular Aβ deposits in the Tg2576 AD mouse model. Although these effects were associated with increased microglial phagocytosis of Aβ, the exact mechanism(s) of action is not clear (Nikolic et al., 2008).

Bone Marrow Transplantation

Since microglia and mononuclear phagocytes play an important role in Aβ clearance, and since these cells are derived from the bone marrow, several groups have suggested that bone marrow transplantation with microglial and monocyte precursors is a viable strategy to reduce the amyloid burden (Simard and Rivest, 2006; Simard et al., 2006; El Khoury and

Luster, 2008). No definitive experiment has been published yet to support this possibility. However, when mice injected with Aβ into their hippocampus, were transplanted with bone marrow-derived mesenchymal stem cells, they exhibited reduced Aβ levels as compared to sham-transplanted animals. The enhanced clearance of injected Aβ was accompanied by activation of microglia located near the Aβ deposits, and a change in their morphology from ramified to ameboid suggesting microglial phagocytosis of Aβ (Lee et al., 2009).

Peripheral Activation of Microglia and Mononuclear Phagocytes

Recently, Frenkel and colleagues assessed whether peripheral activation of microglia by a nasal proteosome-based adjuvant (Protollin) can prevent amyloid deposition in young transgenic AD mice and affect amyloid deposition and memory function in old mice with a large amyloid load. The authors found significant reductions in the level of Aβ in protollin-treated AD mice and improved memory function. These improvements in AD-like pathology correlated with microglial activation and upregulation of the Aβ receptor SRA (Frenkel et al., 2005; Frenkel et al., 2008). These results demonstrate that antibody-independent immunotherapy mediated by peripheral activation of microglia is a promising therapeutic modality for AD.

Gene Therapy with Aβ-Degrading Enzymes

Overexpression of IDE or NEP in neurons significantly reduced brain Aβ levels, delayed amyloid plaque formation, and improved survival in APP mice (Leissring et al., 2003b). Marr and colleagues used a lentiviral vector to deliver human NEP into the brains of transgenic AD mice. Unilateral injection of this vector reduced Aβ deposits by half relative to the untreated side, and ameliorated neurodegeneration in the frontal cortex and hippocampus of these transgenic mice (Marr et al., 2003; Spencer et al., 2008). A similar approach with other Aβ-degrading enzymes has been proposed but no definitive experiment has been published yet (Eckman and Eckman, 2005). Gene therapy with Aβ-degrading enzymes has potential for the development of alternative therapies for AD.

Gaps in Knowledge and Future Directions

Specific upregulation of Aβ clearing pathways appears to have great potential to be a novel therapeutic strategy to delay/stop the progression of AD. Several hurdles need to be overcome before this modality becomes a viable approach to treat AD. First, with regard to Aβ-degrading enzymes, better targeting methods that will cross the BBB and deliver the enzymes to sites of Aβ deposition, where they are most needed, would likely enhance the therapeutic potential for these enzymes. In this regard, gene therapy may be a very promising approach. As for upregulating Aβ phagocytosis and clearance by microglia and monocytes, identifying the most important receptor involved in this process (SRA vs. SRB vs. RAGE etc.) will go a long way in determining which pathway may be of the best therapeutic relevance. Another very promising approach would be to enhance Aβ clearance through efflux across the BBB. Some questions to consider here are whether upregulating efflux pumps (LRP1 or PgP) or downregulating influx pumps (RAGE or other receptors) will be the most effective. Another question is whether other receptors on BBB endothelial cells are involved in this process. Finally is the use of recombinant Aβ receptors as peripheral sinks an effective and realistic strategy for chelating Aβ in the blood and reducing its intracerebral levels. The possibilities raised are very exciting and one can envision the development of new approaches to enhance Aβ clearance as viable and effective therapies for AD in the not-so-distant future.

References

Abumrad NA, el-Maghrabi MR, Amri EZ, Lopez E, Grimaldi PA (1993) Cloning of a rat adipocyte membrane protein implicated in binding or transport of long-chain fatty acids that is induced during preadipocyte differentiation. Homology with human CD36. *J Biol Chem* 268:17665-17668.

Acton S, Rigotti A, Landschulz KT, Xu S, Hobbs HH, Krieger M (1996) Identification of scavenger receptor SR-BI as a high density lipoprotein receptor. *Science* 271:518-520.

Alarcon R, Fuenzalida C, Santibanez M, von Bernhardi R (2005) Expression of scavenger receptors in glial cells. Comparing the adhesion of astrocytes and microglia from neonatal rats to surface-bound beta-amyloid. *J Biol Chem* 280:30406-30415.

Allinson TM, Parkin ET, Turner AJ, Hooper NM (2003) ADAMs family members as amyloid precursor protein alpha-secretases. *J Neurosci Res* 74:342-352.

Arendash GW, Gordon MN, Diamond DM, Austin LA, Hatcher JM, Jantzen P, DiCarlo G, Wilcock D, Morgan D (2001) Behavioral assessment of Alzheimer's transgenic mice following long-term Abeta vaccination: task specificity and correlations between Abeta deposition and spatial memory. *DNA Cell Biol* 20:737-744.

Authier F, Posner BI, Bergeron JJ (1996) Insulin-degrading enzyme. *Clin Invest Med* 19:149-160.

Azarani A, Boileau G, Crine P (1998) Recombinant human endothelin-converting enzyme ECE-1b is located in an intracellular compartment when expressed in polarized Madin-Darby canine kidney cells. *Biochem J* 333 (Pt 2):439-448.

Backstrom JR, Lim GP, Cullen MJ, Tokes ZA (1996) Matrix metalloproteinase-9 (MMP-9) is synthesized in neurons of the human hippocampus and is capable of degrading the amyloid-beta peptide (1-40). *J Neurosci* 16:7910-7919.

Bacskai BJ, Kajdasz ST, McLellan ME, Games D, Seubert P, Schenk D, Hyman BT (2002) Non-Fc-mediated mechanisms are involved in clearance of amyloid-beta in vivo by immunotherapy. *J Neurosci* 22:7873-7878.

Barnes K, Turner AJ, Kenny AJ (1992) Membrane localization of endopeptidase-24.11 and peptidyl dipeptidase A (angiotensin converting enzyme) in the pig brain: a study using subcellular fractionation and electron microscopic immunocytochemistry. *J Neurochem* 58:2088-2096.

Buck MR, Karustis DG, Day NA, Honn KV, Sloane BF (1992) Degradation of extracellular-matrix proteins by human cathepsin B from normal and tumour tissues. *Biochem J* 282 (Pt 1):273-278.

Cacquevel M, Launay S, Castel H, Benchenane K, Cheenne S, Buee L, Moons L, Delacourte A, Carmeliet P, Vivien D (2007) Ageing and amyloid-beta peptide deposition contribute to an impaired brain tissue plasminogen activator activity by different mechanisms. *Neurobiol Dis* 27:164-173.

Cataldo AM, Barnett JL, Pieroni C, Nixon RA (1997) Increased neuronal endocytosis and protease delivery to early endosomes in sporadic Alzheimer's disease: neuropathologic evidence for a mechanism of increased beta-amyloidogenesis. *J Neurosci* 17:6142-6151.

Chandler S, Miller KM, Clements JM, Lury J, Corkill D, Anthony DC, Adams SE, Gearing AJ (1997) Matrix metalloproteinases, tumor necrosis factor and multiple sclerosis: an overview. *J Neuroimmunol* 72:155-161.

Chapman HA, Riese RJ, Shi GP (1997) Emerging roles for cysteine proteases in human biology. *Annu Rev Physiol* 59:63-88.

Chen G, Chen KS, Kobayashi D, Barbour R, Motter R, Games D, Martin SJ, Morris RG (2007) Active beta-amyloid immunization restores spatial learning in PDAPP mice displaying very low levels of beta-amyloid. *J Neurosci* 27:2654-2662.

Chung H, Brazil MI, Irizarry MC, Hyman BT, Maxfield FR (2001) Uptake of fibrillar beta-amyloid by microglia isolated from MSR-A (type I and type II) knockout mice. *Neuroreport* 12:1151-1154.

Cirrito JR, Deane R, Fagan AM, Spinner ML, Parsadanian M, Finn MB, Jiang H, Prior JL, Sagare A, Bales KR, Paul SM, Zlokovic BV, Piwnica-Worms D, Holtzman DM (2005) P-glycoprotein deficiency at the blood-brain barrier increases amyloid-beta deposition in an Alzheimer disease mouse model. *J Clin Invest* 115:3285-3290.

Clifford PM, Zarrabi S, Siu G, Kinsler KJ, Kosciuk MC, Venkataraman V, D'Andrea MR, Dinsmore S, Nagele RG (2007) Abeta peptides can enter the brain through a defective blood-brain barrier and bind selectively to neurons. *Brain Res* 1142:223-236.

Coates D (2003) The angiotensin converting enzyme (ACE). *Int J Biochem Cell Biol* 35:769-773.

Cook DG, Leverenz JB, McMillan PJ, Kulstad JJ, Ericksen S, Roth RA, Schellenberg GD, Jin LW, Kovacina KS, Craft S (2003) Reduced hippocampal insulin-degrading enzyme in late-onset Alzheimer's disease is associated with the apolipoprotein E-epsilon4 allele. *Am J Pathol* 162:313-319.

Coraci IS, Husemann J, Berman JW, Hulette C, Dufour JH, Campanella GK, Luster AD, Silverstein SC, El-Khoury JB (2002) CD36, a class B scavenger receptor, is expressed on microglia in Alzheimer's disease brains and can mediate production of reactive oxygen species in response to beta-amyloid fibrils. *Am J Pathol* 160:101-112.

Crocker SJ, Frausto RF, Whitton JL, Milner R (2008) A novel method to establish microglia-free astrocyte cultures: comparison of matrix metalloproteinase expression profiles in pure cultures of astrocytes and microglia. *Glia* 56:1187-1198.

Cross AK, Woodroofe MN (1999) Chemokine modulation of matrix metalloproteinase and TIMP production in adult rat brain microglia and a human microglial cell line in vitro. *Glia* 28:183-189.

D'Andrea MR, Cole GM, Ard MD (2004) The microglial phagocytic role with specific plaque types in the Alzheimer disease brain. *Neurobiol Aging* 25:675-683.

Das P, Howard V, Loosbrock N, Dickson D, Murphy MP, Golde TE (2003) Amyloid-beta immunization effectively reduces amyloid deposition in FcRgamma-/- knock-out mice. *J Neurosci* 23:8532-8538.

Davenport AP, Kuc RE, Mockridge JW (1998) Endothelin-converting enzyme in the human vasculature: evidence for differential conversion of big endothelin-3 by endothelial and smooth-muscle cells. *J Cardiovasc Pharmacol* 31 Suppl 1:S1-3.

Deane R, Zlokovic BV (2007) Role of the blood-brain barrier in the pathogenesis of Alzheimer's disease. *Curr Alzheimer Res* 4:191-197.

Deane R, Wu Z, Zlokovic BV (2004) RAGE (yin) versus LRP (yang) balance regulates alzheimer amyloid beta-peptide clearance through transport across the blood-brain barrier. *Stroke* 35:2628-2631.

Deane R, Du Yan S, Submamaryan RK, LaRue B, Jovanovic S, Hogg E, Welch D, Manness L, Lin C, Yu J, Zhu H, Ghiso J, Frangione B, Stern A, Schmidt AM, Armstrong DL, Arnold B, Liliensiek B, Nawroth P, Hofman F, Kindy M, Stern D, Zlokovic B (2003) RAGE mediates amyloid-beta peptide transport across the blood-brain barrier and accumulation in brain. *Nat Med* 9:907-913.

Deb S, Wenjun Zhang J, Gottschall PE (2003) Beta-amyloid induces the production of active, matrix-degrading proteases in cultured rat astrocytes. *Brain Res* 970:205-213.

Deuss M, Reiss K, Hartmann D (2008) Part-time alpha-secretases: the functional biology of ADAM 9, 10 and 17. *Curr Alzheimer Res* 5:187-201.

Donahue JE, Flaherty SL, Johanson CE, Duncan JA, 3rd, Silverberg GD, Miller MC, Tavares R, Yang W, Wu Q, Sabo E, Hovanesian V, Stopa EG (2006) RAGE, LRP-1, and amyloid-beta protein in Alzheimer's disease. *Acta Neuropathol* 112:405-415.

Dorfman VB, Pasquini L, Riudavets M, Lopez-Costa JJ, Villegas A, Troncoso JC, Lopera F, Castano EM, Morelli L (2008) Differential cerebral deposition of IDE and NEP in sporadic and familial Alzheimer's disease. *Neurobiol Aging.*

Duffy PE, Rapport M, Graf L (1980) Glial fibrillary acidic protein and Alzheimer-type senile dementia. *Neurology* 30:778-782.

Eckman EA, Eckman CB (2005) Abeta-degrading enzymes: modulators of Alzheimer's disease pathogenesis and targets for therapeutic intervention. *Biochem Soc Trans* 33:1101-1105.

Eckman EA, Reed DK, Eckman CB (2001) Degradation of the Alzheimer's amyloid beta peptide by endothelin-converting enzyme. *J Biol Chem* 276:24540-24548.

Eckman EA, Watson M, Marlow L, Sambamurti K, Eckman CB (2003) Alzheimer's disease beta-amyloid peptide is increased in mice deficient in endothelin-converting enzyme. *J Biol Chem* 278:2081-2084.

Eckman EA, Adams SK, Troendle FJ, Stodola BA, Kahn MA, Fauq AH, Xiao HD, Bernstein KE, Eckman CB (2006) Regulation of steady-state beta-amyloid levels in the brain by neprilysin and endothelin-converting enzyme but not angiotensin-converting enzyme. *J Biol Chem* 281:30471-30478.

El Khoury J, Luster AD (2008) Mechanisms of microglia accumulation in Alzheimer's disease: therapeutic implications. *Trends Pharmacol Sci* 29:626-632.

El Khoury J, Hickman SE, Thomas CA, Loike JD, Silverstein SC (1998) Microglia, scavenger receptors, and the pathogenesis of Alzheimer's disease. *Neurobiol Aging* 19:S81-84.

El Khoury J, Thomas CA, Loike JD, Hickman SE, Cao L, Silverstein SC (1994) Macrophages adhere to glucose-modified basement membrane collagen IV via their scavenger receptors. *J Biol Chem* 269:10197-10200.

El Khoury J, Hickman SE, Thomas CA, Cao L, Silverstein SC, Loike JD (1996) Scavenger receptor-mediated adhesion of microglia to beta-amyloid fibrils. *Nature* 382:716-719.

El Khoury J, Toft M, Hickman SE, Means TK, Terada K, Geula C, Luster AD (2007) Ccr2 deficiency impairs microglial accumulation and accelerates progression of Alzheimer-like disease. *Nat Med* 13:432-438.

El Khoury JB, Moore KJ, Means TK, Leung J, Terada K, Toft M, Freeman MW, Luster AD (2003) CD36 mediates the innate host response to beta-amyloid. *J Exp Med* 197:1657-1666.

Elkins JS, Douglas VC, Johnston SC (2004) Alzheimer disease risk and genetic variation in ACE: a meta-analysis. *Neurology* 62:363-368.

Emoto N, Yanagisawa M (1995) Endothelin-converting enzyme-2 is a membrane-bound, phosphoramidon-sensitive metalloprotease with acidic pH optimum. *J Biol Chem* 270:15262-15268.

Endemann G, Stanton LW, Madden KS, Bryant CM, White RT, Protter AA (1993) CD36 is a receptor for oxidized low density lipoprotein. *J Biol Chem* 268:11811-11816.

Exley C, Korchazhkina OV (2001) Plasmin cleaves Abeta42 in vitro and prevents its aggregation into beta-pleated sheet structures. *Neuroreport* 12:2967-2970.

Falkevall A, Alikhani N, Bhushan S, Pavlov PF, Busch K, Johnson KA, Eneqvist T, Tjernberg L, Ankarcrona M, Glaser E (2006) Degradation of the amyloid beta-protein by the novel mitochondrial peptidasome, PreP. *J Biol Chem* 281:29096-29104.

Farris W, Mansourian S, Chang Y, Lindsley L, Eckman EA, Frosch MP, Eckman CB, Tanzi RE, Selkoe DJ, Guenette S (2003) Insulin-degrading enzyme regulates the levels of insulin, amyloid beta-protein, and the beta-amyloid precursor protein intracellular domain in vivo. *Proc Natl Acad Sci U S A* 100:4162-4167.

Frautschy SA, Yang F, Irrizarry M, Hyman B, Saido TC, Hsiao K, Cole GM (1998a) Microglial response to amyloid plaques in APPsw transgenic mice. *Am J Pathol* 152:307-317.

Frautschy SA, Horn DL, Sigel JJ, Harris-White ME, Mendoza JJ, Yang F, Saido TC, Cole GM (1998b) Protease inhibitor coinfusion with amyloid beta-protein results in enhanced deposition and toxicity in rat brain. *J Neurosci* 18:8311-8321.

Frenkel D, Maron R, Burt DS, Weiner HL (2005) Nasal vaccination with a proteosome-based adjuvant and glatiramer acetate clears beta-amyloid in a mouse model of Alzheimer disease. *J Clin Invest* 115:2423-2433.

Frenkel D, Puckett L, Petrovic S, Xia W, Chen G, Vega J, Dembinsky-Vaknin A, Shen J, Plante M, Burt DS, Weiner HL (2008) A nasal proteosome adjuvant activates microglia and prevents amyloid deposition. *Ann Neurol* 63:591-601.

Fukami S, Watanabe K, Iwata N, Haraoka J, Lu B, Gerard NP, Gerard C, Fraser P, Westaway D, St George-Hyslop P, Saido TC (2002) Abeta-degrading endopeptidase, neprilysin, in mouse brain: synaptic and axonal localization inversely correlating with Abeta pathology. *Neurosci Res* 43:39-56.

Goodwin JL, Kehrli ME, Jr., Uemura E (1997) Integrin Mac-1 and beta-amyloid in microglial release of nitric oxide. *Brain Res* 768:279-286.

Gottschall PE (1996) beta-Amyloid induction of gelatinase B secretion in cultured microglia: inhibition by dexamethasone and indomethacin. *Neuroreport* 7:3077-3080.

Gurney KJ, Estrada EY, Rosenberg GA (2006) Blood-brain barrier disruption by stromelysin-1 facilitates neutrophil infiltration in neuroinflammation. *Neurobiol Dis* 23:87-96.

Hemming ML, Selkoe DJ (2005) Amyloid beta-protein is degraded by cellular angiotensin-converting enzyme (ACE) and elevated by an ACE inhibitor. *J Biol Chem* 280:37644-37650.

Hemming ML, Selkoe DJ, Farris W (2007) Effects of prolonged angiotensin-converting enzyme inhibitor treatment on amyloid beta-protein metabolism in mouse models of Alzheimer disease. *Neurobiol Dis* 26:273-281.

Heneka MT, O'Banion MK (2007) Inflammatory processes in Alzheimer's disease. J *Neuroimmunol* 184:69-91.

Henkin J, Marcotte P, Yang HC (1991) The plasminogen-plasmin system. *Prog Cardiovasc Dis* 34:135-164.

Hickman SE, Allison EK, El Khoury J (2008) Microglial dysfunction and defective beta-amyloid clearance pathways in aging Alzheimer's disease mice. *J Neurosci* 28:8354-8360.

Hu J, Igarashi A, Kamata M, Nakagawa H (2001) Angiotensin-converting enzyme degrades Alzheimer amyloid beta-peptide (A beta); retards A beta aggregation, deposition, fibril formation; and inhibits cytotoxicity. *J Biol Chem* 276:47863-47868.

Huang F, Buttini M, Wyss-Coray T, McConlogue L, Kodama T, Pitas RE, Mucke L (1999) Elimination of the class A scavenger receptor does not affect amyloid plaque formation or neurodegeneration in transgenic mice expressing human amyloid protein precursors. *Am J Pathol* 155:1741-1747.

Husemann J, Loike JD, Kodama T, Silverstein SC (2001) Scavenger receptor class B type I (SR-BI) mediates adhesion of neonatal murine microglia to fibrillar beta-amyloid. *J Neuroimmunol* 114:142-150.

Iribarren P, Zhou Y, Hu J, Le Y, Wang JM (2005) Role of formyl peptide receptor-like 1 (FPRL1/FPR2) in mononuclear phagocyte responses in Alzheimer disease. *Immunol Res* 31:165-176.

Iwata N, Takaki Y, Fukami S, Tsubuki S, Saido TC (2002) Region-specific reduction of A beta-degrading endopeptidase, neprilysin, in mouse hippocampus upon aging. *J Neurosci Res* 70:493-500.

Iwata N, Tsubuki S, Takaki Y, Shirotani K, Lu B, Gerard NP, Gerard C, Hama E, Lee HJ, Saido TC (2001) Metabolic regulation of brain Abeta by neprilysin. *Science* 292:1550-1552.

Iwata N, Mizukami H, Shirotani K, Takaki Y, Muramatsu S, Lu B, Gerard NP, Gerard C, Ozawa K, Saido TC (2004) Presynaptic localization of neprilysin contributes to efficient clearance of amyloid-beta peptide in mouse brain. *J Neurosci* 24:991-998.

Iwata N, Tsubuki S, Takaki Y, Watanabe K, Sekiguchi M, Hosoki E, Kawashima-Morishima M, Lee HJ, Hama E, Sekine-Aizawa Y, Saido TC (2000) Identification of the major Abeta1-42-degrading catabolic pathway in brain parenchyma: suppression leads to biochemical and pathological deposition. *Nat Med* 6:143-150.

Jiang Q, Lee CY, Mandrekar S, Wilkinson B, Cramer P, Zelcer N, Mann K, Lamb B, Willson TM, Collins JL, Richardson JC, Smith JD, Comery TA, Riddell D, Holtzman DM, Tontonoz P, Landreth GE (2008) ApoE promotes the proteolytic degradation of Abeta. *Neuron* 58:681-693.

Johnstone M, Gearing AJ, Miller KM (1999) A central role for astrocytes in the inflammatory response to beta-amyloid; chemokines, cytokines and reactive oxygen species are produced. *J Neuroimmunol* 93:182-193.

Kanemitsu H, Tomiyama T, Mori H (2003) Human neprilysin is capable of degrading amyloid beta peptide not only in the monomeric form but also the pathological oligomeric form. *Neurosci Lett* 350:113-116.

Kehoe PG, Russ C, McIlory S, Williams H, Holmans P, Holmes C, Liolitsa D, Vahidassr D, Powell J, McGleenon B, Liddell M, Plomin R, Dynan K, Williams N, Neal J, Cairns NJ, Wilcock G, Passmore P, Lovestone S, Williams J, Owen MJ (1999) Variation in DCP1, encoding ACE, is associated with susceptibility to Alzheimer disease. *Nat Genet* 21:71-72.

Kingston IB, Castro MJ, Anderson S (1995) In vitro stimulation of tissue-type plasminogen activator by Alzheimer amyloid beta-peptide analogues. *Nat Med* 1:138-142.

Koenigsknecht-Talboo J, Meyer-Luehmann M, Parsadanian M, Garcia-Alloza M, Finn MB, Hyman BT, Bacskai BJ, Holtzman DM (2008) Rapid microglial response around amyloid pathology after systemic anti-Abeta antibody administration in PDAPP mice. *J Neurosci* 28:14156-14164.

Koenigsknecht J, Landreth G (2004) Microglial phagocytosis of fibrillar beta-amyloid through a beta1 integrin-dependent mechanism. *J Neurosci* 24:9838-9846.

Koistinaho M, Lin S, Wu X, Esterman M, Koger D, Hanson J, Higgs R, Liu F, Malkani S, Bales KR, Paul SM (2004) Apolipoprotein E promotes astrocyte colocalization and degradation of deposited amyloid-beta peptides. *Nat Med* 10:719-726.

Krieger M, Herz J (1994) Structures and functions of multiligand lipoprotein receptors: macrophage scavenger receptors and LDL receptor-related protein (LRP). *Annu Rev Biochem* 63:601-637.

Kuo WL, Montag AG, Rosner MR (1993) Insulin-degrading enzyme is differentially expressed and developmentally regulated in various rat tissues. *Endocrinology* 132:604-611.

Lee JK, Jin HK, Bae JS (2009) Bone marrow-derived mesenchymal stem cells reduce brain amyloid-beta deposition and accelerate the activation of microglia in an acutely induced Alzheimer's disease mouse model. *Neurosci Lett* 450:136-141.

Lefterov I, Bookout A, Wang Z, Staufenbiel M, Mangelsdorf D, Koldamova R (2007) Expression profiling in APP23 mouse brain: inhibition of Abeta amyloidosis and inflammation in response to LXR agonist treatment. *Mol Neurodegener* 2:20.

Leissring MA (2008) The AbetaCs of Abeta-cleaving proteases. *J Biol Chem* 283:29645-29649.

Leissring MA, Lu A, Condron MM, Teplow DB, Stein RL, Farris W, Selkoe DJ (2003a) Kinetics of amyloid beta-protein degradation determined by novel fluorescence- and fluorescence polarization-based assays. *J Biol Chem* 278:37314-37320.

Leissring MA, Farris W, Chang AY, Walsh DM, Wu X, Sun X, Frosch MP, Selkoe DJ (2003b) Enhanced proteolysis of beta-amyloid in APP transgenic mice prevents plaque formation, secondary pathology, and premature death. *Neuron* 40:1087-1093.

Liu Y, Walter S, Stagi M, Cherny D, Letiembre M, Schulz-Schaeffer W, Heine H, Penke B, Neumann H, Fassbender K (2005) LPS receptor (CD14): a receptor for phagocytosis of Alzheimer's amyloid peptide. *Brain* 128:1778-1789.

Lucas M, Stuart LM, Zhang A, Hodivala-Dilke K, Febbraio M, Silverstein R, Savill J, Lacy-Hulbert A (2006) Requirements for apoptotic cell contact in regulation of macrophage responses. *J Immunol* 177:4047-4054.

Malm T, Ort M, Tahtivaara L, Jukarainen N, Goldsteins G, Puolivali J, Nurmi A, Pussinen R, Ahtoniemi T, Miettinen TK, Kanninen K, Leskinen S, Vartiainen N, Yrjanheikki J, Laatikainen R, Harris-White ME, Koistinaho M, Frautschy SA, Bures J, Koistinaho J (2006) beta-Amyloid infusion results in delayed and age-dependent learning deficits without role of inflammation or beta-amyloid deposits. *Proc Natl Acad Sci U S A* 103:8852-8857.

Marr RA, Rockenstein E, Mukherjee A, Kindy MS, Hersh LB, Gage FH, Verma IM, Masliah E (2003) Neprilysin gene transfer reduces human amyloid pathology in transgenic mice. *J Neurosci* 23:1992-1996.

Martel CL, Mackic JB, McComb JG, Ghiso J, Zlokovic BV (1996) Blood-brain barrier uptake of the 40 and 42 amino acid sequences of circulating Alzheimer's amyloid beta in guinea pigs. *Neurosci Lett* 206:157-160.

McGeer PL, Itagaki S, Tago H, McGeer EG (1987) Reactive microglia in patients with senile dementia of the Alzheimer type are positive for the histocompatibility glycoprotein HLA-DR. *Neurosci Lett* 79:195-200.

Means TK, Mylonakis E, Tampakakis E, Colvin RA, Seung E, Puckett L, Tai MF, Stewart CR, Pukkila-Worley R, Hickman SE, Moore KJ, Calderwood SB, Hacohen N, Luster AD, El Khoury J (2009) Evolutionarily conserved recognition and innate immunity to fungal pathogens by the scavenger receptors SCARF1 and CD36. *J Exp Med* 206:637-653.

Meilandt WJ, Cisse M, Ho K, Wu T, Esposito LA, Scearce-Levie K, Cheng IH, Yu GQ, Mucke L (2009) Neprilysin overexpression inhibits plaque formation but fails to reduce pathogenic Abeta oligomers and associated cognitive deficits in human amyloid precursor protein transgenic mice. *J Neurosci* 29:1977-1986.

Melchor JP, Pawlak R, Strickland S (2003) The tissue plasminogen activator-plasminogen proteolytic cascade accelerates amyloid-beta (Abeta) degradation and inhibits Abeta-induced neurodegeneration. *J Neurosci* 23:8867-8871.

Miners JS, Baig S, Palmer J, Palmer LE, Kehoe PG, Love S (2008a) Abeta-degrading enzymes in Alzheimer's disease. *Brain Pathol* 18:240-252.

Miners JS, Ashby E, Van Helmond Z, Chalmers KA, Palmer LE, Love S, Kehoe PG (2008b) Angiotensin-converting enzyme (ACE) levels and activity in Alzheimer's disease, and relationship of perivascular ACE-1 to cerebral amyloid angiopathy. *Neuropathol Appl Neurobiol* 34:181-193.

Morgan D, Diamond DM, Gottschall PE, Ugen KE, Dickey C, Hardy J, Duff K, Jantzen P, DiCarlo G, Wilcock D, Connor K, Hatcher J, Hope C, Gordon M, Arendash GW (2000) A beta peptide vaccination prevents memory loss in an animal model of Alzheimer's disease. *Nature* 408:982-985.

Morita M, Kurochkin IV, Motojima K, Goto S, Takano T, Okamura S, Sato R, Yokota S, Imanaka T (2000) Insulin-degrading enzyme exists inside of rat liver peroxisomes and degrades oxidized proteins. *Cell Struct Funct* 25:309-315.

Mort JS, Buttle DJ (1997) Cathepsin B. Int J Biochem Cell Biol 29:715-720.

Mouri A, Noda Y, Hara H, Mizoguchi H, Tabira T, Nabeshima T (2007) Oral vaccination with a viral vector containing Abeta cDNA attenuates age-related Abeta accumulation and memory deficits without causing inflammation in a mouse Alzheimer model. *Faseb J* 21:2135-2148.

Mueller-Steiner S, Zhou Y, Arai H, Roberson ED, Sun B, Chen J, Wang X, Yu G, Esposito L, Mucke L, Gan L (2006) Antiamyloidogenic and neuroprotective functions of cathepsin B: implications for Alzheimer's disease. *Neuron* 51:703-714.

Nicoll JA, Wilkinson D, Holmes C, Steart P, Markham H, Weller RO (2003) Neuropathology of human Alzheimer disease after immunization with amyloid-beta peptide: a case report. *Nat Med* 9:448-452.

Nielsen HM, Veerhuis R, Holmqvist B, Janciauskiene S (2008) Binding and uptake of Abeta1-42 by primary human astrocytes in vitro. *Glia.*

Nikolic WV, Hou H, Town T, Zhu Y, Giunta B, Sanberg CD, Zeng J, Luo D, Ehrhart J, Mori T, Sanberg PR, Tan J (2008) Peripherally administered human umbilical cord blood cells reduce parenchymal and vascular beta-amyloid deposits in Alzheimer mice. *Stem Cells Dev* 17:423-439.

Oba R, Igarashi A, Kamata M, Nagata K, Takano S, Nakagawa H (2005) The N-terminal active centre of human angiotensin-converting enzyme degrades Alzheimer amyloid beta-peptide. *Eur J Neurosci* 21:733-740.

Ockenhouse CF, Magowan C, Chulay JD (1989) Activation of monocytes and platelets by monoclonal antibodies or malaria-infected erythrocytes binding to the CD36 surface receptor in vitro. *J Clin Invest* 84:468-475.

Perez A, Morelli L, Cresto JC, Castano EM (2000) Degradation of soluble amyloid beta-peptides 1-40, 1-42, and the Dutch variant 1-40Q by insulin degrading enzyme from Alzheimer disease and control brains. *Neurochem Res* 25:247-255.

Perlmutter LS, Barron E, Chui HC (1990) Morphologic association between microglia and senile plaque amyloid in Alzheimer's disease. *Neurosci Lett* 119:32-36.

Postina R (2008) A closer look at alpha-secretase. *Curr Alzheimer Res* 5:179-186.

Qiu WQ, Ye Z, Kholodenko D, Seubert P, Selkoe DJ (1997) Degradation of amyloid beta-protein by a metalloprotease secreted by microglia and other neural and non-neural cells. *J Biol Chem* 272:6641-6646.

Ramos-DeSimone N, Hahn-Dantona E, Sipley J, Nagase H, French DL, Quigley JP (1999) Activation of matrix metalloproteinase-9 (MMP-9) via a converging plasmin/stromelysin-1 cascade enhances tumor cell invasion. *J Biol Chem* 274:13066-13076.

Rosenberg GA (2002) Matrix metalloproteinases in neuroinflammation. *Glia* 39:279-291.

Rozemuller JM, Eikelenboom P, Stam FC (1986) Role of microglia in plaque formation in senile dementia of the Alzheimer type. An immunohistochemical study. *Virchows Arch B Cell Pathol Incl Mol Pathol* 51:247-254.

Sagare A, Deane R, Bell RD, Johnson B, Hamm K, Pendu R, Marky A, Lenting PJ, Wu Z, Zarcone T, Goate A, Mayo K, Perlmutter D, Coma M, Zhong Z, Zlokovic BV (2007) Clearance of amyloid-beta by circulating lipoprotein receptors. *Nat Med* 13:1029-1031.

Savaskan E, Hock C, Olivieri G, Bruttel S, Rosenberg C, Hulette C, Muller-Spahn F (2001) Cortical alterations of angiotensin converting enzyme, angiotensin II and AT1 receptor in Alzheimer's dementia. *Neurobiol Aging* 22:541-546.

Schmidt-Ott KM, Tuschick S, Kirchhoff F, Verkhratsky A, Liefeldt L, Kettenmann H, Paul M (1998) Single-cell characterization of endothelin system gene expression in the cerebellum in situ. *J Cardiovasc Pharmacol 31 Suppl* 1:S364-366.

Schweizer A, Valdenaire O, Nelbock P, Deuschle U, Dumas Milne Edwards JB, Stumpf JG, Loffler BM (1997) Human endothelin-converting enzyme (ECE-1): three isoforms with distinct subcellular localizations. *Biochem J* 328 (Pt 3):871-877.

Selkoe DJ (2000) The origins of Alzheimer disease: a is for amyloid. *Jama* 283:1615-1617.

Shaftel SS, Kyrkanides S, Olschowka JA, Miller JN, Johnson RE, O'Banion MK (2007) Sustained hippocampal IL-1 beta overexpression mediates chronic neuroinflammation and ameliorates Alzheimer plaque pathology. *J Clin Invest* 117:1595-1604.

Shibata M, Yamada S, Kumar SR, Calero M, Bading J, Frangione B, Holtzman DM, Miller CA, Strickland DK, Ghiso J, Zlokovic BV (2000) Clearance of Alzheimer's amyloid-ss(1-40) peptide from brain by LDL receptor-related protein-1 at the blood-brain barrier. *J Clin Invest* 106:1489-1499.

Shimizu E, Kawahara K, Kajizono M, Sawada M, Nakayama H (2008) IL-4-induced selective clearance of oligomeric beta-amyloid peptide(1-42) by rat primary type 2 microglia. *J Immunol* 181:6503-6513.

Simard AR, Rivest S (2006) [Bone marrow stem cells to the rescue of Alzheimer's disease]. *Med Sci* (Paris) 22:822-824.

Simard AR, Soulet D, Gowing G, Julien JP, Rivest S (2006) Bone marrow-derived microglia play a critical role in restricting senile plaque formation in Alzheimer's disease. *Neuron* 49:489-502.

Skidgel RA, Erdos EG (1987) The broad substrate specificity of human angiotensin I converting enzyme. *Clin Exp Hypertens* A 9:243-259.

Spencer B, Marr RA, Rockenstein E, Crews L, Adame A, Potkar R, Patrick C, Gage FH, Verma IM, Masliah E (2008) Long-term neprilysin gene transfer is associated with reduced levels of intracellular Abeta and behavioral improvement in APP transgenic mice. *BMC Neurosci* 9:109.

Tamaki C, Ohtsuki S, Iwatsubo T, Hashimoto T, Yamada K, Yabuki C, Terasaki T (2006) Major involvement of low-density lipoprotein receptor-related protein 1 in the clearance of plasma free amyloid beta-peptide by the liver. *Pharm Res* 23:1407-1416.

Thinakaran G, Koo EH (2008) Amyloid precursor protein trafficking, processing, and function. *J Biol Chem* 283:29615-29619.

Thomas CA, Li Y, Kodama T, Suzuki H, Silverstein SC, El Khoury J (2000) Protection from lethal gram-positive infection by macrophage scavenger receptor-dependent phagocytosis. *J Exp Med* 191:147-156.

Town T, Laouar Y, Pittenger C, Mori T, Szekely CA, Tan J, Duman RS, Flavell RA (2008) Blocking TGF-beta-Smad2/3 innate immune signaling mitigates Alzheimer-like pathology. *Nat Med* 14:681-687.

Tsirka SE, Rogove AD, Bugge TH, Degen JL, Strickland S (1997) An extracellular proteolytic cascade promotes neuronal degeneration in the mouse hippocampus. *J Neurosci* 17:543-552.

Tucker HM, Kihiko-Ehmann M, Wright S, Rydel RE, Estus S (2000a) Tissue plasminogen activator requires plasminogen to modulate amyloid-beta neurotoxicity and deposition. *J Neurochem* 75:2172-2177.

Tucker HM, Simpson J, Kihiko-Ehmann M, Younkin LH, McGillis JP, Younkin SG, Degen JL, Estus S (2004) Plasmin deficiency does not alter endogenous murine amyloid beta levels in mice. *Neurosci Lett* 368:285-289.

Tucker HM, Kihiko M, Caldwell JN, Wright S, Kawarabayashi T, Price D, Walker D, Scheff S, McGillis JP, Rydel RE, Estus S (2000b) The plasmin system is induced by and degrades amyloid-beta aggregates. *J Neurosci* 20:3937-3946.

Turner AJ, Murphy LJ (1996) Molecular pharmacology of endothelin converting enzymes. Biochem Pharmacol 51:91-102.

Turner AJ, Tanzawa K (1997) Mammalian membrane metallopeptidases: NEP, ECE, KELL, and PEX. *Faseb J* 11:355-364.

Turner AJ, Isaac RE, Coates D (2001) The neprilysin (NEP) family of zinc metalloendopeptidases: genomics and function. *Bioessays* 23:261-269.

Vartak DG, Gemeinhart RA (2007) Matrix metalloproteases: underutilized targets for drug delivery. *J Drug Target* 15:1-20.

Vasilevko V, Xu F, Previti ML, Van Nostrand WE, Cribbs DH (2007) Experimental investigation of antibody-mediated clearance mechanisms of amyloid-beta in CNS of Tg-SwDI transgenic mice. *J Neurosci* 27:13376-13383.

Vekrellis K, Ye Z, Qiu WQ, Walsh D, Hartley D, Chesneau V, Rosner MR, Selkoe DJ (2000) Neurons regulate extracellular levels of amyloid beta-protein via proteolysis by insulin-degrading enzyme. *J Neurosci* 20:1657-1665.

Vostrikov VM (1985) [Electron-cytochemical study of microglia in Alzheimer's disease and senile dementia]. *Zh Nevropatol Psikhiatr Im S S Korsakova* 85:974-976.

Weeraratna AT, Kalehua A, Deleon I, Bertak D, Maher G, Wade MS, Lustig A, Becker KG, Wood W, 3rd, Walker DG, Beach TG, Taub DD (2007) Alterations in immunological and neurological gene expression patterns in Alzheimer's disease tissues. *Exp Cell Res* 313:450-461.

Wnendt S, Wetzels I, Gunzler WA (1997) Amyloid beta peptides stimulate tissue-type plasminogen activator but not recombinant prourokinase. *Thromb Res* 85:217-224.

Wyss-Coray T, Loike JD, Brionne TC, Lu E, Anankov R, Yan F, Silverstein SC, Husemann J (2003) Adult mouse astrocytes degrade amyloid-beta in vitro and in situ. *Nat Med* 9:453-457.

Xu D, Emoto N, Giaid A, Slaughter C, Kaw S, deWit D, Yanagisawa M (1994) ECE-1: a membrane-bound metalloprotease that catalyzes the proteolytic activation of big endothelin-1. *Cell* 78:473-485.

Yan P, Hu X, Song H, Yin K, Bateman RJ, Cirrito JR, Xiao Q, Hsu FF, Turk JW, Xu J, Hsu CY, Holtzman DM, Lee JM (2006) Matrix metalloproteinase-9 degrades amyloid-beta fibrils in vitro and compact plaques in situ. *J Biol Chem* 281:24566-24574.

Yan SD, Chen X, Fu J, Chen M, Zhu H, Roher A, Slattery T, Zhao L, Nagashima M, Morser J, Migheli A, Nawroth P, Stern D, Schmidt AM (1996) RAGE and amyloid-beta peptide neurotoxicity in Alzheimer's disease. *Nature* 382:685-691.

Yang Y, Estrada EY, Thompson JF, Liu W, Rosenberg GA (2007) Matrix metalloproteinase-mediated disruption of tight junction proteins in cerebral vessels is reversed by synthetic matrix metalloproteinase inhibitor in focal ischemia in rat. *J Cereb Blood Flow Metab* 27:697-709.

Yasojima K, Akiyama H, McGeer EG, McGeer PL (2001) Reduced neprilysin in high plaque areas of Alzheimer brain: a possible relationship to deficient degradation of beta-amyloid peptide. *Neurosci Lett* 297:97-100.

Yesner LM, Huh HY, Pearce SF, Silverstein RL (1996) Regulation of monocyte CD36 and thrombospondin-1 expression by soluble mediators. *Arterioscler Thromb Vasc Biol* 16:1019-1025.

Yin KJ, Cirrito JR, Yan P, Hu X, Xiao Q, Pan X, Bateman R, Song H, Hsu FF, Turk J, Xu J, Hsu CY, Mills JC, Holtzman DM, Lee JM (2006) Matrix metalloproteinases expressed by astrocytes mediate extracellular amyloid-beta peptide catabolism. *J Neurosci* 26:10939-10948.

Zhao J, Li L, Leissring MA (2009a) Insulin-degrading enzyme is exported via an unconventional protein secretion pathway. *Mol Neurodegener* 4:4.

Zhao L, Lin S, Bales KR, Gelfanova V, Koger D, Delong C, Hale J, Liu F, Hunter JM, Paul SM (2009b) Macrophage-mediated degradation of beta-amyloid via an apolipoprotein E isoform-dependent mechanism. *J Neurosci* 29:3603-3612.

Zhou SF (2008) Structure, function and regulation of P-glycoprotein and its clinical relevance in drug disposition. *Xenobiotica* 38:802-832.

Zlokovic BV (2008) The blood-brain barrier in health and chronic neurodegenerative disorders. *Neuron* 57:178-201.

Zlokovic BV, Martel CL, Matsubara E, McComb JG, Zheng G, McCluskey RT, Frangione B, Ghiso J (1996) Glycoprotein 330/megalin: probable role in receptor-mediated transport of apolipoprotein J alone and in a complex with Alzheimer disease amyloid beta at the blood-brain and blood-cerebrospinal fluid barriers. *Proc Natl Acad Sci U S A* 93:4229-4234.

Acknowledgments

This work was supported by NIH grants NS059005 and AG032349 and a grant from the Dana foundation to JEK. We thank Elizabeth Allison for assistance with imaging and for a critical read of the manuscript and Dr. Lingzhi Zhao for helpful comments and suggestions.

In: Alzheimer's Disease and Dementia (Vol. 4)
Editor: Miao-Kun Sun
ISBN:978-1-60876-152-4

Chapter III

Synaptic Transmission Regulates Amyloid-β Dynamics

John R. Cirrito
Department of Neurology, Washington University School of Medicine,
St. Louis, Missouri, 63110, USA

Abstract

Aggregation of amyloid-β (Aβ) within the brain extracellular space into soluble and insoluble forms is central to the pathogenesis of Alzheimer's disease. While a substantial amount is known about how Aβ is generated, the mechanisms that regulate Aβ release and that modulate soluble extracellular Aβ levels are less clear. Neuronal activity modulates Aβ generation and levels via several pathways. Postsynaptic receptor activation can alter the non-amyloidogenic processing of the amyloid precursor protein, thereby affecting Aβ generation. The process of synaptic transmission also directly modulates Aβ generation and release from neurons into the extracellular space. Synaptic transmission increases endocytosis of APP from the plasma membrane, thus driving formation and release of Aβ. The cellular pathways underlying the link between neuronal activity and Aβ generation have been demonstrated in culture as well as in living mouse models of Alzheimer's disease. There is parallel evidence in humans that neuronal activity impacts Aβ levels as well as Aβ accumulation as plaques. Brain areas with high levels of metabolic and neuronal activity are the most vulnerable to Aβ deposition as plaques. Synaptic transmission is critical for life and cannot be blocked completely. However, understanding the pathways linking synaptic activity and Aβ may provide opportunities to interrupt this relationship in ways that marginally alter transmission but still reduce Aβ levels.

Abbreviation List

amyloid-β, Aβ; amyloid precursor protein, APP; Alzheimer's disease, AD; Tetrodotoxin, TTX; Electroencephalography, EEG; metabotropic glutamate receptors type 2/3, mGluR2/3; α-latrotoxin,LTX

Introduction

Accumulation of amyloid-β (Aβ) within the brain extracellular space is a key step in the pathogenesis and progression of Alzheimer's disease (AD). Insoluble amyloid plaques, composed primarily of the Aβ peptide, are one pathological hallmark of AD. Growing evidence suggests that soluble Aβ oligomers within the brain interstitial fluid (ISF) may also participate in the disease. In vitro experiments suggest that conversion of Aβ from a monomeric peptide to either an oligomeric or fibrillar forms is concentration-dependent. Thus, higher concentrations of soluble, extracellular Aβ may lead directly to potentially toxic and disruptive Aβ species. Consequently, understanding factors that regulate Aβ levels within the brain has implications for disease pathogenesis and may suggest methods to modulate disease progression.

Aβ is a 38-42 amino acid peptide that is produced by cleavage of the amyloid precursor protein (APP). APP is synthesized in the endoplasmic reticulum and transported through the secretory pathway to the plasma membrane. Evidence suggests that a limited amount of Aβ is produced in these compartments (Hartmann et al., 1997; Xu et al., 1997). It appears that the majority of Aβ is produced within the endocytic pathway (Koo and Squazzo, 1994). Full length APP on the cell surface is internalized by clathrin-mediated endocytosis into endosomes. Within endosomes, β-secretase cleaves APP to produce a membrane-bound C-terminal fragment of APP. γ-secretase then cleaves this fragment to release Aβ into the lumen of the endocytic vesicle. A portion of Aβ is then returned to the cell surface, presumably via recycling endosomes, and released into the brain ISF. The percentage of Aβ that is secreted from neurons as opposed to retained in the cell in unknown. Aβ is present in a soluble form throughout life at highest concentrations in the central nervous system.

Extracellular Aβ can impact disease onset and progression by contributing to toxic aggregates. It is unknown where the seed of a plaque forms however evidence suggests that it could occur intracellularly (Takahashi et al., 2002) or extracellularly (Meyer-Luehmann et al., 2003). While the location of seed formation is controversial, growth of existing plaques will occur extracellularly (Meyer-Luehmann et al., 2003); once a plaque has formed, it expands as Aβ within the ISF polymerizes onto existing insoluble structures. High ISF Aβ levels are particularly important because they can promote conversion into species that contribute to plaque formation and growth.

Regulation of Aβ Levels

Steady-state levels of a protein are determined by a balance of production and elimination. Aβ is cleared from the brain via a variety of pathways including proteolytic degradation, cellular uptake, transport across the blood-brain barrier, and passive bulk transport into lymph (Shibata et al., 2000; Cirrito et al., 2005b; Yin et al., 2006; Farris et al., 2007). While a substantial amount is known about how Aβ is produced (secretases, subcellular localization, etc), much less is known about what regulates its production. Several studies in 2002 suggested that synaptic transmission was one regulator of Aβ levels. Two independent groups lesioned the perforant pathway and demonstrated reduced Aβ plaque load in the hippocampus of APP transgenic mice (Lazarov et al., 2002; Sheng et al., 2002). The perforant pathway is the major afferent projection into the hippocampus. Lesions of this pathway should reduce transport of APP from the entorhinal cortex to the dentate gyrus as well as reduce neuronal activity in the hippocampus. While these studies were not conclusive, they did strongly suggest that neuronal activity might be a contributing factor to Aβ levels and plaque formation.

Postsynaptic Activation Modulates APP Processing

In animal models and in humans, the relationship between synaptic transmission and Aβ levels has been demonstrated at a molecular level. Postsynaptic receptor activation leads to alteration of Aβ levels by modulating the activity of proteases involved in APP cleavage. APP is cleaved by β-secretase and γ-secretase to produce Aβ. Alternatively, α-secretase can cleave APP within the Aβ sequence, a cleavage that precludes Aβ production. Activation of muscarinic M1 acetylcholine receptors in animal models and in humans increases α-secretase cleavage of APP, thus decreasing Aβ levels in the brain and CSF (Nitsch et al., 2000; Beach et al., 2001). Chronic treatment with M1 selective agonists such as AF267B reduces plaque pathology in a mouse model of AD (Caccamo et al., 2006). Animals with fewer plaques also had improved cognitive function compared to control mice. In contrast, NMDA receptor activation can increase α-secretase activity thus decreasing extracellular Aβ levels in dissociated neuronal cultures (Hoey et al., 2009). The effect of both M1 receptor and NMDA receptor-mediated modulation of APP processing and Aβ levels occurs over hours to days.

Neuronal activity also modulates extracellular Aβ levels in organotypic brain slices that overexpress mutated forms of human APP transgenically or following virally-driven expression. Picrotoxin, a non-competitive $GABA_A$ receptor antagonist, increases synaptic activity and elevates extracellular Aβ levels by 70% whereas decreasing transmission with tetrodotoxin, a sodium channel blocker, depresses Aβ levels by 50% (Kamenetz et al., 2003). These in vitro studies assessed Aβ levels in media after 24-72 hours of treatment. The picrotoxin-dependent increase in extracellular Aβ levels is accompanied by elevated β-CTF levels in the brain slice. This may suggest a change in β-secretase cleavage of APP. Whether this effect is driven by postsynaptic or presynaptic mechanisms, however, remains unclear.

While it is clear that postsynaptic effects can modulate APP processing, it remains possible that presynaptic effects can affect Aβ production and release as well.

Increased Synaptic Activity Elevates ISF Aβ Levels in Vivo

In vitro experiments provide convenient model systems to test the role of neuronal activity on Aβ generation; however the role of these mechanisms in a living animal is unknown. In order to determine the relationship between synaptic activity and Aβ in vivo, our research group utilized a microdialysis technique to measure ISF Aβ levels longitudinally in awake, behaving mice. Microdialysis has been used for decades to assess small molecules within extracellular fluids of living animals and humans. Microdialysis probes with a 38 kilo-Dalton molecular weight cut-off membrane are stereotaxically implanted into the hippocampus of Tg2576 APP transgenic mice. This size membrane permits recovery of small peptides, such as Aβ (molecular weight 4.4 kDa), from the brain extracellular space. Microdialysis enables serial sampling of ISF Aβ every thirty minutes for up to 36 hours (Cirrito et al., 2003; Cirrito et al., 2005a). By attaching field potential recording electrodes to the microdialysis guide cannula, we are able to assess extracellular field potentials (depth EEG) at the same time and location that we assess Aβ levels. In order to study normal Aβ metabolism, we utilized three to five month old Tg2576$^{+/-}$, which is an age prior to Aβ plaque accumulation. Experiments on mice of this age permit us to evaluate the effect of synaptic activity on Aβ without complications from Aβ deposits.

To determine if increased synaptic activity alters ISF Aβ levels, we implanted Tg2576 mice with microdialysis probes and recording electrodes within the hippocampus, as well as an ipsilateral stimulating electrode into the perforant pathway. High frequency electrical stimulation of the perforant pathway generates seizures within the hippocampal formation, evident in extracellular field potential recordings (Sloviter et al., 1996; Cirrito et al., 2005a). Hippocampal seizures increased ISF Aβ levels by 25% within the first 30 minutes of stimulation compared to pre-stimulation Aβ levels (Fig. 1A). In fact, as long as seizures continued, ISF Aβ levels remained elevated.

To determine if a more subtle increase in synaptic activity can also modulate ISF Aβ levels, we administered 25 μM picrotoxin directly into the hippocampus via reverse microdialysis. While high doses of picrotoxin can cause seizures (>200 μM), this low dose of the $GABA_A$ receptor antagonist caused occasional synchronous spikes in electroencephalography (EEG) activity, but did not cause seizures (data not shown). Picrotoxin treatment increased ISF Aβ levels by 20% within the first 30 minutes of treatment with levels reaching a maximum increase of 45% by 4 hours compared to basal levels (Fig. 1A). Interestingly, a low dose of picrotoxin elevated ISF Aβ more than electrically stimulated seizures did. Stimulation-induced seizures cause brief bursts of very high levels of EEG activity (fast frequency and high amplitude) followed by interictal suppression of activity whereas picrotoxin caused a sustained, low level of elevated activity (spikes of spontaneous activity a 2-4 Hz). It is possible that the distinct kinetics and overall change in synaptic activity in these two paradigms account for the varying degrees of ISF Aβ alteration.

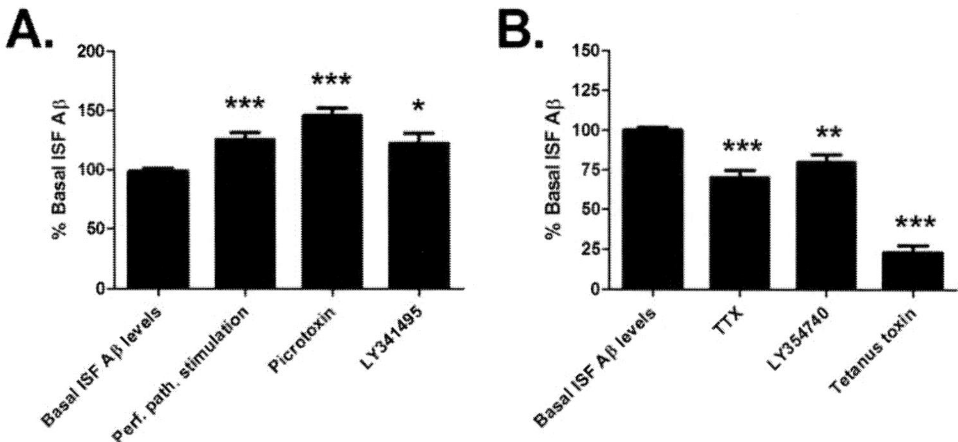

Figure 1. Synaptic activity dynamically modulates ISF Aβ levels in vivo. (A) Electrical stimulation of the perforant pathway induced hippocampal seizures and increased ISF Aβ levels by 25.5 ± 5.4% within 30 minutes compared to baseline ($p<0.0001$). Similarly, 25μM picrotoxin via reverse microdialysis increased ISF Aβ levels by 45.4 ± 6.8% after four hours of treatment ($p<0.0001$) and 100 μM LY341495 increased Aβ levels by 22.2 ± 8.4% ($p<0.05$) (B) Decreased synaptic transmission lowered ISF Aβ levels. Direct administration of TTX (5 μM) to the hippocampus gradually lowered ISF Aβ levels to 70.4 ± 4.5% after eight hours ($p<0.0001$). LY354740 (30 μM) inhibition of endogenous, glutamatergic synaptic transmission within the hippocampus decreased ISF Aβ levels by 20.0 ± 4.6% over 6 hours ($p<0.01$). And tetanus toxin (0.2 μg) blockade of synaptic vesicle exocytosis dramatically depressed ISF Aβ levels by 76.7 ± 4.6% of basal levels by 18 hours after treatment ($p<0.0001$). Data expressed as mean ± SEM.

Picrotoxin increases neuronal activity by reducing inhibition imposed by GABA receptors. In contrast, blockade of metabotropic glutamate receptors type 2/3 (mGluR2/3) directly increases neuronal activity by promoting presynaptic glutamate release. These G-protein coupled receptors are located presynaptically and serve in a negative feedback loop so that less activation actually augments glutamate release from those terminals. Administration of LY341495, an mGluR2/3 antagonist, directly to the hippocampus increased synaptic activity and increased ISF Aβ levels (Fig. 1A). Three distinct mechanisms that increase neuronal activity (perforant pathway stimulation, GABA inhibitors, and mGluR2/3 antagonists) all lead to a rapid and sustained increase in ISF Aβ levels in living mice.

Decreased Synaptic Activity Depresses ISF Aβ Levels in Vivo

As a complementary test of the relationship between synaptic activity and extracellular Aβ levels, we sought to determine if depressed activity would have the opposite effect of seizures and picrotoxin treatment. Tetrodotoxin (TTX) is a sodium channel blocker produced in puffer fish. If ingested in food or administered peripherally, TTX is lethal. If TTX is administered directly to the brain however, it blocks action potential propagation and locally inhibits neuronal activity. After establishing basal ISF Aβ levels by microdialysis, mice were continuously administered TTX via reverse microdialysis directly into the hippocampus for 8 hours. During this treatment, EEG activity within the hippocampus gradually declined to zero with a concurrent decrease in ISF Aβ levels (Cirrito et al., 2005a). By 8 hours of treatment, ISF Aβ levels reached 70% of basal levels (Fig. 1B). The effect of TTX was reversible. Four hours of TTX treatment reduced EEG activity and Aβ levels, however both of these measures gradually returned to baseline levels when the drug was removed from the microdialysis perfusion buffer (Cirrito et al., 2005a).

We also tested whether a manipulation of synaptic vesicle release modulates Aβ release. When activated, mGluR2/3 receptors lower glutamate release by direct effects within the presynaptic terminal. We administered an agonist to mGluR2/3, LY354740, directly into the hippocampus. This drug decreased ISF Aβ levels by 20% over 6 hours of treatment suggesting that endogenous synaptic activity contributes significantly to normal ISF Aβ levels (Fig. 1B).

TTX and LY354740 reduce, but do not completely prevent, neuronal activity. For instance, these drugs inhibit evoked synaptic transmission, but do not block spontaneous activity. In order to block synaptic transmission to a greater extent, we administered a bolus injection of tetanus toxin directly into the hippocampus surrounding a microdialysis probe. Tetanus toxin is taken into the presynaptic terminal and cleaves VAMP2, which is necessary for synaptic vesicle exocytosis. This does not interfere with upstream action potential formation and propagation but does prevent exocytosis of synaptic vesicles, thereby blocking all types of local synaptic activity. Tetanus toxin reduced the levels of ISF Aβ by almost 75 % (Fig. 1B). This dramatic reduction in Aβ levels strongly suggests that synaptic vesicle exocytosis may be a critical event involved in Aβ release from neurons.

Synaptic Vesicle Exocytosis is Critical for Aβ Release in Acute Brain Slices

Presynaptic neurotransmission involves fusion of the synaptic vesicle with the plasma membrane, release of neurotransmitter into the synaptic cleft, and subsequent recycling of the vesicle membrane. We hypothesized that synaptic vesicle cycling alone, in the absence of neuronal depolarization could cause Aβ release. To test this premise directly, we developed an acute brain slice model that was amenable to complex pharmacological treatments. Living brain slices (300μm thick) were produced from 3-4 week old Tg2576 mice and placed into medium at 37°C for three hours to recover. Media from these slices contains molecules secreted from the brain slice and in many ways is analogous to extracellular brain fluid. Following recovery, slices were incubated with either vehicle or α-latrotoxin (LTX), which acts presynaptically to cause synaptic vesicle exocytosis without directly depolarizing the neuron. LTX caused a 35% increase in extracellular Aβ levels (Fig. 2). The neurotransmitter released in response to the toxin, however induced downstream activation of the postsynaptic neuron. To isolate the role of vesicle cycling in the absence of depolarization, we co-administered LTX with a cocktail of activity blockers that included TTX, APV, and NBQX to inhibit sodium channels, NMDA receptors, and AMPA receptors, respectively. The cocktail of inhibitors alone reduced Aβ levels by 20% compared to the untreated condition (Fig. 2). This is comparable to our in vivo results using TTX alone (Fig. 1B). When LTX and the inhibitor cocktail were co-applied to brain slices, extracellular Aβ levels were still significantly elevated (Fig. 2). This demonstrates that synaptic vesicle exocytosis alone, in the absence of postsynaptic depolarization, is sufficient to drive Aβ release from neurons. Aβ released following latrotoxin and inhibitors demonstrates a presynaptic mechanism for Aβ generation. Interestingly, there is an even greater increase in Aβ caused by latrotoxin when inhibitors are not present. This suggests that activation of postsynaptic receptors in dendrites may further drive Aβ production in this system.

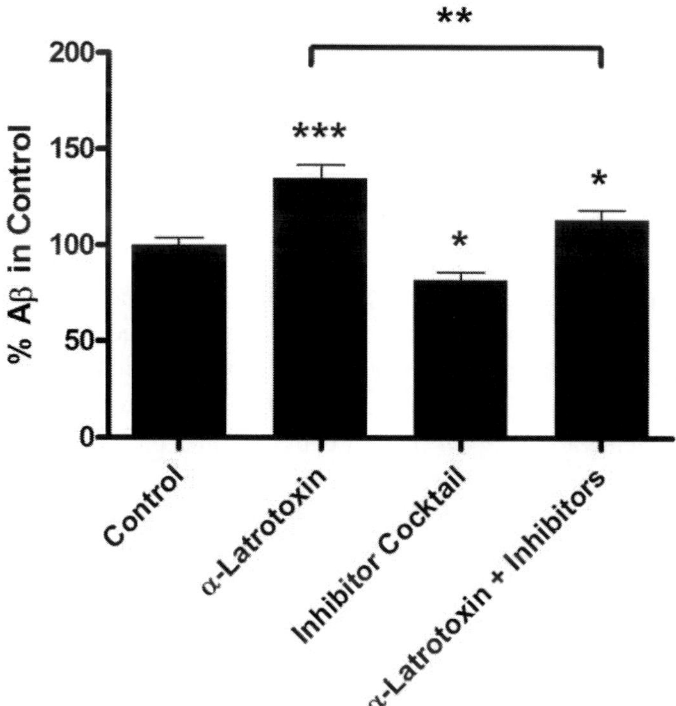

Figure 2. Synaptic vesicle exocytosis alone is sufficient to elevate ISF Aβ levels in vitro. Acute brain slices were generated from 3-4 week old Tg2576$^{+/-}$ mice and maintained at 37°C in culture media for up to 12 hours. After recovering from slicing for three hours, slices were treated for two hours with 1) vehicle, 2) α-latrotoxin (0.5nM), 3) an inhibitor cocktail containing TTX (100nM), APV (50μM), and NBQX (10μM), or 4) a combination of the inhibitor cocktail and α-latrotoxin. Co-treatment with LTX and the inhibitor cocktail caused a 13.3 ± 5.1% increase in Aβ levels within the media compared to untreated slices ($p<0.05$) while latrotoxin alone increased Aβ levels by 35.0 ± 6.9%. Data expressed as mean ± SEM.

Synaptic Activity Regulates Endocytosis of APP and Aβ Generation

Synaptic activity rapidly and dynamically modulates ISF Aβ levels in vivo. In as little as thirty minutes, seizure activity significantly increased hippocampal ISF Aβ levels whereas a complete blockade of synaptic transmission lowered ISF Aβ levels by 75%. Data from acute brain slices demonstrate that synaptic vesicle cycling is critical for Aβ release. Studies employing biochemical and immuno-electron microscopy techniques have not found Aβ within synaptic vesicles (Ikin et al., 1996; Marquez-Sterling et al., 1997). Instead, Aβ exists primarily within the endocytic compartment. This suggests that synaptic vesicle exocytosis does not directly cause Aβ release, though it is likely a closely associated event that is directly responsible for neuronal Aβ generation and release.

Full length APP is synthesized in the endoplasmic reticulum and is trafficked through the secretory pathway to the plasma membrane. During this journey and at the cell surface, APP is available primarily for cleavage by α-secretase (Hartmann et al., 1997; Xu et al., 1997). If full length APP remains on the cell surface, it undergoes clathrin-mediated endocytosis into the endocytic pathway where it can interact with β- and γ-secretase (Peraus et al., 1997). Most Aβ is generated within the endocytic pathway and inhibition of endocytosis reduces Aβ production and secretion in vitro (Koo and Squazzo, 1994). Once produced in endosomes, Aβ can be shunted to the lysosome for degradation or trafficked back to the plasma membrane to be secreted from the cell.

When synaptic vesicles release their neurotransmitter, the synaptic vesicle membrane typically fuses with the plasma membrane. Some of that vesicle membrane and the associated proteins are then recycled from the plasma membrane and used to replenish the pool of synaptic vesicles. One mechanism used to remove synaptic membrane from the cell surface is clathrin-mediated endocytosis (Newton et al., 2006). With increased synaptic activity, more synaptic vesicle membrane will be endocytosed from the plasma membrane. Given that endocytosis of APP is a critical step in Aβ generation, this is a likely place for synaptic transmission and Aβ generation to intersect. Within clathrin-coated vesicles, APP co-localizes with several synaptic vesicle markers, namely SV2, synaptotagmin I and synaptophysin (Marquez-Sterling et al., 1997). This is consistent with the notion that synaptic vesicle membrane recycling is linked to APP endocytosis.

We tested in vivo the effect of inhibiting endocytosis on ISF Aβ levels. Dynamin interaction with amphiphysin is necessary for scission of clathrin coated vesicles from the plasma membrane. Blocking this interaction with a dominant negative peptide has been used to inhibit endocytosis in culture for years in a variety of studies. This approach has also been shown to reduce APP internalization and reduce Aβ generation (Carey et al., 2005). A dominant negative peptide of dynamin (dynamin-DN) was infused into the brains of wildtype mice using reverse microdialysis. Inhibiting endocytosis reduced ISF Aβ levels by 70% in vivo (Fig. 3) (Cirrito et al., 2008). Similar to transgenic mice, a low dose of picrotoxin infused into the hippocampus of wildtype mice also increases ISF Aβ levels. Inhibiting endocytosis first however blocked this synaptic-dependent increase in ISF Aβ levels. Endocytosis appears to only affect Aβ production since elimination of Aβ from the brain is not altered in the presence of dynamin-DN (Cirrito et al., 2008). While our studies do not directly assess where Aβ is produced or released, it is likely that Aβ generation that is caused by events within the synaptic terminal would occur at or near the synapse. It is possible that activity and APP are not functionally linked, but that APP is only coincidentally endocytosed as synaptic vesicle membrane is recycled.

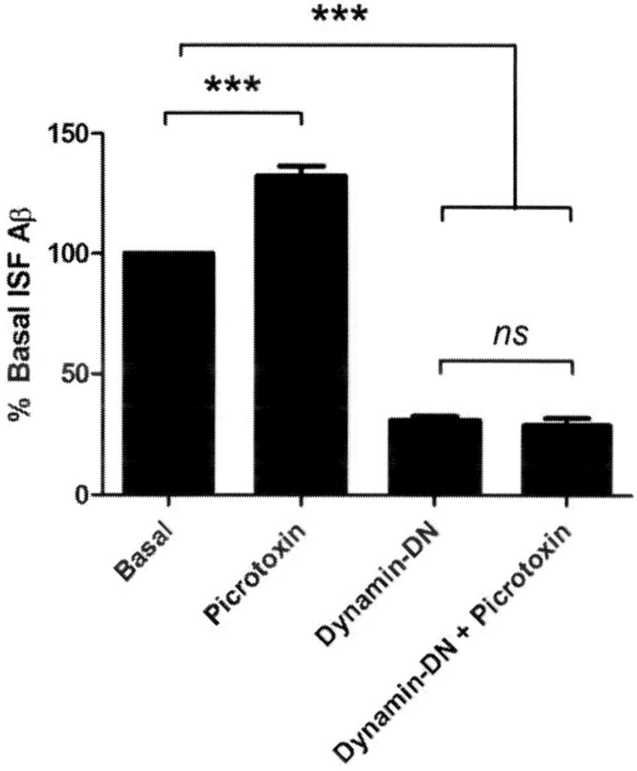

Figure 3. Endocytosis is required for synaptic-dependent regulation of Aβ levels. In C57Bl6 mice, 25μM picrotoxin increased ISF murine Aβ levels by 32.4 ± 4.1% of baseline over 12 hours ($p<0.0001$). 200μM dynamin-DN reduced murine Aβ levels to 31.1 ± 1.7% of baseline ($p<0.0001$). Pretreatment with dynamin-DN for 1 hour then co-administration of dynamin-DN and picrotoxin caused ISF Aβ levels to decrease to 29.0 ± 2.9% of baseline which was not statistically different from dynamin-DN treatment alone. Data presented as mean ± SEM. *** represents $p<0.0001$.

Underlying Pathways for Aβ Generation

The data suggest there are at least three cellular mechanisms that contribute to ISF Aβ production (Cirrito et al., 2008). One, a pathway that is synaptic activity-dependent and endocytosis-dependent which contributes to approximately 60% of ISF Aβ levels in Tg2576 mice. Two, a pool of ISF Aβ exists that requires endocytosis, but is independent of synaptic activity. This pathway is responsible for another 10% of ISF Aβ levels. Interestingly, inhibition of endocytosis does not reduce ISF Aβ levels to zero. The third remaining pool of Aβ, comprising 30% of total ISF Aβ levels, may be the product of several mechanisms, including Aβ produced within the secretory pathway or Aβ diffusing from brain areas that are not affected by inhibition of endocytosis or TTX. Alternatively, this last pool may be a factor of incomplete inhibition of endocytosis or some small contribution of altered Aβ elimination. These values provide rough estimates for each of these pools and provide an interesting framework to consider the various pathways that contribute to the overall pool of ISF Aβ. Given the need for efficient recycling of synaptic vesicle membrane, the synaptic terminal is likely a specialized cellular compartment with very high levels of clathrin-mediated endocytosis. We propose that of the endocytosis-dependent pool of ISF Aβ, the synaptic-dependent portion (60%) is produced at or near the synaptic terminal whereas the synaptic-independent portion (10%) is likely from Aβ being produced by constitutive endocytosis elsewhere in the neuron. There is a substantial amount of APP in dendrites however how much Aβ is produced there and by what cellular mechanisms is unknown. A source of 70% of ISF Aβ in vivo is a tantalizing target for therapeutic development. While inhibiting all clathrin-mediated endocytosis is unlikely to be a feasible strategy for lowering extracellular Aβ levels, it may be possible to modulate individual components of the endocytic machinery or synaptic transmission to selectively affect Aβ generation.

Several molecules influence the rate and amount of APP endocytosis. LRP1 expression increases the rate of APP endocytosis from the plasma membrane whereas LRP1b expression reduces the rate of internalization (Cam et al., 2004; Cam et al., 2005). Recent evidence also implicates another LDL-R family member, LR11 or SorLa, in modulating APP trafficking through the endosomal compartment (Andersen et al., 2005; Dodson et al., 2006; Offe et al., 2006; Rogaeva et al., 2007). LR11 overexpression increases APP co-localization within the Golgi and reduces Aβ generation in culture whereas deletion of the *LR11* gene in mice increases brain Aβ levels (Andersen et al., 2005). Given that several LDL-R family members modulate Aβ endocytosis, it will be important to elucidate if and how these molecules affect synaptic activity-dependent Aβ generation.

Physiological Alterations in Neuronal Activity Alter ISF Aβ Levels in Mice and Humans

Evidence in both humans and animals suggests that environmental stressors may increase risk for AD or AD pathology. In humans, persons without dementia who are prone to psychological distress are more likely to develop AD (Wilson et al., 2003; Wilson et al., 2005). Also, plasma levels of the stress hormone, cortisol, are correlated with the rate of dementia progression in patients with AD (Csernansky et al., 2006). In mouse models of AD, animals subjected to isolation stress over months had decreased learning performance and accelerated Aβ deposition (Dong et al., 2004). The same mouse model when subjected to acute restraint stress and chronic isolation stress had significantly elevated levels of ISF Aβ (Kang et al., 2007). This acute increase in Aβ was blocked by pre-administration of TTX to the hippocampus to block neuronal activity, thus it appears that stress-induced elevations neuronal activity increase ISF Aβ levels. Taken together with previous studies, this elevation in Aβ levels seems to increase risk of developing amyloid plaques which could increase the risk of developing AD.

Recent studies in humans by Drs. David Brody, Sandra Magnoni and colleagues demonstrated that brain ISF Aβ levels correlate with cognitive function in traumatic brain injury patients (Brody et al., 2008). Patients that had suffered acute brain injury and were undergoing invasive intracranial monitoring for clinical purposes were also outfitted with intracerebral microdialysis probes to measure ISF Aβ levels. Given their severe injury, many of these patients began the study in a comatose state. ISF Aβ was detectable in all patients and sampled longitudinally over several days. Interestingly, the trend was for ISF Aβ levels to gradually increase over time. The fluctuations in Aβ were tightly correlated with each patient's cognitive status; as the patient recovered and became more conscious ISF Aβ levels also increased. In patients that did not recover, ISF Aβ levels remained low and steady whereas patients that suffered a secondary injury, such as ischemia, had Aβ levels decline over time. While only correlative, this study strongly suggests that even in humans neuronal activity can rapidly and dynamically modulate ISF Aβ levels.

High Levels of Neuronal Activity Correlate with Aβ Deposition in Humans

Several studies in humans suggest that neuronal activity may be linked to Aβ deposition as plaques. For instance, 10% of individuals with temporal lobe epilepsy (TLE) develop diffuse Aβ plaques throughout the temporal lobe at ages when AD pathology would otherwise be very rare (Mackenzie and Miller, 1994; Gouras et al., 1997). Although the epileptic tissue where the plaques occur is not necessarily normal, these individuals share dramatically elevated neuronal activity compared to activity in the same brain regions of normal individuals. Individuals as young as 30 years old already exhibited diffuse Aβ plaques at autopsy. Interestingly, even though Aβ plaques are present, TLE does not confer a greater risk of developing AD.

Other studies linking neuronal activity with Aβ deposition come from recent brain imaging work. Studies by Buckner and colleagues demonstrate that brain areas that have a high level of basal metabolic activity are the same brain areas that are most vulnerable to Aβ deposition in human AD patients (Buckner et al., 2005; Buckner et al., 2009). Fluorodeoxyglucose-positron emission tomography (FDG-PET) demonstrated that when individuals are cognitively idle, meaning that they are not focusing on a particular task, a stereotypical pattern of brain regions are active including prefrontal, lateral temporal, precuneus, and lateral parietal cortices. These areas comprise what is referred to as the "default state" brain regions (Raichle et al., 2001). When individuals begin performing a particular mental task (e.g. reading a word), the default state brain regions generally decrease in metabolic activity while different areas increase in activity. Over the course of a lifetime, it is likely that the default state brain regions are some of the most metabolically active areas in the brain (Gusnard et al., 2001). FDG-PET measures of metabolic activity are believed to be a close corollary of neuronal activity. Interestingly, a cortical map of the default state regions and a map of brain regions that develop Aβ pathology in Alzheimer's disease are remarkably similar (Buckner et al., 2005). This suggests that in humans, areas that have the most overall neuronal activity are particularly vulnerable to Aβ deposition.

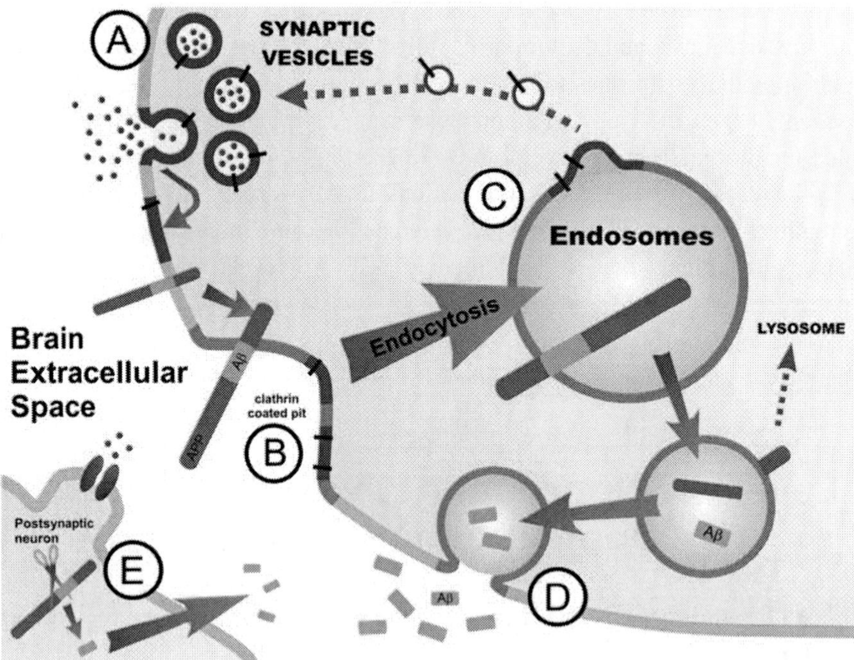

Figure 4. Model of activity-dependent regulation of Aβ release from neurons. (A) Synaptic vesicle exocytosis causes vesicular membrane to fuse with the plasma membrane. (B) Synaptic vesicle membrane is recycled from the cell surface, at least in part via clathrin-mediated endocytosis. Full length APP resides on the plasma membrane and is endocytosed via clathrin-mediated endocytosis. Increased synaptic activity leads to more vesicle membrane recycling and more coincident APP endocytosis. (C) Within the endocytic compartment, APP is cleaved to produce Aβ. (D) Aβ is brought back to the cell surface within recycling endosomes and secreted into the brain ISF. (E) Additionally, activation of receptors on the postsynaptic neuron can modulate downstream synaptic transmission as well as alter processing of APP.

Synaptic Activity has Several Independent Effects on Aβ Levels

Evidence in humans suggests that elevated neuronal activity may be linked with accumulation of Aβ as plaques (Mackenzie and Miller, 1994; Buckner et al., 2005; Brody et al., 2008). Additionally, experiments in dissociated neuronal culture and in organotypic brain slices demonstrate that modulation of synaptic activity alters extracellular Aβ levels. Studies by our group demonstrate in awake, behaving mice that synaptic transmission dynamically modulates ISF Aβ levels within minutes. There appears to be at least two mechanisms linking activity and Aβ levels however. The first mechanism involves postsynaptic receptors, namely M1 acetylcholine receptors and NMDA receptors, which activate signaling pathways resulting in altered processing of APP, thereby affecting Aβ production (Beach et al., 2001;

Lesne et al., 2005). It is likely that this mechanism appreciably affects Aβ levels over a time course of hours to days. The second mechanism is directly linked to the presynaptic machinery necessary for synaptic transmission. Both increases and decreases in synaptic activity can modulate ISF Aβ levels. This phenomenon is linked directly to synaptic vesicle cycling and occurs on a time scale of minutes. Given that postsynaptic receptor activation can lead to presynaptic vesicle release, these mechanisms may work concurrently within the same neuron.

The Complex Relationship Between Synaptic Transmission and Aβ

A growing literature demonstrates that certain forms of Aβ can inhibit synaptic plasticity (Hartley et al., 1999; Townsend et al., 2006; Shankar et al., 2008). Additionally, viral-expressed APP depresses synaptic activity in nearby neurons in organotypic brain slices (Kamenetz et al., 2003). This occurs at least in part by Aβ inducing AMPA receptor and NMDA receptor internalization from the postsynaptic membrane (Hsieh et al., 2006). Because synaptic transmission directly contributes to Aβ release and because extracellular Aβ can modulate synaptic transmission, it is possible that a feedback loop exists between these phenomena. In the future, it will be important to determine the precise conformations of Aβ that alter synaptic plasticity, the temporal and physical locations of these species, and the root cellular and molecular targets of these species. Are modulatory Aβ species released presynaptically or do they convert into active species following release? Does this feedback loop occur under basal conditions or only in the setting of Alzheimer's disease? Understanding these questions may address fundamental processes involved in Alzheimer's disease pathogenesis and progression.

References

Andersen OM, Reiche J, Schmidt V, Gotthardt M, Spoelgen R, Behlke J, von Arnim CA, Breiderhoff T, Jansen P, Wu X, Bales KR, Cappai R, Masters CL, Gliemann J, Mufson EJ, Hyman BT, Paul SM, Nykjaer A, Willnow TE (2005) Neuronal sorting protein related receptor sorLA/LR11 regulates processing of the amyloid precursor protein. *Proc Natl Acad Sci U S A* 102:13461-13466.

Beach TG, Kuo YM, Schwab C, Walker DG, Roher AE (2001) Reduction of cortical amyloid beta levels in guinea pig brain after systemic administration of physostigmine. *Neurosci Lett* 310:21-24.

Brody DL, Magnoni S, Schwetye KE, Spinner ML, Esparza TJ, Stocchetti N, Zipfel GJ, Holtzman DM (2008) Amyloid-beta dynamics correlate with neurological status in the injured human brain. *Science* 321:1221-1224.

Buckner RL, Sepulcre J, Talukdar T, Krienen FM, Liu H, Hedden T, Andrews-Hanna JR, Sperling RA, Johnson KA (2009) Cortical hubs revealed by intrinsic functional connectivity: mapping, assessment of stability, and relation to Alzheimer's disease. *J Neurosci* 29:1860-1873.

Buckner RL, Snyder AZ, Shannon BJ, LaRossa G, Sachs R, Fotenos AF, Sheline YI, Klunk WE, Mathis CA, Morris JC, Mintun MA (2005) Molecular, structural, and functional characterization of Alzheimer's disease: evidence for a relationship between default activity, amyloid, and memory. *J Neurosci* 25:7709-7717.

Caccamo A, Oddo S, Billings LM, Green KN, Martinez-Coria H, Fisher A, LaFerla FM (2006) M1 receptors play a central role in modulating AD-like pathology in transgenic mice. *Neuron* 49:671-682.

Cam JA, Zerbinatti CV, Li Y, Bu G (2005) Rapid endocytosis of the low density lipoprotein receptor-related protein modulates cell surface distribution and processing of the beta-amyloid precursor protein. *J Biol Chem* 280:15464-15470.

Cam JA, Zerbinatti CV, Knisely JM, Hecimovic S, Li Y, Bu G (2004) The low density lipoprotein receptor-related protein 1B retains beta-amyloid precursor protein at the cell surface and reduces amyloid-beta peptide production. *J Biol Chem* 279:29639-29646.

Carey RM, Balcz BA, Lopez-Coviella I, Slack BE (2005) Inhibition of dynamin-dependent endocytosis increases shedding of the amyloid precursor protein ectodomain and reduces generation of amyloid beta protein. *BMC cell biology* 6:30.

Cirrito JR, Kang JE, Lee J, Stewart FR, Verges DK, Silverio LM, Bu G, Mennerick S, Holtzman DM (2008) Endocytosis is required for synaptic activity-dependent release of amyloid-beta in vivo. *Neuron* 58:42-51.

Cirrito JR, Yamada KA, Finn MB, Sloviter RS, Bales KR, May PC, Schoepp DD, Paul SM, Mennerick S, Holtzman DM (2005a) Synaptic Activity Regulates Interstitial Fluid Amyloid-beta Levels In Vivo. *Neuron* 48:913-922.

Cirrito JR, May PC, O'Dell MA, Taylor JW, Parsadanian M, Cramer JW, Audia JE, Nissen JS, Bales KR, Paul SM, DeMattos RB, Holtzman DM (2003) In vivo assessment of brain interstitial fluid with microdialysis reveals plaque-associated changes in amyloid-beta metabolism and half-life. *J Neurosci* 23:8844-8853.

Cirrito JR, Deane R, Fagan AM, Spinner ML, Parsadanian M, Finn MB, Jiang H, Prior JL, Sagare A, Bales KR, Paul SM, Zlokovic BV, Piwnica-Worms D, Holtzman DM (2005b) P-glycoprotein deficiency at the blood-brain barrier increases amyloid-beta deposition in an Alzheimer disease mouse model. *J Clin Invest* 115:3285-3290.

Csernansky JG, Dong H, Fagan AM, Wang L, Xiong C, Holtzman DM, Morris JC (2006) Plasma cortisol and progression of dementia in subjects with Alzheimer-type dementia. *The American journal of psychiatry* 163:2164-2169.

Dodson SE, Gearing M, Lippa CF, Montine TJ, Levey AI, Lah JJ (2006) LR11/SorLA expression is reduced in sporadic Alzheimer disease but not in familial Alzheimer disease. *J Neuropathol Exp Neurol* 65:866-872.

Dong H, Goico B, Martin M, Csernansky CA, Bertchume A, Csernansky JG (2004) Modulation of hippocampal cell proliferation, memory, and amyloid plaque deposition in APPsw (Tg2576) mutant mice by isolation stress. *Neuroscience* 127:601-609.

Farris W, Schutz SG, Cirrito JR, Shankar GM, Sun X, George A, Leissring MA, Walsh DM, Qiu WQ, Holtzman DM, Selkoe DJ (2007) Loss of neprilysin function promotes amyloid plaque formation and causes cerebral amyloid angiopathy. *Am J Pathol* 171:241-251.

Gouras GK, Relkin NR, Sweeney D, Munoz DG, Mackenzie IR, Gandy S (1997) Increased apolipoprotein E epsilon 4 in epilepsy with senile plaques. *Ann Neurol* 41:402-404.

Gusnard DA, Raichle ME, Raichle ME (2001) Searching for a baseline: functional imaging and the resting human brain. *Nat Rev Neurosci* 2:685-694.

Hartley DM, Walsh DM, Ye CP, Diehl T, Vasquez S, Vassilev PM, Teplow DB, Selkoe DJ (1999) Protofibrillar intermediates of amyloid beta-protein induce acute electrophysiological changes and progressive neurotoxicity in cortical neurons. *J Neurosci* 19:8876-8884.

Hartmann T, Bieger SC, Bruhl B, Tienari PJ, Ida N, Allsop D, Roberts GW, Masters CL, Dotti CG, Unsicker K, Beyreuther K (1997) Distinct sites of intracellular production for Alzheimer's disease A beta40/42 amyloid peptides. *Nat Med* 3:1016-1020.

Hoey SE, Williams RJ, Perkinton MS (2009) Synaptic NMDA Receptor Activation Stimulates α-secretase Amyloid Precursor Protein Processing and Inhibits Amyloid-β Production. *Journal of Neuroscience* 29:1442-1460.

Hsieh H, Boehm J, Sato C, Iwatsubo T, Tomita T, Sisodia S, Malinow R (2006) AMPAR removal underlies Abeta-induced synaptic depression and dendritic spine loss. *Neuron* 52:831-843.

Ikin AF, Annaert WG, Takei K, De Camilli P, Jahn R, Greengard P, Buxbaum JD (1996) Alzheimer amyloid protein precursor is localized in nerve terminal preparations to Rab5-containing vesicular organelles distinct from those implicated in the synaptic vesicle pathway. *J Biol Chem* 271:31783-31786.

Kamenetz F, Tomita T, Hsieh H, Seabrook G, Borchelt D, Iwatsubo T, Sisodia S, Malinow R (2003) APP Processing and Synaptic Function. *Neuron* 37:925-937.

Kang JE, Cirrito JR, Dong H, Csernansky JG, Holtzman DM (2007) Acute stress increases interstitial fluid amyloid-beta via corticotropin-releasing factor and neuronal activity. *Proc Natl Acad Sci U S A* 104:10673-10678.

Koo EH, Squazzo SL (1994) Evidence that production and release of amyloid beta-protein involves the endocytic pathway. *J Biol Chem* 269:17386-17389.

Lazarov O, Lee M, Peterson DA, Sisodia SS (2002) Evidence that synaptically released beta-amyloid accumulates as extracellular deposits in the hippocampus of transgenic mice. *J Neurosci* 22:9785-9793.

Mackenzie IR, Miller LA (1994) Senile plaques in temporal lobe epilepsy. *Acta Neuropathol* (Berl) 87:504-510.

Marquez-Sterling NR, Lo AC, Sisodia SS, Koo EH (1997) Trafficking of cell-surface beta-amyloid precursor protein: evidence that a sorting intermediate participates in synaptic vesicle recycling. *J Neurosci* 17:140-151.

Meyer-Luehmann M, Stalder M, Herzig MC, Kaeser SA, Kohler E, Pfeifer M, Boncristiano S, Mathews PM, Mercken M, Abramowski D, Staufenbiel M, Jucker M (2003) Extracellular amyloid formation and associated pathology in neural grafts. *Nat Neurosci* 6:370-377.

Newton AJ, Kirchhausen T, Murthy VN (2006) Inhibition of dynamin completely blocks compensatory synaptic vesicle endocytosis. Proc Natl Acad Sci U S A 103:17955-17960.

Nitsch RM, Deng M, Tennis M, Schoenfeld D, Growdon JH (2000) The selective muscarinic M1 agonist AF102B decreases levels of total Abeta in cerebrospinal fluid of patients with Alzheimer's disease. *Ann Neurol* 48:913-918.

Offe K, Dodson SE, Shoemaker JT, Fritz JJ, Gearing M, Levey AI, Lah JJ (2006) The lipoprotein receptor LR11 regulates amyloid beta production and amyloid precursor protein traffic in endosomal compartments. *J Neurosci* 26:1596-1603.

Peraus GC, Masters CL, Beyreuther K (1997) Late compartments of amyloid precursor protein transport in SY5Y cells are involved in beta-amyloid secretion. *J Neurosci* 17:7714-7724.

Raichle ME, MacLeod AM, Snyder AZ, Powers WJ, Gusnard DA, Shulman GL (2001) A default mode of brain function. *Proc Natl Acad Sci U S A* 98:676-682.

Rogaeva E et al. (2007) The neuronal sortilin-related receptor SORL1 is genetically associated with Alzheimer disease. *Nat Genet* 39:168-177.

Shankar GM, Li S, Mehta TH, Garcia-Munoz A, Shepardson NE, Smith I, Brett FM, Farrell MA, Rowan MJ, Lemere CA, Regan CM, Walsh DM, Sabatini BL, Selkoe DJ (2008) Amyloid-beta protein dimers isolated directly from Alzheimer's brains impair synaptic plasticity and memory. *Nat Med* 14:837-842.

Sheng JG, Price DL, Koliatsos VE (2002) Disruption of corticocortical connections ameliorates amyloid burden in terminal fields in a transgenic model of Abeta amyloidosis. *J Neurosci* 22:9794-9799.

Shibata M, Yamada S, Kumar SR, Calero M, Bading J, Frangione B, Holtzman DM, Miller CA, Strickland DK, Ghiso J, Zlokovic BV (2000) Clearance of Alzheimer's amyloid-ss(1-40) peptide from brain by LDL receptor-related protein-1 at the blood-brain barrier. *J Clin Invest* 106:1489-1499.

Sloviter RS, Dichter MA, Rachinsky TL, Dean E, Goodman JH, Sollas AL, Martin DL (1996) Basal expression and induction of glutamate decarboxylase and GABA in excitatory granule cells of the rat and monkey hippocampal dentate gyrus. *J Comp Neurol* 373:593-618.

Takahashi RH, Milner TA, Li F, Nam EE, Edgar MA, Yamaguchi H, Beal MF, Xu H, Greengard P, Gouras GK (2002) Intraneuronal Alzheimer abeta42 accumulates in multivesicular bodies and is associated with synaptic pathology. *Am J Pathol* 161:1869-1879.

Townsend M, Shankar GM, Mehta T, Walsh DM, Selkoe DJ (2006) Effects of secreted oligomers of amyloid beta-protein on hippocampal synaptic plasticity: a potent role for trimers. *J Physiol* 572:477-492.

Wilson RS, Evans DA, Bienias JL, Mendes de Leon CF, Schneider JA, Bennett DA (2003) Proneness to psychological distress is associated with risk of Alzheimer's disease. *Neurology* 61:1479-1485.

Wilson RS, Barnes LL, Bennett DA, Li Y, Bienias JL, Mendes de Leon CF, Evans DA (2005) Proneness to psychological distress and risk of Alzheimer disease in a biracial community. *Neurology* 64:380-382.

Xu H, Sweeney D, Wang R, Thinakaran G, Lo AC, Sisodia SS, Greengard P, Gandy S (1997) Generation of Alzheimer beta-amyloid protein in the trans-Golgi network in the apparent absence of vesicle formation. *Proc Natl Acad Sci U S A* 94:3748-3752.

Yin KJ, Cirrito JR, Yan P, Hu X, Xiao Q, Pan X, Bateman R, Song H, Hsu FF, Turk J, Xu J, Hsu CY, Mills JC, Holtzman DM, Lee JM (2006) Matrix metalloproteinases expressed by astrocytes mediate extracellular amyloid-beta peptide catabolism. *J Neurosci* 26:10939-10948.

Acknowledgments

This work was supported by the National Institutes of Health (AG029524) and the Cure Alzheimer's Fund.

In: Alzheimer's Disease and Dementia (Vol. 4) ISBN:978-1-60876-152-4
Editor: Miao-Kun Sun

Chapter IV

Anti-Aβ Antibodies for the Treatment of Alzheimer's Disease

***Bin Liu*[*]*, Hongjun Fu*[*]*, Jeffrey L. Frost, and Cynthia A. Lemere*[**]**
Center for Neurologic Disease, Department of Neurology, Brigham & Women's Hospital and Harvard Medical School, Boston, MA, 02115, USA

Abstract

Alzheimer's disease (AD) is the most common form of dementia in individuals, becoming an even greater problem as the average life expectancy increases. While current pharmacological treatments for AD provide transient symptomatic benefit for some patients, no treatments have been shown to reverse or slow disease progression. Immunotherapy targeting the amyloid-beta (Aß) peptide has shown promise in animal models (mice, non-human primates and canines) and human studies. Although preclinical efficacy was seen in AD transgenic mouse models, the initial human clinical trial of an active Aß vaccine was halted because of the appearance of meningoencephalitis in ~6% of the vaccinated AD patients. Nevertheless, some encouraging improvements, including limited cognitive stabilization and plaque clearance, were obtained in subset of patients who generated antibody titers. Currently, numerous efforts are underway to develop refined, highly effective and possibly safer active and passive immunotherapeutic approaches. The active immunotherapeutic strategies focus on developing B cell epitope-specific immunogens with a Th2-type immune-biased adjuvant, or display of an Aß immunogen by gene manipulation. Passive immunotherapy, using N-, mid-region- and C-teminal-specific Aß antibodies, as well as conformation-specific antibodies that target toxic soluble Aß oligomers, is under investigation. Preclinical studies in transgenic mice, non-human primates and canines, as well as new human clinical trials, for both active and passive immunotherapy are ongoing.

---

*These authors contributed equally
**Correspondence to: Cynthia A. Lemere, Ph.D. clemere@rics.bwh.harvard.edu

Abbreviation List

Aβ, amyloid-β; AD, Alzheimer's Disease; ADDLs, Aß-derived diffusible ligands; APP, amyloid precursor protein; BBB, blood-brain barrier; CAA, cerebral amyloid angiopathy; CFA, Complete Freund's Adjuvant; CNS, central nervous system; CSF, cerebrospinal fluid; FcR, Fc receptor; HSV, herpes simplex virus; IAPP, islet amyloid polypeptide; i.c.v, intracerebroventricular; IFN-γ, interferon-gamma; IVIg, intravenous immunoglobulin; LTP, long-term potentiation; MPL, monophosphoryl lipid A; MRI, Magnetic Resonance Imaging; MWM, Morris water maze; NFT, neurofibrillary tangles; ODN, oligodeoxynucleotides; PADRE, pan human leukocyte antigen DR-binding peptide; PEDI, Pseudomonas exotoxin A; PLG, poly (D,L-lactide co-glycolide); PS, presenilin; scFv, single-chain variable fragment; TDM, trehalose dicorynomycolate; 3xTg, triple transgenic; TMG, TiterMax Gold; TxFC, tetanus toxin Fragment C.

1. Introduction

Alzheimer's disease (AD) is a devastating neurodegenerative condition that affects more than 18 million people worldwide (www.ahaf.org). The average life expectancy is roughly 7 to 15 years after the clinical diagnosis, however, diseae progression varies significantly from patient to patient. Clinical symptoms of AD are characterized by progressive memory loss and the gradual inability to learn and carry out daily activities. The pathologic hallmarks of AD include: extracellular neuritic plaques and cerebral amyloid angiopathy (CAA) formed by amyloid-beta (Aß) deposits, intracellular aggregation of hyperphosphorylated tau as paired helical filaments in neurofibrillary tangles, neuritic dystrophy, neuronal loss, gliosis, and inflammation (Dickson, 1997; Selkoe, 2001; Hardy and Selkoe, 2002). Although the precise mechanism of the disease is still elusive, accumulating evidence suggests that the "Aß hypothesis", which hypothesizes that overproduction and/or insufficient clearance of Aß peptide is the major cause of neuronal loss and dysfunction underlying dementia in AD (Hardy and Selkoe, 2002), is responsible for the pathogenesis of AD.

Aß protein is a 39-43 residue, soluble peptide that is generated by cleavage from amyloid precursor protein (APP) by ß- and γ-secretases (Kang et al., 1987). Genetic studies indicate that missense mutations in the APP or in the presenilin (PS) 1 and 2 (which protein expression is an important subunit of γ-secretase) genes cause early-onset, familial forms of AD. Recent *in vitro* and *in vivo* studies imply that once water-soluble Aß reaches a crucial concentration, at which point a conformational change occurs, it initiates a neurodegenerative cascade including: impairment of long-term potentiation (LTP) (Knobloch et al., 2007; Winklhofer et al., 2008), alteration of synaptic function (Shankar et al., 2008; Chiba et al., 2009; Nikolaev et al., 2009), and accelerated formation of neurofibrillary tangles (NFT) that will ultimately lead to synaptic failure and neuronal death (Selkoe, 2000). This compelling evidence supports the speculation that Aß processing and aggregation are central to the pathogenesis of AD. As a result, the Aß protein has become a crucial therapeutic target and lowering the Aß burden in brain by immunotherapy is considered a promising strategy for AD clinical treatment.

2. A Historical View of Aß Immunotherapy

Current pharmacological treatments for AD provide modest symptomatic benefit for some patients, but do little to modify disease progression (Lleo et al., 2006). In turn, interest in Aß immunotherapy has grown as a potentially useful strategy against pathogenic changes in AD.

2.1 Active Aβ Vaccination in Transgenic Mice and Non-Human Primates

Typically, active immunization is performed by co-administration of an antigen with an adjuvant. In 1999, Schenk et al of ELAN Pharmaceuticals reported the first preclinical study of $Aß_{1-42}$ active immunization in PDAPP transgenic mice (Schenk et al., 1999). Mice that were immunized prior to the onset of pathology and were immunized monthly thereafter had reduced levels of cerebral amyloid and high serum antibody titers. Furthermore, plaque burden was reduced even when mice were immunized after the onset of plaque deposition. In 2000, Schenk's work was confirmed by active intranasal immunization using a mixture of $Aß_{1-40}$ and $Aß_{1-42}$ peptides without adjuvant in PDAPP transgenic (tg) mice (Lemere et al., 2000; Weiner et al., 2000). Quickly thereafter, two additional reports demonstrated that immunization with Aß peptide in Tg CRND8 (Janus et al., 2000) or APP/PS1 (Morgan et al., 2000) tg mice strongly improved behavioral performance in learning and memory tasks by employing the radial-arm water maze test or the Morris water maze (MWM) test, respectively. Since then, numerous studies have been published that confirm the Aß lowering effect of Aß immunotherapy in AD-like tg mouse models. An example of this effect is illustrated in Figure 1. We intranasally immunized J20 APP tg mice with full-length Aß1-40/42 and adjuvant *E. coli* heat labile enterotoxin LT(R192G) from 1 to 12 months of age. Untreated age-matched control J20 mice had abundant plaque deposition in hippocampus (shown here) and cortex, whereas Aß immunized J20 mice had almost no plaque deposition. Instead, only small punctate dots of Aß immunoreactivity remained, often adjacent to blood vessels. Thus, immunizing APP tg mice prior to plaque deposition strongly prevented plaque deposition.

Limitations exist with the use of AD transgenic mouse models in Aß immunotherapy due to the fact that when AD tg mice are immunized the immune response elicited is one of removal of humanized Aß protein but when AD patients are immunized with the same immunogen the target is the endogenous Aß protein in brain. Hence the need for a preclinical model that genetically homologous and ages similar to humans, exhibits AD pathology with normal aging as well as displays a comparable immune system and response (Foster et al., 2009). Such a model would be ideal to test preclinical anti-Aß immunotherapies for efficacy, and importantly, safety before transitioning to clinical trials. Fortunately, it has been shown that several species of non-human primates, including rhesus monkeys (Macaca mulatta) and Caribbean vervets (*Chlorocebus aethiops*, SK) exhibit age-related Aß deposition similar to AD in humans (Gandy et al., 2004; Lemere et al., 2004). In a pilot study, Aß vaccination in 5 aged vervets with 1mg aged Aß1-40/42 in Complete Freund's Adjuvant (CFA) followed by 7 boosts with Aß1-40/42 in Incomplete Freund's Adjuvant (IFA) over ten months, it was demonstrated that immunized vervets produced appreciable titers of plasma Aß antibodies that recognized plaques in human, vervet, and APP tg mouse brains (Lemere et al., 2004). Lower anti-Aß titers were detected in cerebrospinal fluid (CSF). Furthermore, Aß immunization led to increased Aß levels in plasma and decreased Aß levels in CSF and brain tissues in the vaccinated vervets. No T cell response or inflammation was observed in the brain tissues of immunized vervets.

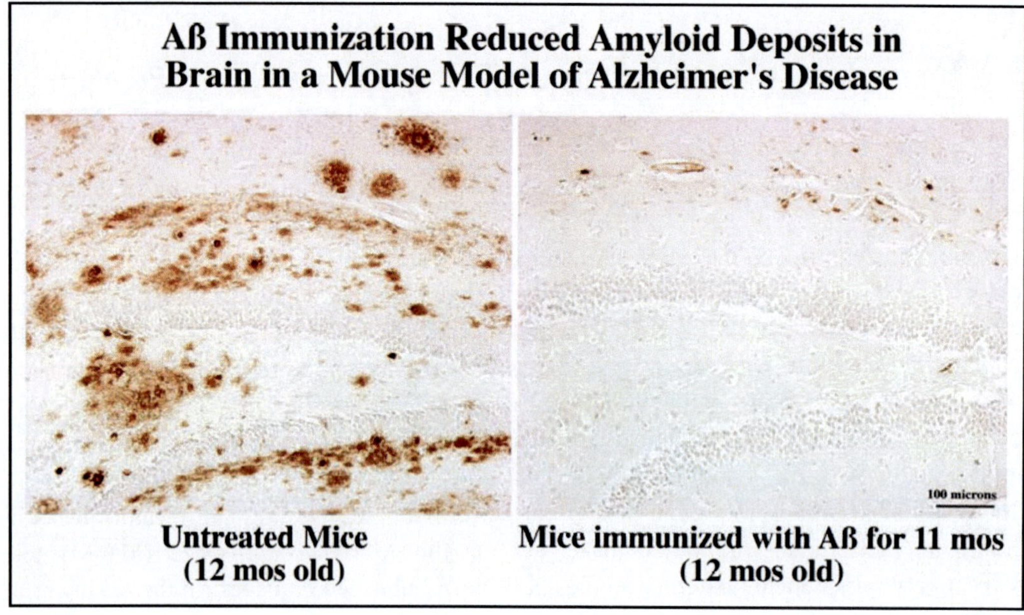

Figure 1. Immunization with full-length Aß dramatically reduced cerebral Aß plaque burden in J20 APP transgenic mice, a mouse model of Alzheimer's disease. In this study, 1 mo-old mice were primed by giving an intraperitoneal injection of 100 µg Aß40/42 synthetic peptide plus 50 µg Complete Freund's adjuvant. The mice were then boosted weekly by intranasal application of 100 µg Aß40/42 plus 5 µg adjuvant LT(R192G) for a total of 11 months and euthanized at 12 months, an age in which these mice typically accumulate many plaques in cortex and hippocampus (left panel). Immunohistochemical analysis with an Aß-specific polyclonal antibody, R1282 (gift of Dennis Selkoe, CND, Boston, MA), revealed a significant reduction in plaque burden in cortex and hippocampus (shown in right panel). Scale bar: 100 µm. [Reprinted with permission from Lemere, C.A., Maier, M., Jiang, L., Peng, Y., Seabrook, T.J. Amyloid-beta immunotherapy for the prevention and treatment of Alzheimer's disease: Lessons from mice, monkeys and men. Rejuvenation Research 9:77-84, 2006.]

A similar active vaccine with aggregated $Aß_{1-42}$ or aggregated islet amyloid polypeptide (IAPP) and CFA was investigated in rhesus monkeys. The monkeys received 2 initial vaccinations (10mg of peptide per injection with CFA) and subsequent boost for 6 months. Moderate anti-Aß titers were noted in rhesus monkeys that received aggregated $Aß_{1-42}$, as well as a 5-10 fold increase of Aß levels in plasma, as compared with the rhesus monkeys that were vaccinated with aggregated IAPP (Gandy et al., 2004). However, in contrast to previous vaccination studies in vervets (Lemere et al., 2004), Aß levels in these younger monkeys did not decrease in the brain even though plasma Aß levels were elevated after vaccination (Gandy et al., 2004), possibly because they had not reached plaque-bearing age. Thus, these two studies demonstrate that non-human primates display natural Aß deposition with aging and when actively vaccinated with an Aß peptide, anti-Aß antibodies with biological activity were generated.

2.2 Active AN1792 Aß Vaccination Clinical Trial in Humans

Based on the promising preclinical transgenic mouse data of active Aß immunotherapy, this approach was translated rapidly to Phase I and Phase II human clinical trials by ELAN/Wyeth in 2000 and 2001. In a Phase I clinical trial, the safety, tolerability and immunogenicity of multiple-dose immunization of the $Aß_{1-42}$ peptide (AN1792) in combination with the adjuvant QS-21 was evaluated in 80 patients with mild to moderate AD in the United Kingdom. After 4 immunizations, 23% of patients developed anti-Aß titers, whereas after re-formulation with polysorbate 80 and additional injections, close to 59% percent of the patients developed an anti-Aß humoral response (Bayer et al., 2005). There were few adverse effects and some signs of possible improvement in one of the clinical measurements. Based on the promising results of Phase I trial, a multi-center Phase II human clinical trial in 372 mild to moderate AD patients was initiated, with 300 patients receiving the AN1792 (QS-21) and the remainder, receiving placebo. However, this Phase II trial was halted after 18 (6%) of 300 patients immunized with the AN1792 (QS-21) developed meningoencephalitis (Orgogozo et al., 2003; Gilman et al., 2005). The exact cause of this adverse event in 6% of the patients is not clear, however, it was unrelated to serum anti-Aß antibody titers as not all of the patients that developed meningoencephalitis generated anti-Aß antibodies, and it may have been due to the activation of cytotoxic T cells and/or autoimmune reactions (Cribbs et al., 2003; Nicoll et al., 2003; Orgogozo et al., 2003; Ferrer et al., 2004). Despite the Phase II human clinical trial being halted, reports of the clinical, cognitive and neuropathological consequences of AN1792 (QS-21) immunization have been useful for the development of new strategies for Aß immunotherapy. The autopsies of two AN1792 (QS-21) vaccinated patients that developed meningoencephalitis and one vaccinated patient without side effects showed a localized dramatic reduction in Aß plaque deposition, as well as the appearance of activated microglia and multinuclear giant cells surrounding the collapsed Aß plaques in brain (Nicoll et al., 2003; Ferrer et al., 2004; Masliah et al., 2005). This evidence supports the validity of Aß immunization for amyloid clearance in humans and the underlying role of phagocytosis induced by microglia. While only about 20% of vaccinated patients developed anti-Aß antibodies, those patients had modest but statistically significant slower rates of decline of cognitive functions as compared to patients without such antibodies (Hock et al., 2002; Hock et al., 2003; Bayer et al., 2005). In addition, a year after immunization with AN1792, antibody-responders had reduced tau levels in CSF and a slowing of cognitive decline in the neurological test battery (Gilman et al., 2005). An unexpected outcome of the Phase II human clinical trial of AN1792 came from a one-year volumetric Magnetic Resonance Imaging (MRI) study (Fox et al., 2005). Brain volume was significantly reduced in immunized patients that made anti-Aß antibodies; titers correlated with brain volume loss. However, reduction of brain volume was not reflected in worsening of cognitive performance. The reasons for the dissociation between brain volume loss and cognitive function observed in antibody responders remain unclear but it has been suggested that the brain volume changes were due to amyloid removal and associated cerebral fluid shifts. This effect was transient as brain volumes were closer to baseline levels 2 years after dosing was stopped.

Active immunization with AN1792, albeit for only a short period, has produced some evidence that this treatment approach succeeded to some degree in generating an anti-Aß antibody response, Aß clearance, and benefits in cognitive functions. However, long-term effects of the AN1792 trial showed that at least in a small group of AD patients who came to autopsy several years after the trial was stopped, there were no significant differences between placebo and AN1792 vaccinated groups in survival outcomes or time to severe dementia, or in cognitive measures, despite having large areas of cortex devoid of amyloid plaques (Holmes et al., 2008). It is possible that the disease process, including frank neuronal loss, was too far along when these patients entered the trial, suggesting that Aß vaccination may have its best effects if given prior to or in the very early stages of AD. Because vascular amyloid (Nicoll et al., 2003; Ferrer et al., 2004) and tau-related pathologies (Holmes et al., 2008) were still observed in deceased AN1792 antibody-responders, it has been suggested that active vaccination needs to be initiated before the development of significant AD-related clinical pathology (Wisniewski and Konietzko, 2008). Interest in active immunization has not diminished, and multiple new human clinical trials with active Aß immunization are currently in the pipeline or underway by pharmaceutical companies such as ELAN/Wyeth, Novartis, Merck and Affiris.

2.3 Passive Aβ Antibody Immunization in Transgenic Mice

Passive immunization involves direct injection of antibodies into the body, avoiding the need for a humoral immune response to generate antibodies as in active immunization. Antibodies, which were designed to recognize specific epitopes of the Aß molecule, were investigated in transgenic mice with AD-like pathology. Many of the Aß antibodies used in preclinical passive immunization studies were designed to recognize epitopes in the N-terminus of Aß peptide such as 3D6 ($Aß_{1-5}$) (Bard et al., 2000; Bard et al., 2003), 10D5 ($Aß_{3-7}$) (Bard et al., 2003; Hartman et al., 2005), BAM-10 ($Aß_{1-12}$) (Kotilinek et al., 2002), and 20.1 ($Aβ_{1-8}$) (Oddo et al., 2006b). Other antibodies used for passive vaccination studies in mice targeted the Aß mid-domain, such as m266 ($Aß_{13-28}$) (DeMattos et al., 2001) or the C-terminus of Aß, such as 2286 ($Aβ_{28-40}$) (Wilcock et al., 2004a) and 2H6 ($Aß_{33-40}$) (Wilcock et al., 2006).

Bard and colleagues first reported the effects of passive immunization in PDAPP mice using several different monoclonal anti-Aß antibodies that targeted various Aß epitopes, and represented different IgG isotypes (Bard et al., 2000). Passively administered antibodies were able to enter the central nervous system (CNS), bind plaques and induce clearance of pre-existing amyloid. Their follow-up study indicated that antibodies against the N-terminus of Aß (3D6 against $Aß_{1-5}$ or 10D5 against $Aß_{3-7}$) were the most effective at lowering cerebral Aß and indicated that an IgG_{2a}-Fcγ receptor-mediated phagocytic mechanism by microglia might be involved in this process (Bard et al., 2003). Immunization of PDAPP tg mice with the 10D5 antibody resulted in reduced plaque deposition, increased plasma Aß, improved hippocampal LTP, and improved behavioral performance (Hartman et al., 2005). Intraperitoneal injection of BAM-10, a monoclonal antibody against $Aß_{1-12}$, fully reversed memory loss in Tg2576 APP tg mice, however, the beneficial effect was not associated with a significant Aß reduction (Kotilinek et al., 2002).

N-terminal antibodies have been shown to be effective at removing Aß from plaques, however, one potential concern associated with the administration of these antibodies is cerebral microhemorrhage. The occurrence of microhemorrhages after immunization with N-terminal Aß antibodies was first reported in a study of aged APP23 mice (Pfeifer et al., 2002). Since then, CAA-associated microhemorrhage, as well as acute hematomas, have been observed in the brains of other passively immunized mice as confirmed by several groups (Wilcock et al., 2004b; Racke et al., 2005).

DeMattos and colleagues reported that bi-weekly passive immunization with a central-domain Aβ antibody, m226, for 5 months significantly attenuated Aß plaque pathology in PDAPP transgenic mice (DeMattos et al., 2001). A subsequent study by this group showed that even a single injection of this antibody in aged PDAPP mice produced beneficial effects on cognition as well as a significantly increased serum Aß levels that were detectable the day after immunization (Dodart et al., 2002). While this antibody has a high affinity for soluble, monomeric Aß, it does not directly bind plaque deposits in brain suggesting that the m266 antibody reduced cerebral Aß levels via peripheral clearance as opposed to a central phagocytic mechanism. Another beneficial effect of m266 is that unlike the N-terminal antibodies (3D6 and 10D5) that caused a significant increase in CAA-associated microhemorrhage, this mid-domain antibody did not cause microhemorrhage in transgenic mouse brains (Racke et al., 2005).

The first study of passive immunization with a C-terminal Aß antibody (16C11) was reported by Bard in 2000 (Bard et al., 2000). However, in her study, the 16C11 antibody (against $Aß_{33-42}$) failed to lower plaque burden or improve cognitive deficits. In 2004, Wilcock and colleagues described a study using an IgG_1 C-terminal Aß antibody called 2286 (against $Aß_{28-40}$) for passive immunization in mice. Tg2576 transgenic mice that were immunized with 2286 for 3 months showed an improvement in alternation performance in the Y maze, a reduction in both diffuse and compact amyloid deposits, and transient but significant microglial activation (Wilcock et al., 2004a). However, this anti-Aß antibody was also shown to significantly increase CAA-associated microhemorrhage (Wilcock et al., 2004b). Thereafter, an IgG_{2b} C-terminal antibody (2H6) and its de-glycosylated version (de-2H6) were examined and both showed considerable capacity to reduce Aß pathology and significantly improve performance in a radial arm water maze (Carty et al., 2006; Wilcock et al., 2006). Also, significantly fewer vascular amyloid deposits and microhemorrhages, in the absence of enhanced microglial activation, were observed in de-2H6-vaccinated mice which might due to a decreased affinity for Fcγ receptor of this antibody by deglycosylation.

2.4 Passive Immunization Clinical Trials Using Intravenous Immunoglobulin (IVIg)

Passive transfer of exogenous anti-Aß antibodies may be a simple and relatively safe method to provide antibodies without eliciting Th1-mediated autoimmunity. Intravenous immunoglobulin (IVIg) is a purified mixture of endogenous human immunoglobulins that include natural human autoantibodies against Aß. IVIg antibodies were shown to interfere with the oligomerization and fibrillization of Aß peptide (Du et al., 2003; Ma et al., 2006), protect neurons exposed to toxic concentrations of Aß peptide (Du et al., 2003), and promote the clearance of Aß peptide from the brain (Istrin et al., 2006), suggesting that IVIg may be useful in humans as a type of passive immunotherapy to treat AD. A pilot clinical trial using this promising strategy was conducted (Dodel et al., 2004) and showed that IVIg markedly reduced the concentration of Aß peptide in the CSF and significantly increased the Aβ levels in blood, suggesting that the antibody mixture induced efflux of Aß from the brain to the periphery. Furthermore, those passively immunized patients exhibited some improvement in cognitive function without adverse events. Interestingly, anti-Aß antibodies were detected in CSF of the patients subsequent to IVIg treatment, indicating that IVIg antibodies may cross the blood-brain barrier (BBB) and induce the decrease in the concentration of Aß in the brain (Foster et al., 2009).

The potential of IVIg immunotherapy for AD has been supported by additional small clinical trials, however, further validation is needed as these studies were carried out only in a relatively small number of AD patients (reviewed in Relkin et al., 2008; Foster et al., 2009). A larger phase III clinical IVIg trial in AD patients, supported by Baxter Biosciences, is currently underway. In addition, pharmaceutical companies such as ELAN/Wyeth, Eli Lilly, Pfizer, GlaxoSmithKline, Neuroimmune, are currently carrying out human clinical trials using passive Aß immunization.

3. Ongoing Studies and Future Directions

3.1 Second-Generation Active Aß Vaccines in Murine Models

The initial clinical trial of AN1792 (using adjuvant QS21) resulted in an unexpected side effect of meningoencephalitis in 6% of AN1792 vaccinated patients thought to be elicited by Th1-mediated autoimmunity, thereby raising concerns regarding the safety and efficacy of active immunization. Recent alternative strategies for boosting antibody generation after Aβ administration, as well as eliminating the Th1 response are focused on: (1) generating epitope-specific Aβ immunogens to eliminate Aß-specific T cell responses, (2) testing various adjuvants that favor a Th2 immune response to avoid adverse side effects, (3) producing the Aβ peptide by DNA vaccines or phage-display system and, (4) using different routes of vaccine administration.

3.1a Epitope-Specific Aβ Fragments

The dominant B cell epitope for anti-Aß antibodies generated by active immunization with full-length Aß was found to reside within the first 15 amino acids of the Aß N-terminus (Lemere et al., 2000). Later studies reported refinement of the B cell epitope to Aß1-5, 1-7, 1-8, 1-9, 1-11, 1-16, 4-10, and 3-7 in mice (Town et al., 2001; McLaurin et al., 2002; Bard et al., 2003; Cribbs et al., 2003; Seabrook et al., 2004), Aß1-7 in vervets (Lemere et al., 2004), and Aß1-8 in humans (Lee et al., 2005). Dominant Aß T cell epitopes have been mapped to Aß6-28 (Cribbs et al, 2003) or beyond Aß1-15 (Monsonego et al, 2001) in mice and Aß16-33 in humans (Monsonego et al., 2003). Therefore, the use of N-terminal Aβ derivatives as immunogens, was hypothesized to generate a strong humoral immune response while avoiding a deleterious Aß-specific T cell response.

In 2001, Sigurdsson and colleagues reported that an Aß derivative vaccine containing 6 lysines linked to the first 30 residues of Aß (K6Aß1-30-NH_2) induced anti-Aß antibodies and reduced plaque burden and inflammation in brains of Tg2576 APP tg mice (Sigurdsson et al., 2001). This soluble non-amyloid, non-toxic Aß derivative was designed to avoid the potential for toxicity using aggregated full-length Aß, a peptide conformation known to be neurotoxic *in vitro*. In a subsequent study, Aß residues were mutated at positions 18 and 19, to maintain solubility of the immunogen, and at least in theory, avoid T cell recognition. The immunogen, K6Aß1-30[$E_{18}E_{19}$] was shown to induce low anti-Aß antibody titers that were enough to protect against cognitive impairment of Tg2676 mice in a radial arm maze (Sigurdsson et al., 2004).

In 2005, Agadjanyan and colleagues designed a prototype epitope vaccine that contains the $A\beta_{1-15}$ in tandem with the synthetic pan HLADR-binding peptide (PADRE) in order to reduce the risk of an adverse T cell-mediated immune response and found that immunization of BALB/c mice with the PADRE-$A\beta_{1-15}$ epitope vaccine produced high antibody titers (Agadjanyan et al., 2005). Two years later, the same group described another epitope vaccine composed of two copies of $A\beta_{1-11}$ fused with PADRE that completely abolished autoreactive T cell responses and induced humoral immune responses in Tg2576 mice with pre-existing AD-like pathology (Petrushina et al., 2007). In this study, a positive correlation between the anti-$A\beta_{1-11}$ antibody concentration and a reduction of insoluble Aß (but not soluble Aβ) and reduced cerebral Aβ plaque load were reported.

In our own studies, we found that while $A\beta_{1-15}$ peptide was less immunogenic than $A\beta_{1-40/42}$ for antibody production in wild-type mice (Leverone et al., 2003), intranasal boosting with dendrimeric $A\beta_{1-15}$ (16 copies of Aß1-15 on a lysine tree, dAß1-15) mucosal adjuvant after a single injection of $A\beta_{1-40/42}$ in J20 APP mice produced significant antibody titers and lowered amyloid plaque burden in brain by approximately 60% (Seabrook et al., 2006a). In a subsequent study, intranasal dosing of dAß1-15 with LT(R192G) without a priming injection, also induced robust anti-Aß titers and lowered cerebral Aß levels and plaques in the brains of J20 APP tg mice in the absence of an Aß-specific cellular immune response (Seabrook et al., 2006b). Intranasal administration of two additional short Aß immunogens, 2xAß1-15 and R2xAß1-15 (tandem repeat of Aß1-15 linked by 2 lysine residues, without or with an RGD motif at the N-terminus, respectively) generated high anti-Aß antibody titers in the absence of an Aß-specific T cell response, reduced plaque load, and in the case of the 2xAß1-15 vaccine, improved memory acquisition in the Morris water maze in J20 APP tg mice (Maier et al.,

2006). Numerous other short Aß fragment active vaccines by many different investigators are described in a review article (Lemere et al., 2007).

3.1b Adjuvants

The adjuvant QS21, a Th1 type adjuvant, used the AN1792 may have contributed to the adverse events observed in that trial by initiating the production of pro-inflammatory cytokines such as interferon-gamma (IFNγ) and stimulating an Aß-specific T-cell reaction. Cribbs and colleagues examined 4 adjuvants CFA, alum, TiterMax Gold (TMG) and QS21 with an $A\beta_{1-42}$ vaccine and found that Th1-type adjuvants, QS21 and CFA, induced the strongest humoral response to Aβ while the Th2-type adjuvant, alum, generated an intermediate humoral response (Cribbs et al., 2003). The Th1-type adjuvant TMG gave the weakest humoral response. Furthermore, this group compared the induction of humoral immune responses with another Th1-type adjuvant, Quil A, and Th2-type adjuvant Alum separately and in combination, using PADRE-$A\beta_{1-15}$ (Ghochikyan et al., 2006a). Interestingly, switching adjuvants from Alum to Quil A induced higher concentrations of antibodies than injections with Alum only, but only slightly lower than Quil A alone. This result suggested that switching from Alum to Quil A after the priming dose might be beneficial for AD patients because anti-Aβ antibody production was enhanced without changing the initially generated and likely beneficial Th2-type humoral response. Although Alum may be less effective in generating as robust a humoral immune response compared with some Th1 type adjuvants, when used with active Aß vaccination, it avoided vascular microhemorrhages observed with some Th1-type adjuvants (Asuni et al., 2006).

In a study from our lab, we compared the humoral and cellular immune responses produced by two different adjuvants used for subcutaneous Aβ vaccination: monophosphoryl lipid A (MPL)/trehalose dicorynomycolate (TDM) and *E. coli* heat-labile enterotoxin LT(R192G). MPL/TDM generated much greater antibody titers than LT(R192G) and was accompanied by a moderate splenocyte proliferation and IFNγ production indicating a cellular response (Maier et al., 2005). In general, LT(R192G), a mucosal adjuvant, was more efficacious for active Aß immunization when given intranasally than subcutaneously, resulting in a Th2-biased antibody response (Lemere et al., 2002).

Agadjanyan and colleagues used mannan, a molecular adjuvant to promote a Th2-mediated immune response, conjugated to $A\beta_{28}$ at low concentrations to immunize wild-type (Ghochikyan et al., 2006b) and Tg2576 mice (Petrushina et al., 2008) without a conventional adjuvant. The mannan-conjugate induced a significant Th2-biased anti-Aβ antibody response in both wild type and Tg2576 mice. Vaccination with mannan-$A\beta_{28}$ prevented Aβ plaque deposition in transgenic mice, but unexpectedly increased microhemorrhages in the brains of aged immunized mice. This effect was likely unrelated to the anti-mannan antibodies, because control mice immunized with mannan-BSA also induced antibodies specific to mannan, but did not have increased levels of cerebral microhemorrhages compared with non-immunized mice.

In 2008, an adjuvant that might be useful to generate an oral Aβ peptide vaccine was suggested by Rajkannan and colleagues. Aβ peptides ($A\beta_{1-12}$, $A\beta_{29-40}$ and $A\beta_{1-42}$) were loaded separately onto poly(D,L-lactide co-glycolide) (PLG) microparticles using W/O/W double emulsion solvent evaporation method. Oral immunization of Aβ peptide-loaded microparticles in female BALB/c mice elicited a strong immune response, inducing anti-Aβ antibodies for a prolonged time (24 weeks) (Rajkannan et al., 2008). Somewhat surprisingly, the C-terminal fragment ($A\beta_{29-40}$) served as a better epitope to stimulate anti-Aβ antibodies in mice than the N-terminal fragment ($A\beta_{1-12}$).

An alternative strategy has focused on engaging the immune system to direct the humoral immune response to antibody production in the absence of classical adjuvants. Both IL-4 and GM-CSF are cytokines that drive dendritic cell differentiation and direct a Th2-type response. DaSilva and colleagues used these cytokines in combination with Aß to elicit a Th2-type humoral response in TgCRND8 mice. This combination elicited high anti-Aß antibody titers and significantly reduced amyloid deposition in mouse brain (DaSilva et al., 2006).

3.1C PHAGE Display and DNA Vaccines

Solomon and colleagues first showed in 1997 that N-terminal anti-Aß antibodies bound to amyloid fibrils, causing them to disaggregate and neutralizing their toxicity (Solomon et al., 1997). Soon thereafter, they determined that the EFRH amino acid sequence of Aß (residues 3-6) was a key anti-aggregation epitope (Frenkel et al., 1998; Frenkel et al., 1999). They used a filamentous phage to display the EFRH peptide for Aß vaccination in wildtype (Frenkel et al., 2000a) and APP(V717I) transgenic mice (Frenkel et al., 1999). In both studies, the EFRH phage vaccine resulted in anti-Aß antibody generation which, in the APP tg mice, led to a 50% reduction in cerebral plaque burden.

Gene gun-mediated $A\beta_{1-42}$ gene vaccination with (Ghochikyan et al., 2003; Kim et al., 2005; Dasilva et al., 2009) or without (Qu et al., 2006; Dasilva et al., 2009) adjuvants has been shown to be efficient for breaking host Aβ42 tolerance and inducing a Th2 immune response. $A\beta_{1-42}$ DNA vaccination significantly reduced the cerebral Aβ burden in different AD-like transgenic mouse models (Ghochikyan et al., 2003; Qu et al., 2006; Dasilva et al., 2009) and, reduced CAA, high-molecular-weight oligomers, and Aβ trimers in TgCRND8 mice (Dasilva et al., 2009).

In 2005, Kim and colleagues showed that an adenovirus vector encoding 11 tandem repeats of $A\beta_{1-6}$ induced an immune response against Aβ peptide (Kim et al., 2005). When an adenovirus vector encoding GM-CSF (Kim et al., 2005) or receptor-binding domain (Ia) of Pseudomonas exotoxin A (PEDI) (Kim et al., 2007b) was co-administered with their Aß vaccine, antibody titers against Aβ protein were enhanced, leading to a significant reduction in Aβ load in the brain. Immunoglobulin isotyping revealed a predominant IgG_1 response, indicating an anti-inflammatory Th2 type response. To elicit a more robust Th2 response, they employed a DNA prime-adenovirus boost regimen in the AdPEDI-($A\beta_{1-6}$)11 vaccine study (Kim et al., 2007a). The average anti-Aβ antibody titer (predominantly of the IgG_1 isotype) induced by the DNA prime-adenovirus boost regimen was approximately 7-fold greater than that by AdPEDI-($A\beta_{1-6}$)11 alone. The beneficial effect of enhancing the Th2-type humoral immune response by heterologous prime-boost strategies was also suggested by Subramanian et al (Subramanian and Divya Shree, 2008). In addition, they reported that anti-Aβ antibody titers may be further enhanced when co-administrating CpG oligodeoxynucleotides (ODN) as an adjuvant.

Movsesyan and colleagues recently developed and tested a DNA epitope vaccine composed of three copies of the gene encoding the B cell epitope Aβ_{1-11} fused with a foreign T helper epitope, PADRE (Movsesyan et al., 2008a; Movsesyan et al., 2008b). To enhance immune responses, they linked this DNA vaccine with an adjuvant encoding macrophage-derived chemokine (MDC/CCL22) (Movsesyan et al., 2008a) or an adjuvant encoding three copies of Complement 3d (3C3d) (Movsesyan et al., 2008b). They demonstrated that 3xTg-AD mice (encoding mutant human APP, PS1 and Tau) immunized with their pMDC-3Aβ_{1-11}-PADRE construct generated a robust Th2 immune response that induced high titers of anti-Aβ antibodies. Importantly, Aβ pathology and glial activation were reduced without increasing the incidence of microhemorrhages in the brains of immunized 3xTg-AD mice, and behavioral deficits were attenuated (Movsesyan et al., 2008a). Similar beneficial effects on antibody response and Aβ burden were also observed in mice immunized with the 3Aβ_{1-11}-PADRE-3C3d construct (Movsesyan et al., 2008b).

Recently, Zou et al. developed a novel adenovirus vaccine, which expresses quadrivalent foldable Aβ_{1-15} (4xAβ_{1-15}) plus gene adjuvant GM-CSF *in vivo* (Zou et al., 2008). The 4xAβ_{1-15} adenovirus vaccine induced an Aβ-specific IgG_1-predominant humoral immune response and reduced brain Aβ deposition and cognition deficits in Tg2576 mice. Detection of IL-4 and IFN-γ in restimulated splenocytes showed a significant Th2-biased immune response.

In 2005, Bowers and colleagues used another viral vector, herpes simplex virus (HSV)-derived amplicons, to elicit distinctive immune responses against Aβ. An amplicon vector coding for Aβ, with and without a tetanus toxin Fragment C (TxFC) adjuvant, was packaged in an HSV amplicon and then administered monthly to Tg2576 mice for 3 months. Although antibody titers were elevated after vaccination, only moderate cerebral amyloid reductions were observed with this method (Bowers et al., 2005). In addition, HSV-Aβ resulted in a significant T-cell response and some T-cell infiltration into the brain. Recently, the authors improved this approach by co-delivering Aβ with IL-4, a cytokine that promotes the generation of Th2-like T-cell responses, in the expression vector. When administered to 3xTg-AD mice, HSV-Aβ-IL-4 initiated a Th2 response, generated anti-Aß titers, and reduced cerebral Aβ to undetectable levels (Frazer et al., 2008). In addition, tau pathological progression was prevented, and learning and memory were improved in the HSV-Aβ-IL-4 vaccinated mice versus the other experimental groups.

A non-viral Aβ DNA vaccine was reported by Okura and colleagues (Okura et al., 2006; Okura et al., 2008a). In their study, APP23 tg mice were vaccinated prior to Aß deposition (protective treatment) or after the onset of Aβ deposition (therapeutic treatment) in the brain. A mild to moderate reduction of Aβ burden in immunized mice was observed following the protective treatment. Therapeutic treatment reduced cerebral Aβ burden to approximately 50% by the age of 18 months. Importantly, this therapy avoided neuroinflammation and T cell responses to Aβ peptide in both APP23 and wildtype mice, even after long-term vaccination (Okura et al., 2006).

3.1d Novel Routes for Administration of Active Aß Vaccines

Alternate delivery routes of an Aß vaccine enlist different populations of antigen presenting cells and cellular immune responses thereby providing another possibility for improving the safety and efficacy of such a vaccine. In 2000, we reported the first use of intranasal administration of Aβ peptides which, in the absence of adjuvant, induced a modest anti-Aß antibody response sufficient enough to significantly reduce cerebral Aβ levels in PDAPP mice (Lemere et al., 2000; Weiner et al., 2000). Subsequent studies were conducted using a mucosal adjuvant described earlier, *E. coli* heat labile enterotoxin LT(R192G), which significantly enhanced anti-Aß antibody generation in wildtype and APP tg mice when administered intranasally with short Aß peptide immunogens, dAß1-15 (Seabrook et al., 2006b) and 2xAß1-15 (Maier et al., 2006). In both studies, intranasal Aß immunization using LT(R192G) led to a predominantly Th2-type immune response and lowering of cerebral Aß without any adverse effects.

Transcutaneous immunization is another approach under investigation for administration of an Aß vaccine as it utilizes antigen presentation by Langerhans cells in the skin. In 2006, we reported that transcutaneous immunization with dAß1-15, but not Aß1-40/42, together with *E. coli* heat labile enterotoxin LT(R192G) resulted in moderately high anti-Aß antibody titers, mainly consisting of IgG1 antibodies, in wildtype mice (Seabrook et al., 2006b). Soon thereafter, Town and colleagues demonstrated that transcutaneous immunization with Aß1-42 combined with a cholera toxin adjuvant led to robust anti-Aß antibody titers, reduced cerebral Aß levels, and increased Aß in blood, all in the absence of T cell infiltration into brain or cerebral microhemorrhage (Nikolic et al., 2007).

Oral administration of a DNA vaccine (adeno-associated viral vector carrying Aß cDNA, AAV/Aβ) without adjuvant has been reported. The oral vaccine induced the expression and secretion of $A\beta_{1-43}$ or $A\beta_{1-21}$ in Tg2576 transgenic mice (Hara et al., 2004). Serum antibody levels were elevated for more than six months. In another study, a single oral administration of AAV/Aβ to Tg2576 mice at 10 months of age alleviated progressive cognitive impairment and decreased Aβ deposition, insoluble Aβ, soluble Aβ oligomers (Aβ56), microgliosis, and synaptic degeneration (Mouri et al., 2007).

As described earlier, an oral Aβ peptide vaccine was made by using an Aβ peptide-loaded microparticles. Although, the immunization with these microparticles has been conducted only in wildtype mice thus far, the advantage of this formula is that it induces long-term anti-Aβ antibody production (Rajkannan et al., 2008).

3.2 Second-Generation Passive Immunotherapy in Murine Models

A number of studies have shown that Aβ oligomers (dimers, trimers, tetramers, etc.) rather than monomers or fibrils may be the major toxic agents that specifically inhibit synaptic plasticity and LTP in AD (Walsh and Selkoe, 2007). Therefore, some passive Aß immunotherapies have focused on inhibiting or reversing Aβ oligomerization using specific anti-oligomer antibodies. One example of an oligomer conformation-specific monoclonal antibody, NAB61, has been shown to preferentially recognize a conformational epitope present in dimeric, small oligomeric, and higher order Aβ structures but not full-length or C-terminal Aβ peptides. Passive immunization of aged Tg2576 mice with NAB61 resulted in significant improvement in spatial learning and memory, without altering brain amyloid deposition or APP processing (Lee et al., 2006). This result provided further evidence that cognitive deficits in APP tg mice is at least partially caused by toxic soluble Aβ oligomers. In addition, Lambert and co-workers have generated monoclonal antibodies against Aß-derived diffusible ligands (ADDLs) that recognize pathological Aß assemblies in human Alzheimer's disease brain tissue and neutralized Aβ oligomers *in vitro* suggesting that they may be useful candidates for passive immunotherapy (Lambert et al., 2007).

Wang et al. reported recently that four single-chain variable fragment (scFv) antibodies isolated from the naive human scFv library by phage display specifically recognized Aβ oligomers but not monomers and fibrils (Wang et al., 2009). These conformation-dependent scFv antibodies inhibited both Aβ fibrillization and cytotoxicity, and bound to the same type of eptitope displayed on the Aβ oligomers. They suggested that the scFv antibodies specifically targeting toxic Aβ oligomers may have potential therapeutic and diagnostic applications for AD.

A novel approach to inhibit Aβ production via antibodies against the beta-secretase cleavage site of the APP was proposed by Arbel et al (Arbel et al., 2005). Anti-APP beta-site antibodies, were previously tested *in vitro* and were found to bind full-length APP, interfere with BACE activity and inhibit both intracellular and extracellular Aβ peptide formation (Arbel et al., 2005). Later, they investigated the effect of anti-beta-site antibody in Tg2576 mice and showed that long-term systemic administration of this antibody to Tg2576 mice improved cognitive deficits, reduced inflammation, and decreased the incidence of microhemorrhage without inducing any peripheral autoimmunity responses. In spite of the beneficial effects observed in antibody-treated mice, cerebral Aβ levels were not changed as a result of antibody treatment (Rakover et al., 2007).

Beneficial effects of passive Aß immunization on synaptic plasticity and neuronal function have been reported. Chauhan and colleagues showed that intracerebroventricular (i.c.v.) infusion of Aβ antibodies was able to protect APP transgenic mice from synaptic loss and gliosis (Chauhan and Siegel, 2002; Chauhan and Siegel, 2003). Klyubin and co-workers reported that i.c.v. infusion of 4G8, a monoclonal antibody directed to the mid-region of Aß ($A\beta_{17-24}$), prevented synaptic plasticity disruption induced by naturally-occurring, cell-derived Aβ oligomers (Klyubin et al., 2005). Subsequently, this group demonstrated that systemic infusion of 4G8 in rat prevented the inhibition of hippocampal LTP induced by i.c.v. infusion of human CSF containing Aβ dimers (Klyubin et al., 2008). Recently, Spires-Jones et al. examined dendritic spine morphology and found that immunization with an Aß monoclonal antibody recognizing the free N-terminus, 3D6, rapidly increased structural plasticity in PDAPP mouse brain (Spires-Jones et al., 2009). Moreover, Chiba and coworkers reported that an age-dependent decrease of p-STAT, thought to be involved in memory, was observed in hippocampus of Tg2576 mice and AD patients (Chiba et al., 2009). This finding was further confirmed by showing that i.c.v. administration of $A\beta_{1-42}$ resulted in a down-regulation of p-STAT3 level in mouse brain. Passive immunization with an Aβ monoclonal antibody, 6E10, restored hippocampal p-STAT3 levels in Tg2576 mice, paralleling a decrease in the brain Aβ burden.

Several reports describe alternative strategies that might improve the efficacy of passive immunization and reduce its side effects. Prolonged i.c.v. infusions of 6E10 (by osmotic mini-pump) dose-dependently reduced the parenchymal plaque burden, astrogliosis, and dystrophic neurites at doses 10- to 50-fold lower than used with systemic delivery of the same antibody (Thakker et al., 2009). Moreover, side effects observed after administration of some N-terminal Aß antibodies can be attenuated by modulating antibody dose (Schroeter et al., 2008), deglycosylating whole IgG Aß antibody (Wilcock et al., 2006), removing the Fc portion by proteolysis to produce Fab'2 (Tamura et al., 2005), or designing recombinant Fab (rFab) or scFv (Robert et al., 2009).

3.3 Second-Generation Aβ Vaccines in Non-Human Primates and Canines

The halting of the human AN1792 phase II clinical trial demonstrated the need for a safer and more effective form of Aß immunotherapy. As described earlier, many efforts are underway to develop novel Aß vaccines that will elicit strong humoral immune responses while avoiding Aß-specific cellular immune responses that might contribute to adverse events such as those observed in the AN1792 trial. Second-generation Aß vaccines have been reported in three different species of non-human primates to date including baboons, Cynomolgus macaques, and lemurs. In general, non-human primates develop Aß plaque deposition with aging, although to varying degrees depending on species. In a vaccination study performed in baboons and macaques, an active Aß vaccine using UBITh yielded promising results (Wang et al., 2007). UBITh is composed of two designer peptides used to generate N-terminal-specific $A\beta_{1-14}$ antibodies using a proprietary Th2-biased delivery platform. The vaccine was shown to be effective in both non-human primate species, providing evidence for the vaccines' potential versatility. Vaccinated monkeys generated anti-Aß antibodies that sequestered toxic Aβ from the CNS into the periphery. In addition, repeat dosing with the UBITh vaccine was well-tolerated and non-toxic in macaques, boding well for the vaccine's safety factor (Wang et al., 2007).

A recent active Aβ vaccination study using several Aβ derivatives described above, K6Aß1-30 and K6Aß1-30[$E_{18}E_{19}$], with alum adjuvant demonstrated that lemurs generated moderate to robust anti-Aβ IgM and IgG titers that were thought to bind to Aβ in the brain and draw it to the periphery, as shown by an increase of $A\beta_{1-40}$ in plasma (Trouche et al., 2009). Interestingly, the anti-Aß antibody levels generated by the Aß derivative vaccines (but not full-length Aß) dropped to pre-immune levels 22 weeks after the 3rd immunization, suggesting the potential for reversibility of this active vaccine.

In contrast to non-human primates that develop both diffuse and compacted, mature plaques, aged canines, and in particular, beagles, accumulate primarily Aβ diffuse plaques in the brain with normal aging. Like non-human primates, Aß in dogs is homologous to human Aß. Furthermore, in dogs, Aβ plaque burden has been shown to parallel cognitive decline. Immunization with fibrillar $A\beta_{1-42}$ and alum, a Th2-biased adjuvant, generated a strong anti-Aß antibody response in beagles with pre-existing Aβ deposition (Head et al., 2008). Although Aβ plaque burden was decreased in several brain regions, especially in prefrontal cortex, Aß vaccination did not improve cognitive performance in tests of learning and spatial attention. Thus, Aß immunotherapy may not be effective after robust plaque deposition, suggesting that the best cognitive benefit may come from Aß vaccination given prior to or in the early stages of plaque deposition, i.e. via prevention.

4. Potential Mechanisms Underlying Aβ Immunotherapy

The mechanisms underlying the removal of Aβ from the brain via active or passive immunization are not yet clear. Several hypotheses have been proposed, however, these mechanisms do not exclude one another and may act concomitantly or sequentially for Aβ immunotherapy at different stages of AD.

4.1 Fc Receptor(FcR)-Dependent Phagocytosis

Bard and co-workers found that passive immunization with anti-Aβ monoclonal antibodies in PDAPP mice resulted in the clearance of Aβ and the presence of activated microglia filled with Aß protein suggesting that Aß antibodies crossed the BBB, bound to Aß in plaques and Fc receptors (FcR) on microglia, and induced phagocytosis of Aß by the microglia (Bard et al., 2000; Bard et al., 2003). Furthermore, in an *ex vivo* assay with sections of PDAPP or AD brain tissue, antibodies against Aβ peptide triggered microglial cells to clear plaques through FcR-mediated phagocytosis and subsequent peptide degradation (Bard et al., 2000). Active vaccination with $A\beta_{1-42}$ in PDAPP mice (Schenk et al., 1999) and in AD patients (Nicoll et al., 2003; Ferrer et al., 2004) showed evidence that small and densely stained Aβ plaques were associated with activated microglia. New Aβ non-viral DNA vaccines were also found to lead to enhanced microglial phagocytosis of Aβ deposits (Okura et al., 2008a; Okura and Matsumoto, 2008b). Both the results of active and passive Aβ immunotherapy suggest that FcR-mediated activation of microglia and subsequent clearance of Aβ plaques by phagocytosis could be a central mechanism.

4.2 FcR-Independent Phagocytosis

FcR-independent activation of microglia and subsequent degradation of Aβ plaques via phagocytosis is a second mechanism thought to be involved in Aβ immunotherapy. Following active $A\beta_{1-42}$ immunization, the reduction in cerebral Aβ burden in FcRγ-/-Tg2576 mice was equivalent to that seen in age-matched, FcR-sufficient Tg2576 mice (Das et al., 2003). Because FcRγ-/- mice have complete impairment of phagocytosis of Aβ immune complexes via FcR, this result suggests that the Fc portion of Aβ antibodies is not necessary for Aβ clearance. Furthermore, direct application of F(ab')2 fragments of the anti-Aβ antibody 3D6 (which lack the Fc region of the antibody) to APP transgenic mouse brain led to clearance of Aβ deposits similar to that following application of the full-length 3D6 antibody (Bacskai et al., 2002; Tamura et al., 2005). These findings demonstrate that Fc-independent mechanisms, in addition to Fc-dependent mechanisms, appear to be able to mediate the effects of active and passive Aβ immunization.

4.3 Peripheral Sink

A third mechanism by which Aß immunotherapy effectively lowers cerebral Aß levels and may prevent plaque deposition is the "peripheral sink" effect, in which plasma Aß antibodies sequester Aβ from the brain by promoting efflux of Aß from brain to peripheral blood. The peripheral sink mechanism was first described by DeMattos and colleagues in an elegant series of experiments involving both *in vitro* and *in vivo* studies in PDAPP tg mice (DeMattos et al., 2001). An Aß monoclonal antibody, m266, was able to sequester Aß from brain to blood. This mechanism was later confirmed by active immunization (Lemere et al., 2003; Sigurdsson et al., 2004) and passive immunization (Dodart et al., 2002; Dodel et al., 2002; Deane et al., 2003; Deane et al., 2005) studies. The mechanism of Aβ clearance from the brain into the blood have been investigated further (Deane et al., 2003), and net clearance was shown to involve both a peripheral sink effect and an active FcR-mediated process at the BBB (Deane et al., 2005).

4.4 Antibody-Mediated Aß Disaggregation and Neutralization of Aß Toxicity

Some anti-Aβ antibodies have been shown to prevent (Solomon et al., 1996; McLaurin et al., 2002; Legleiter et al., 2004) or reverse (Solomon et al., 1997; Frenkel et al., 2000a) the aggregation of Aβ fibrils and inhibit the toxicity of Aβ peptide (Frenkel et al., 2000b; McLaurin et al., 2002) *in vitro*. Conformation-specific Aß antibodies might target existing plaques in the brain and induce dissembly of Aß aggregates (Bacskai et al., 2001). Thus, these observations suggest that direct interaction of anti-Aβ antibodies with Aβ deposits could potentially cause the disaggregation of Aβ fibrils both *in vitro* and *in vivo*, suggesting another possible mechanism for Aβ immunotherapy. There is some experimental evidence that passive immunization with specific Aβ antibodies targeting Aβ peptide oligomers may reverse or prevent the learning and memory deficits caused by Aβ oligomers *in vivo* (Klyubin et al., 2005; Lee et al., 2006; Oddo et al., 2006a; Oddo et al., 2006b; Brody and Holtzman, 2008), indicating that the blockade of the neurotoxicity induced by Aβ oligomers may be another potential mechanism underlying the effects of Aβ immunotherapy.

Overall, as stated above, there may be many mechanisms underlying Aβ plaque removal and cognitive improvement resulting from active and passive immunization. These mechanisms may act independently, concomitantly or sequentially for Aß immunotherapy depending on the severity of disease, antibody type, or the specific animal model under investigation. In addition, antibody-independent immune cell-mediated plaque clearance, effects on Aβ-mediated vasoconstriction, and modulation of CNS cytokine production as well as IgM-mediated hydrolysis of Aβ may be other possible mechanisms involved in Aβ immunotherapy (Brody and Holtzman, 2008; Wisniewski and Konietzko, 2008).

5. Conclusions

Aß immunotherapy in AD-like tg mouse models, non-human primates, dogs, and to some degree, human AD patients, has resulted in anti-Aß antibody generation, the lowering of cerebral Aβ levels, and in some studies, cognitive stabilization or improvement. Although, the first clinical trial of the active Aβ vaccine (AN1792) was halted due to an unexpected adverse side effect of meningoencephalitis in 6% of patients, follow-up studies demonstrated that Aβ deposition was reduced focally in brain of a small number of patients that have come to autopsy and in some cases, there was evidence of cognitive stabilization in the vaccinated patients who generated anti-Aß titers (Nicoll et al., 2003; Hock et al., 2003; Gilman et al., 2005). More recently, many groups, both academic and commercial, have focused on generating novel Aß vaccines by targeting specific Aß epitopes and avoid Aß-specific cellular immune responses, directing a Th2-biased immune response using certain adjuvants and routes of immunization, and reducing the need for repeated vaccines by using DNA vaccines. Multiple active and passive Aß immunotherapy clinical trials are underway. In addition to Aβ immunotherapeutic strategies, studies of tau-related vaccines are also underway in tangle-bearing tau tg mouse models (Asuni et al., 2007). Due to the ever-increasing number of AD patients worldwide suffering from this devastating neurological disorder, it is of the utmost importance to find a safe and effective way to prevent the disease and slow its progression. We remain hopeful that Aß immunotherapy, either alone or in combination with other therapies, will succeed in reaching this goal.

Reference List

Agadjanyan, M.G., Ghochikyan, A., Petrushina, I., Vasilevko, V., Movsesyan, N., Mkrtichyan, M., Saing, T., Cribbs, D.H. Prototype Alzheimer's disease vaccine using the immunodominant B cell epitope from beta-amyloid and promiscuous T cell epitope pan HLA DR-binding peptide. *J. Immunol.* 174: 1580-1586, 2005.

Arbel, M., Yacoby, I., Solomon, B. Inhibition of amyloid precursor protein processing by beta-secretase through site-directed antibodies. *Proc. Natl. Acad. Sci. U. S. A.* 102: 7718-7723, 2005.

Asuni, A.A., Boutajangout, A., Scholtzova, H., Knudsen, E., Li, Y.S., Quartermain, D., Frangione, B., Wisniewski, T., Sigurdsson, E.M. Vaccination of Alzheimer's model mice with Abeta derivative in alum adjuvant reduces Abeta burden without microhemorrhages. *Eur. J. Neurosci.* 24: 2530-2542, 2006.

Asuni, A.A., Boutajangout, A., Quartermain, D., Sigurdsson, E.M. Immunotherapy targeting pathological tau conformers in a tangle mouse model reduces brain pathology with associated functional improvements. *J. Neurosci.* 27:9115-9129, 2007.

Bacskai, B.J., Kajdasz, S.T., Christie, R.H., Carter, C., Games, D., Seubert, P., Schenk, D., Hyman, B.T. Imaging of amyloid-beta deposits in brains of living mice permits direct observation of clearance of plaques with immunotherapy. *Nat. Med.* 7: 369-372, 2001.

Bacskai, B.J., Kajdasz, S.T., McLellan, M.E., Games, D., Seubert, P., Schenk, D., Hyman, B.T. Non-Fc-mediated mechanisms are involved in clearance of amyloid-beta in vivo by immunotherapy. *J. Neurosci.* 22: 7873-7878, 2002.

Bard, F., Cannon, C., Barbour, R., Burke, R.L., Games, D., Grajeda, H., Guido, T., Hu, K., Huang, J., Johnson-Wood, K., Khan, K., Kholodenko, D., Lee, M., Lieberburg, I., Motter, R., Nguyen, M., Soriano, F., Vasquez, N., Weiss, K., Welch, B., Seubert, P., Schenk, D., Yednock, T. Peripherally administered antibodies against amyloid beta-peptide enter the central nervous system and reduce pathology in a mouse model of Alzheimer disease. *Nat. Med.* 6: 916-919, 2000.

Bard, F., Barbour, R., Cannon, C., Carretto, R., Fox, M., Games, D., Guido, T., Hoenow, K., Hu, K., Johnson-Wood, K., Khan, K., Kholodenko, D., Lee, C., Lee, M., Motter, R., Nguyen, M., Reed, A., Schenk, D., Tang, P., Vasquez, N., Seubert, P., Yednock, T. Epitope and isotype specificities of antibodies to beta-amyloid peptide for protection against Alzheimer's disease-like neuropathology. *Proc. Natl. Acad. Sci. U. S. A.* 100: 2023-2028, 2003.

Bayer, A.J., Bullock, R., Jones, R.W., Wilkinson, D., Paterson, K.R., Jenkins, L., Millais, S.B., Donoghue, S. Evaluation of the safety and immunogenicity of synthetic Abeta42 (AN1792) in patients with AD. *Neurology* 64: 94-101, 2005.

Bowers, W.J., Mastrangelo, M.A., Stanley, H.A., Casey, A.E., Milo, L.J., Jr., Federoff, H.J. HSV amplicon-mediated Abeta vaccination in Tg2576 mice: differential antigen-specific immune responses. *Neurobiol. Aging* 26: 393-407, 2005.

Brody, D.L., Holtzman, D.M. Active and passive immunotherapy for neurodegenerative disorders. *Annu. Rev. Neurosci.* 31: 175-193, 2008.

Carty, N.C., Wilcock, D.M., Rosenthal, A., Grimm, J., Pons, J., Ronan, V., Gottschall, P.E., Gordon, M.N., Morgan, D. Intracranial administration of deglycosylated C-terminal-specific anti-Abeta antibody efficiently clears amyloid plaques without activating microglia in amyloid-depositing transgenic mice. *J. Neuroinflammation* 3: 11, 2006.

Chauhan, N.B., Siegel, G.J. Reversal of amyloid beta toxicity in Alzheimer's disease model Tg2576 by intraventricular antiamyloid beta antibody. *J. Neurosci. Res.* 69: 10-23, 2002.

Chauhan, N.B., Siegel, G.J. Intracerebroventricular passive immunization with anti-Abeta antibody in Tg2576. *J. Neurosci. Res.* 74: 142-147, 2003.

Chiba, T., Yamada, M., Sasabe, J., Terashita, K., Shimoda, M., Matsuoka, M., Aiso, S. Amyloid-beta causes memory impairment by disturbing the JAK2/STAT3 axis in hippocampal neurons. *Mol. Psychiatry* 14: 206-222, 2009.

Cribbs, D.H., Ghochikyan, A., Vasilevko, V., Tran, M., Petrushina, I., Sadzikava, N., Babikyan, D., Kesslak, P., Kieber-Emmons, T., Cotman, C.W., Agadjanyan, M.G. Adjuvant-dependent modulation of Th1 and Th2 responses to immunization with beta-amyloid. *Int. Immunol.* 15: 505-514, 2003.

Das, P., Howard, V., Loosbrock, N., Dickson, D., Murphy, M.P., Golde, T.E. Amyloid-beta immunization effectively reduces amyloid deposition in FcRgamma-/- knock-out mice. *J. Neurosci.* 23: 8532-8538, 2003.

DaSilva, K., Brown, M.E., Westaway, D., McLaurin, J. Immunization with amyloid-beta using GM-CSF and IL-4 reduces amyloid burden and alters plaque morphology. *Neurobiol. Dis.* 23: 433-444, 2006.

Dasilva, K.A., Brown, M.E., McLaurin, J. Reduced oligomeric and vascular amyloid-beta following immunization of TgCRND8 mice with an Alzheimer's DNA vaccine. *Vaccine* 27: 1365-1376, 2009.

Deane, R., Du Yan, S., Submamaryan, R.K., LaRue, B., Jovanovic, S., Hogg, E., Welch, D., Manness, L., Lin, C., Yu, J., Zhu, H., Ghiso, J., Frangione, B., Stern, A., Schmidt, A.M., Armstrong, D.L., Arnold, B., Liliensiek, B., Nawroth, P., Hofman, F., Kindy, M., Stern, D., Zlokovic, B. RAGE mediates amyloid-beta peptide transport across the blood-brain barrier and accumulation in brain. *Nat. Med.* 9: 907-913, 2003.

Deane, R., Sagare, A., Hamm, K., Parisi, M., LaRue, B., Guo, H., Wu, Z., Holtzman, D.M., Zlokovic, B.V. IgG-assisted age-dependent clearance of Alzheimer's amyloid beta peptide by the blood-brain barrier neonatal Fc receptor. *J. Neurosci.* 25: 11495-11503, 2005.

DeMattos, R.B., Bales, K.R., Cummins, D.J., Dodart, J.C., Paul, S.M., Holtzman, D.M. Peripheral anti-Abeta antibody alters CNS and plasma A beta clearance and decreases brain Abeta burden in a mouse model of Alzheimer's disease. *Proc. Natl. Acad. Sci. U. S. A.* 98: 8850-8855, 2001.

Dickson, D.W. The pathogenesis of senile plaques. *J. Neuropathol. Exp. Neurol.* 56: 321-339, 1997.

Dodart, J.C., Bales, K.R., Gannon, K.S., Greene, S.J., DeMattos, R.B., Mathis, C., DeLong, C.A., Wu, S., Wu, X., Holtzman, D.M., Paul, S.M. Immunization reverses memory deficits without reducing brain Abeta burden in Alzheimer's disease model. *Nat. Neurosci.* 5: 452-457, 2002.

Dodel, R., Hampel, H., Depboylu, C., Lin, S., Gao, F., Schock, S., Jackel, S., Wei, X., Buerger, K., Hoft, C., Hemmer, B., Moller, H., Farlow, M., Oertel, W., Sommer, N., Du, Y. Human antibodies against amyloid beta peptide: a potential treatment for Alzheimer's disease. *Ann. Neurol.* 52: 253-256, 2002.

Dodel, R.C., Du, Y., Depboylu, C., Hampel, H., Frolich, L., Haag, A., Hemmeter, U., Paulsen, S., Teipel, S.J., Brettschneider, S., Spottke, A., Nolker, C., Moller, H.J., Wei, X., Farlow, M., Sommer, N., Oertel, W.H. Intravenous immunoglobulins containing antibodies against beta-amyloid for the treatment of Alzheimer's disease. *J. Neurol. Neurosurg. Psychiatry* 75: 1472-1474, 2004.

Du, Y., Wei, X., Dodel, R., Sommer, N., Hampel, H., Gao, F., Ma, Z., Zhao, L., Oertel, W.H., Farlow, M. Human anti-beta-amyloid antibodies block beta-amyloid fibril formation and prevent beta-amyloid-induced neurotoxicity. *Brain* 126: 1935-1939, 2003.

Ferrer, I., Boada Rovira, M., Sanchez Guerra, M.L., Rey, M.J., Costa-Jussa, F. Neuropathology and pathogenesis of encephalitis following amyloid-beta immunization in Alzheimer's disease. *Brain Pathol.* 14: 11-20, 2004.

Foster, J.K., Verdile, G., Bates, K.A., Martins, R.N. Immunization in Alzheimer's disease: naive hope or realistic clinical potential? *Mol. Psychiatry* 14: 239-251, 2009.

Fox, N.C., Black, R.S., Gilman, S., Rossor, M.N., Griffith, S.G., Jenkins, L., Koller, M. Effects of Abeta immunization (AN1792) on MRI measures of cerebral volume in Alzheimer disease. *Neurology* 64: 1563-1572, 2005.

Frazer, M.E., Hughes, J.E., Mastrangelo, M.A., Tibbens, J.L., Federoff, H.J., Bowers, W.J. Reduced pathology and improved behavioral performance in Alzheimer's disease mice vaccinated with HSV amplicons expressing amyloid-beta and interleukin-4. *Mol. Ther.* 16: 845-853, 2008.

Frenkel, D., Balass, M., Solomon, B. N-terminal EFRH sequence of Alzheimer's beta-amyloid peptide represents the epitope of its anti-aggregating antibodies. *J. Neuroimmunol.* 88: 85-90, 1998.

Frenkel, D., Balass, M., Katchalski-Katzir, E., Solomon, B. High affinity binding of monoclonal antibodies to the sequential epitope EFRH of beta-amyloid peptide is essential for modulation of fibrillar aggregation. *J. Neuroimmunol.* 95: 136-142, 1999.

Frenkel, D., Katz, O., Solomon, B. Immunization against Alzheimer's beta -amyloid plaques via EFRH phage administration. *Proc. Natl. Acad. Sci. U. S. A.* 97: 11455-11459, 2000a.

Frenkel, D., Solomon, B., Benhar, I. Modulation of Alzheimer's beta-amyloid neurotoxicity by site-directed single-chain antibody. *J. Neuroimmunol.* 106: 23-31, 2000b.

Frenkel, D., Dewachter, I., Van Leuven, F., Solomon, B. Reduction of beta-amyloid plaques in brain of transgenic mouse model of Alzheimer's disease by EFRH-phage immunization. *Vaccine* 21: 1060-1065, 2003.

Gandy, S., DeMattos, R.B., Lemere, C.A., Heppner, F.L., Leverone, J., Aguzzi, A., Ershler, W.B., Dai, J., Fraser, P., St George Hyslop, P., Holtzman, D.M., Walker, L.C., Keller, E.T. Alzheimer's Abeta vaccination of rhesus monkeys (Macaca mulatta). *Mech. Ageing Dev.* 125: 149-151, 2004.

Ghochikyan, A., Vasilevko, V., Petrushina, I., Movsesyan, N., Babikyan, D., Tian, W., Sadzikava, N., Ross, T.M., Head, E., Cribbs, D.H., Agadjanyan, M.G. Generation and characterization of the humoral immune response to DNA immunization with a chimeric beta-amyloid-interleukin-4 minigene. Eur. *J. Immunol.* 33: 3232-3241, 2003.

Ghochikyan, A., Mkrtichyan, M., Petrushina, I., Movsesyan, N., Karapetyan, A., Cribbs, D.H., Agadjanyan, M.G. Prototype Alzheimer's disease epitope vaccine induced strong Th2-type anti-Abeta antibody response with Alum to Quil A adjuvant switch. *Vaccine* 24: 2275-2282, 2006a.

Ghochikyan, A., Petrushina, I., Lees, A., Vasilevko, V., Movsesyan, N., Karapetyan, A., Agadjanyan, M.G., Cribbs, D.H. Abeta-immunotherapy for Alzheimer's disease using mannan-amyloid-Beta peptide immunoconjugates. *DNA Cell Biol.* 25: 571-580, 2006b.

Gilman, S., Koller, M., Black, R.S., Jenkins, L., Griffith, S.G., Fox, N.C., Eisner, L., Kirby, L., Boada Rovira, M., Forette, F., Orgogozo, J.M. Clinical effects of Abeta immunization (AN1792) in patients with AD in an interrupted trial. *Neurology* 64: 1553-1562, 2005.

Hara, H., Monsonego, A., Yuasa, K., Adachi, K., Xiao, X., Takeda, S., Takahashi, K., Weiner, H.L., Tabira, T. Development of a safe oral Abeta vaccine using recombinant adeno-associated virus vector for Alzheimer's disease. *J. Alzheimers Dis.* 6: 483-488, 2004.

Hardy, J., Selkoe, D.J. The amyloid hypothesis of Alzheimer's disease: progress and problems on the road to therapeutics. *Science* 297: 353-356, 2002.

Hartman, R.E., Izumi, Y., Bales, K.R., Paul, S.M., Wozniak, D.F., Holtzman, D.M. Treatment with an amyloid-beta antibody ameliorates plaque load, learning deficits, and hippocampal long-term potentiation in a mouse model of Alzheimer's disease. *J. Neurosci.* 25: 6213-6220, 2005.

Head, E., Pop, V., Vasilevko, V., Hill, M., Saing, T., Sarsoza, F., Nistor, M., Christie, L.A., Milton, S., Glabe, C., Barrett, E., Cribbs, D. A two-year study with fibrillar beta-amyloid (Abeta) immunization in aged canines: effects on cognitive function and brain *Abeta. J. Neurosci.* 28: 3555-3566, 2008.

Hock, C., Konietzko, U., Papassotiropoulos, A., Wollmer, A., Streffer, J., von Rotz, R.C., Davey, G., Moritz, E., Nitsch, R.M. Generation of antibodies specific for beta-amyloid by vaccination of patients with Alzheimer disease. *Nat. Med.* 8: 1270-1275, 2002.

Hock, C., Konietzko, U., Streffer, J.R., Tracy, J., Signorell, A., Muller-Tillmanns, B., Lemke, U., Henke, K., Moritz, E., Garcia, E., Wollmer, M.A., Umbricht, D., de Quervain, D.J., Hofmann, M., Maddalena, A., Papassotiropoulos, A., Nitsch, R.M. Antibodies against beta-amyloid slow cognitive decline in Alzheimer's disease. *Neuron* 38: 547-554, 2003.

Holmes, C., Boche, D., Wilkinson, D., Yadegarfar, G., Hopkins, V., Bayer, A., Jones, R.W., Bullock, R., Love, S., Neal, J.W., Zotova, E., Nicoll, J.A. Long-term effects of Abeta42 immunisation in Alzheimer's disease: follow-up of a randomised, placebo-controlled phase I trial. *Lancet* 372: 216-223, 2008.

Istrin, G., Bosis, E., Solomon, B. Intravenous immunoglobulin enhances the clearance of fibrillar amyloid-beta peptide. *J. Neurosci. Res.* 84: 434-443, 2006.

Janus, C., Pearson, J., McLaurin, J., Mathews, P.M., Jiang, Y., Schmidt, S.D., Chishti, M.A., Horne, P., Heslin, D., French, J., Mount, H.T., Nixon, R.A., Mercken, M., Bergeron, C., Fraser, P.E., St George-Hyslop, P., Westaway, D. A beta peptide immunization reduces behavioural impairment and plaques in a model of Alzheimer's disease. *Nature* 408: 979-982, 2000.

Kang, J., Lemaire, H.-G., Unterbeck, A., Salbaum, J.M., Masters, C.L., Grzeschik, K.-H., Multhaup, G., Beyreuther, K., Muller-Hill, B. The precursor of Alzheimer's disease amyloid A4 protein resembles a cell-surface receptor. *Nature* 325: 733-736, 1987.

Kim, H.D., Maxwell, J.A., Kong, F.K., Tang, D.C., Fukuchi, K. Induction of anti-inflammatory immune response by an adenovirus vector encoding 11 tandem repeats of Abeta1-6: toward safer and effective vaccines against Alzheimer's disease. Biochem. Biophys. *Res. Commun.* 336: 84-92, 2005.

Kim, H.D., Jin, J.J., Maxwell, J.A., Fukuchi, K. Enhancing Th2 immune responses against amyloid protein by a DNA prime-adenovirus boost regimen for Alzheimer's disease. Immunol. *Lett.* 112: 30-38, 2007a.

Kim, H.D., Tahara, K., Maxwell, J.A., Lalonde, R., Fukuiwa, T., Fujihashi, K., Van Kampen, K.R., Kong, F.K., Tang, D.C., Fukuchi, K. Nasal inoculation of an adenovirus vector encoding 11 tandem repeats of Abeta1-6 upregulates IL-10 expression and reduces amyloid load in a Mo/Hu APPswe PS1dE9 mouse model of Alzheimer's disease. *J. Gene Med.* 9: 88-98, 2007b.

Klyubin, I., Walsh, D.M., Lemere, C.A., Cullen, W.K., Shankar, G.M., Betts, V., Spooner, E.T., Jiang, L., Anwyl, R., Selkoe, D.J., Rowan, M.J. Amyloid beta protein immunotherapy neutralizes Abeta oligomers that disrupt synaptic plasticity in vivo. *Nat. Med.* 11: 556-561, 2005.

Klyubin, I., Betts, V., Welzel, A.T., Blennow, K., Zetterberg, H., Wallin, A., Lemere, C.A., Cullen, W.K., Peng, Y., Wisniewski, T., Selkoe, D.J., Anwyl, R., Walsh, D.M., Rowan,

M.J. Amyloid beta protein dimer-containing human CSF disrupts synaptic plasticity: prevention by systemic passive immunization. *J. Neurosci.* 28: 4231-4237, 2008.

Knobloch, M., Farinelli, M., Konietzko, U., Nitsch, R.M., Mansuy, I.M. Abeta oligomer-mediated long-term potentiation impairment involves protein phosphatase 1-dependent mechanisms. *J. Neurosci.* 27: 7648-7653, 2007.

Kotilinek, L.A., Bacskai, B., Westerman, M., Kawarabayashi, T., Younkin, L., Hyman, B.T., Younkin, S., Ashe, K.H. Reversible memory loss in a mouse transgenic model of Alzheimer's disease. *J. Neurosci.* 22: 6331-6335, 2002.

Lambert, M.P., Velasco, P.T., Chang, L., Viola, K.L., Fernandez, S., Lacor, P.N., Khuon, D., Gong, Y., Bigio, E.H., Shaw, P., De Felice, F.G., Krafft, G.A., Klein, W.L. Monoclonal antibodies that target pathological assemblies of Abeta. *J. Neurochem.* 100: 23-35, 2007.

Lavie, V., Becker, M., Cohen-Kupiec, R., Yacoby, I., Koppel, R., Wedenig, M., Hutter-Paier, B., Solomon, B. EFRH-phage immunization of Alzheimer's disease animal model improves behavioral performance in Morris water maze trials. *J. Mol. Neurosci.* 24: 105-113, 2004.

Lee, M., Bard, F., Johnson-Wood, K., Lee, C., Hu, K., Griffith, S. G., Black, R. S., Schenk, D., Seubert, P. Abeta42 immunization in Alzheimer's disease generates Abeta N-terminal antibodies. *Ann. Neurol.,* 58:430-435, 2005.

Lee, E.B., Leng, L.Z., Zhang, B., Kwong, L., Trojanowski, J.Q., Abel, T., Lee, V.M. Targeting amyloid-beta peptide (Abeta) oligomers by passive immunization with a conformation-selective monoclonal antibody improves learning and memory in Abeta precursor protein (APP) transgenic mice. *J. Biol. Chem.* 281: 4292-4299, 2006.

Legleiter, J., Czilli, D.L., Gitter, B., DeMattos, R.B., Holtzman, D.M., Kowalewski, T. Effect of different anti-Abeta antibodies on Abeta fibrillogenesis as assessed by atomic force microscopy. *J. Mol. Biol.* 335: 997-1006, 2004.

Lemere, C.A., Maron, R., Spooner, E.T., Grenfell, T.J., Mori, C., Desai, R., Hancock, W.W., Weiner, H.L., Selkoe, D.J. Nasal Abeta treatment induces anti-Abeta antibody production and decreases cerebral amyloid burden in PD-APP mice. *Ann. N. Y. Acad. Sci.* 920: 328-331, 2000.

Lemere, C.A., Spooner, E.T., Leverone, J.F., Mori, C., Clements, J.D. Intranasal immunotherapy for the treatment of Alzheimer's disease: *Escherichia coli* LT and LT(R192G) as mucosal adjuvants. *Neurobiol. Aging* 23:991-1000, 2002.

Lemere, C.A., Spooner, E.T., LaFrancois, J., Malester, B., Mori, C., Leverone, J.F., Matsuoka, Y., Taylor, J.W., DeMattos, R.B., Holtzman, D.M., Clements, J.D., Selkoe, D.J., Duff, K.E. Evidence for peripheral clearance of cerebral Abeta protein following chronic, active Abeta immunization in PSAPP mice. *Neurobiol. Dis.* 14: 10-18, 2003.

Lemere, C.A., Beierschmitt, A., Iglesias, M., Spooner, E.T., Bloom, J.K., Leverone, J.F., Zheng, J.B., Seabrook, T.J., Louard, D., Li, D., Selkoe, D.J., Palmour, R.M., Ervin, F.R. Alzheimer's disease Aß vaccine reduces central nervous system Aß levels in a non-human primate, the Caribbean vervet. *Am. J. Pathol.* 165: 283-297, 2004.

Lemere, C.A., Maier, M., Peng, Y., Jiang, L., Seabrook, T.J. Novel Aß immunogens: Is shorter better? *Current Alzheimer Research* 4:427-436, 2007.

Leverone, J.F., Spooner, E.T., Lehman, H.K., Clements, J.D., Lemere, C.A. Aß1-15 is less immunogenic than Aß1-40/42 for intranasal immunization of wild-type mice but may be effective for "boosting". *Vaccine* 21: 2197-2206, 2003.

Lleo, A., Greenberg, S.M., Growdon, J.H. Current pharmacotherapy for Alzheimer's disease. *Annu. Rev. Med.* 57: 513-533, 2006.

Ma, Q.L., Lim, G.P., Harris-White, M.E., Yang, F., Ambegaokar, S.S., Ubeda, O.J., Glabe, C.G., Teter, B., Frautschy, S.A., Cole, G.M. Antibodies against beta-amyloid reduce Abeta oligomers, glycogen synthase kinase-3beta activation and tau phosphorylation in vivo and in vitro. *J. Neurosci. Res.* 83: 374-384, 2006.

Maier, M., Seabrook, T.J., Lemere, C.A. Modulation of the humoral and cellular immune response in Aß immunotherapy by the adjuvants monophosphoryl lipid A (MPL), cholera toxin B subunit (CTB) and E. coli enterotoxin LT(R192G). *Vaccine* 23: 5149-5159, 2005.

Maier, M., Seabrook, T.J., Lazo, N.D., Jiang, L., Das, P., Janus, C., Lemere, C.A. Short amyloid-ß (Aß) immunogens reduce cerebral Aß load and learning deficits in an Alzheimer's disease mouse model in the absence of an Aß-specific cellular immune response. *J Neurosci* 26:4717-4728, 2006.

Masliah, E., Hansen, L., Adame, A., Crews, L., Bard, F., Lee, C., Seubert, P., Games, D., Kirby, L., Schenk, D. Abeta vaccination effects on plaque pathology in the absence of encephalitis in Alzheimer disease. *Neurology* 64: 129-131, 2005.

McLaurin, J., Cecal, R., Kierstead, M.E., Tian, X., Phinney, A.L., Manea, M., French, J.E., Lambermon, M.H., Darabie, A.A., Brown, M.E., Janus, C., Chishti, M.A., Horne, P., Westaway, D., Fraser, P.E., Mount, H.T., Przybylski, M., St George-Hyslop, P. Therapeutically effective antibodies against amyloid-beta peptide target amyloid-beta residues 4-10 and inhibit cytotoxicity and fibrillogenesis. *Nat. Med.* 8: 1263-1269, 2002.

Monsonego, A., Maron, R., Zota, V., Selkoe, D.,Weiner, H. Immune hyporesponsiveness to amyloid-ß peptide in amyloid precursor protein transgenic mice: Implications for the pathogenesis and treatment of Alzheimer's disease. *Proc. Natl. Acad. Sci. USA,* 98:10273-10278, 2001.

Monsonego A., Zota V., Karni A., Krieger J.I., Bar-Or A., Bitan G., Budson A.E., Sperling R., Selkoe D.J., Weiner H.L. Increased T cell reactivity to amyloid beta protein in older humans and patients with Alzheimer disease. *J. Clin. Invest.* 112:415-422, 2003.

Morgan, D., Diamond, D.M., Gottschall, P.E., Ugen, K.E., Dickey, C., Hardy, J., Duff, K., Jantzen, P., DiCarlo, G., Wilcock, D., Connor, K., Hatcher, J., Hope, C., Gordon, M., Arendash, G.W. A beta peptide vaccination prevents memory loss in an animal model of Alzheimer's disease. *Nature* 408: 982-985, 2000.

Mouri, A., Noda, Y., Hara, H., Mizoguchi, H., Tabira, T., Nabeshima, T. Oral vaccination with a viral vector containing Abeta cDNA attenuates age-related Abeta accumulation and memory deficits without causing inflammation in a mouse Alzheimer model. *FASEB J.* 21: 2135-2148, 2007.

Movsesyan, N., Ghochikyan, A., Mkrtichyan, M., Petrushina, I., Davtyan, H., Olkhanud, P.B., Head, E., Biragyn, A., Cribbs, D.H., Agadjanyan, M.G. Reducing AD-like pathology in 3xTg-AD mouse model by DNA epitope vaccine - a novel immunotherapeutic strategy. *PLoS ONE* 3: e2124, 2008a.

Movsesyan, N., Mkrtichyan, M., Petrushina, I., Ross, T.M., Cribbs, D.H., Agadjanyan, M.G., Ghochikyan, A. DNA epitope vaccine containing complement component C3d enhances anti-amyloid-beta antibody production and polarizes the immune response towards a Th2 phenotype. *J. Neuroimmunol.* 205: 57-63, 2008b.

Nicoll, J.A., Wilkinson, D., Holmes, C., Steart, P., Markham, H., Weller, R.O. Neuropathology of human Alzheimer disease after immunization with amyloid-beta peptide: a case report. *Nat. Med.* 9: 448-452, 2003.

Nikolaev, A., McLaughlin, T., O'Leary, D.D., Tessier-Lavigne, M. APP binds DR6 to trigger axon pruning and neuron death via distinct caspases. *Nature* 457: 981-989, 2009.

Nikolic, W.V., Bai, Y., Obregon, D., Hou, H., Mori, T., Zeng, J., Ehrhart, J., Shytle, R.D., Giunta, B., Morgan, D., Town, T., Tan, J. Transcutaneous ß-amyloid immunization reduces cerebral ß-amyloid deposits without T cell infiltration and microhemorrhage. *PNAS* 104:2507-2512, 2007.

Oddo, S., Billings, L., Kesslak, J.P., Cribbs, D.H., LaFerla, F.M. Abeta immunotherapy leads to clearance of early, but not late, hyperphosphorylated tau aggregates via the proteasome. *Neuron* 43: 321-332, 2004.

Oddo, S., Caccamo, A., Tran, L., Lambert, M.P., Glabe, C.G., Klein, W.L., LaFerla, F.M. Temporal profile of amyloid-beta (Abeta) oligomerization in an in vivo model of Alzheimer disease. A link between Abeta and tau pathology. *J. Biol. Chem.* 281: 1599-1604, 2006a.

Oddo, S., Vasilevko, V., Caccamo, A., Kitazawa, M., Cribbs, D.H., LaFerla, F.M. Reduction of soluble Abeta and tau, but not soluble Abeta alone, ameliorates cognitive decline in transgenic mice with plaques and tangles. *J. Biol. Chem.* 281: 39413-39423, 2006b.

Okura, Y., Miyakoshi, A., Kohyama, K., Park, I.K., Staufenbiel, M., Matsumoto, Y. Nonviral Abeta DNA vaccine therapy against Alzheimer's disease: long-term effects and safety. *Proc. Natl. Acad. Sci. U. S. A.* 103: 9619-9624, 2006.

Okura, Y., Kohyama, K., Park, I.K., Matsumoto, Y. Nonviral DNA vaccination augments microglial phagocytosis of beta-amyloid deposits as a major clearance pathway in an Alzheimer disease mouse model. *J. Neuropathol. Exp. Neurol.* 67: 1063-1071, 2008a.

Okura, Y., Matsumoto, Y. DNA vaccine therapy for Alzheimer's disease: present status and future direction. *Rejuvenation Res.* 11: 301-308, 2008b.

Orgogozo, J.M., Gilman, S., Dartigues, J.F., Laurent, B., Puel, M., Kirby, L.C., Jouanny, P., Dubois, B., Eisner, L., Flitman, S., Michel, B.F., Boada, M., Frank, A., Hock, C. Subacute meningoencephalitis in a subset of patients with AD after Abeta42 immunization. *Neurology* 61: 46-54, 2003.

Petrushina, I., Ghochikyan, A., Mktrichyan, M., Mamikonyan, G., Movsesyan, N., Davtyan, H., Patel, A., Head, E., Cribbs, D.H., Agadjanyan, M.G. Alzheimer's disease peptide epitope vaccine reduces insoluble but not soluble/oligomeric Abeta species in amyloid precursor protein transgenic mice. *J. Neurosci.* 27: 12721-12731, 2007.

Petrushina, I., Ghochikyan, A., Mkrtichyan, M., Mamikonyan, G., Movsesyan, N., Ajdari, R., Vasilevko, V., Karapetyan, A., Lees, A., Agadjanyan, M.G., Cribbs, D.H. Mannan-Abeta28 conjugate prevents Abeta-plaque deposition, but increases microhemorrhages in the brains of vaccinated Tg2576 (APPsw) mice. *J. Neuroinflammation* 5: 42, 2008.

Pfeifer, M., Boncristiano, S., Bondolfi, L., Stalder, A., Deller, T., Staufenbiel, M., Mathews, P.M., Jucker, M. Cerebral hemorrhage after passive anti-Abeta immunotherapy. *Science* 298: 1379, 2002.

Qu, B., Boyer, P.J., Johnston, S.A., Hynan, L.S., Rosenberg, R.N. Abeta42 gene vaccination reduces brain amyloid plaque burden in transgenic mice. *J. Neurol. Sci.* 244: 151-158, 2006.

Racke, M.M., Boone, L.I., Hepburn, D.L., Parsadainian, M., Bryan, M.T., Ness, D.K., Piroozi, K.S., Jordan, W.H., Brown, D.D., Hoffman, W.P., Holtzman, D.M., Bales, K.R., Gitter, B.D., May, P.C., Paul, S.M., DeMattos, R.B. Exacerbation of cerebral amyloid angiopathy-associated microhemorrhage in amyloid precursor protein transgenic mice by immunotherapy is dependent on antibody recognition of deposited forms of amyloid beta. *J. Neurosci.* 25: 629-636, 2005.

Rajkannan, R., Arul, V., Malar, E.J., Jayakumar, R. Preparation, physiochemical characterization, and oral immunogenicity of Abeta(1-12), Abeta(29-40), and Abeta(1-42) loaded PLG microparticles formulations. *J. Pharm. Sci.*, 2008.

Rakover, I., Arbel, M., Solomon, B. Immunotherapy against APP beta-secretase cleavage site improves cognitive function and reduces neuroinflammation in Tg2576 mice without a significant effect on brain abeta levels. *Neurodegener. Dis.* 4: 392-402, 2007.

Relkin, N.R., Szabo, P., Adamiak, B., Burgut, T., Monthe, C., Lent, R.W., Younkin, S., Younkin, L., Schiff, R., Weksler, M.E. 18-Month study of intravenous immunoglobulin for treatment of mild Alzheimer disease. *Neurobiol. Aging,* 2008.

Robert, R., Dolezal, O., Waddington, L., Hattarki, M.K., Cappai, R., Masters, C.L., Hudson, P.J., Wark, K.L. Engineered antibody intervention strategies for Alzheimer's disease and related dementias by targeting amyloid and toxic oligomers. Protein Eng. *Des. Sel.* 22: 199-208, 2009.

Schenk, D., Barbour, R., Dunn, W., Gordon, G., Grajeda, H., Guido, T., Hu, K., Huang, J., Johnson-Wood, K., Khan, K., Kholodenko, D., Lee, M., Liao, Z., Lieberburg, I., Motter, R., Mutter, L., Soriano, F., Shopp, G., Vasquez, N., Vandevert, C., Walker, S., Wogulis, M., Yednock, T., Games, D., Seubert, P. Immunization with amyloid-beta attenuates Alzheimer-disease-like pathology in the PDAPP mouse. *Nature* 400: 173-177, 1999.

Schroeter, S., Khan, K., Barbour, R., Doan, M., Chen, M., Guido, T., Gill, D., Basi, G., Schenk, D., Seubert, P., Games, D. Immunotherapy reduces vascular amyloid-beta in PDAPP mice. *J. Neurosci.* 28: 6787-6793, 2008.

Seabrook, T.J., Bloom, J.K., Iglesias, M., Spooner, E.T., Walsh, D.M., Lemere, C.A. Species-specific immune response to immunization with human vs rodent A□ peptide. *Neurobiol. Aging* 25:1141-1151, 2004.

Seabrook, T.J., Jiang, L., Thomas, K., Lemere, C.A. Boosting with intranasal dendrimeric Aß1-15 but not Aß1-15 peptide leads to an effective immune response following a single injection of Aß1-40/42 in APP-tg mice. *J. Neuroinflammation* 3: 14, 2006a.

Seabrook, T.J., Thomas, K., Jiang, L., Bloom, J., Spooner, E., Maier, M., Bitan, G., Lemere, C.A. Dendrimeric Aß-15 is an effective immunogen in wildtype and APP tg mice. *Neurobiol. Aging* 28: 813-823, 2006b.

Selkoe, D.J. Toward a comprehensive theory for Alzheimer's disease. Hypothesis: Alzheimer's disease is caused by the cerebral accumulation and cytotoxicity of amyloid-beta protein. Annals N.Y. *Acad. of Sci.* 924: 17-25, 2000.

Selkoe, D.J. Alzheimer's disease: genes, proteins, and therapy. *Physiol. Rev.* 81: 741-766, 2001.

Shankar, G.M., Li, S., Mehta, T.H., Garcia-Munoz, A., Shepardson, N.E., Smith, I., Brett, F.M., Farrell, M.A., Rowan, M.J., Lemere, C.A., Regan, C.M., Walsh, D.M., Sabatini, B.L., Selkoe, D.J. Amyloid-beta protein dimers isolated directly from Alzheimer's brains impair synaptic plasticity and memory. *Nat. Med.* 14: 837-842, 2008.

Sigurdsson, E.M., Scholtzova, H., Mehta, P.D., Frangione, B., Wisniewski, T. Immunization with a nontoxic/nonfibrillar amyloid-beta homologous peptide reduces Alzheimer's disease-associated pathology in transgenic mice. *Am. J. Pathol.* 159: 439-447, 2001.

Sigurdsson, E.M., Knudsen, E., Asuni, A., Fitzer-Attas, C., Sage, D., Quartermain, D., Goni, F., Frangione, B., Wisniewski, T. An attenuated immune response is sufficient to enhance cognition in an Alzheimer's disease mouse model immunized with amyloid-beta derivatives. *J. Neurosci.* 24: 6277-6282, 2004.

Solomon, B., Koppel, R., Hanan, E., Katzav, T. Monoclonal antibodies inhibit in vitro fibrillar aggregation of the Alzheimer beta-amyloid peptide. *Proc. Natl. Acad. Sci. U. S. A.* 93: 452-455, 1996.

Solomon, B., Koppel, R., Frenkel, D., Hanan-Aharon, E. Disaggregation of Alzheimer beta-amyloid by site-directed mAb. *Proc. Natl. Acad. Sci. U. S. A.* 94: 4109-4112, 1997.

Spires-Jones, T.L., Mielke, M.L., Rozkalne, A., Meyer-Luehmann, M., de Calignon, A., Bacskai, B.J., Schenk, D., Hyman, B.T. Passive immunotherapy rapidly increases structural plasticity in a mouse model of Alzheimer disease. *Neurobiol. Dis.* 33: 213-220, 2009.

Subramanian, S., Divya Shree, A.N. Enhanced Th2 immunity after DNA prime-protein boost immunization with amyloid beta (1-42) plus CpG oligodeoxynucleotides in aged rats. *Neurosci. Lett.* 436: 219-222, 2008.

Tamura, Y., Hamajima, K., Matsui, K., Yanoma, S., Narita, M., Tajima, N., Xin, K.Q., Klinman, D., Okuda, K. The F(ab)'2 fragment of an Abeta-specific monoclonal antibody reduces Abeta deposits in the brain. *Neurobiol. Dis.* 20: 541-549, 2005.

Thakker, D.R., Weatherspoon, M.R., Harrison, J., Keene, T.E., Lane, D.S., Kaemmerer, W.F., Stewart, G.R., Shafer, L.L. Intracerebroventricular amyloid-beta antibodies reduce cerebral amyloid angiopathy and associated micro-hemorrhages in aged Tg2576 mice. *Proc. Natl. Acad. Sci. U. S. A.* 106: 4501-4506, 2009.

Town, T., Tan, J., Sansone, N., Obregon, D., Klein, T., Mullan, M. Characterization of murine immunoglobulin G antibodies against human amyloid-ß1-42. *Neurosci. Lett.*, 307:101-104, 2001.

Trouche, S.G., Asuni, A., Rouland, S., Wisniewski, T., Frangione, B., Verdier, *J.M., Sigurdsson,*

E.M., Mestre-Frances, N. Antibody response and plasma Abeta1-40 levels in young Microcebus murinus primates immunized with Abeta1-42 and its derivatives. *Vaccine* 27: 957-964, 2009.

Walker, LC. and Cork, LC. The neurobiology of aging in nonhuman primates. In Terry, R.D., et al. (Ed.), *Alzheimer's Disease*. Lippincott, Williams & Wilkins publisher, 1999, pp. 233-243.

Walsh, D.M., Selkoe, D.J. Abeta oligomers - a decade of discovery. *J. Neurochem.* 101: 1172-1184, 2007.

Wang, C.Y., Finstad, C.L., Walfield, A.M., Sia, C., Sokoll, K.K., Chang, T.Y., Fang, X.D., Hung, C.H., Hutter-Paier, B., Windisch, M. Site-specific UBITh amyloid-beta vaccine for immunotherapy of Alzheimer's disease. *Vaccine* 25: 3041-3052, 2007.

Wang, X.P., Zhang, J.H., Wang, Y.J., Feng, Y., Zhang, X., Sun, X.X., Li, J.L., Du, X.T., Lambert, M.P., Yang, S.G., Zhao, M., Klein, W.L., Liu, R.T. Conformation-dependent single-chain variable fragment antibodies specifically recognize beta-amyloid oligomers. *FEBS Lett.* 583: 579-584, 2009.

Weiner, H.L., Lemere, C.A., Maron, R., Spooner, E.T., Grenfell, T.J., Mori, C., Issazadeh, S., Hancock, W.W., Selkoe, D.J. Nasal administration of amyloid-beta peptide decreases cerebral amyloid burden in a mouse model of Alzheimer's disease. *Ann. Neurol.* 48: 567-579, 2000.

Wilcock, D.M., Rojiani, A., Rosenthal, A., Levkowitz, G., Subbarao, S., Alamed, J., Wilson, D., Wilson, N., Freeman, M.J., Gordon, M.N., Morgan, D. Passive amyloid immunotherapy clears amyloid and transiently activates microglia in a transgenic mouse model of amyloid deposition. *J. Neurosci.* 24: 6144-6151, 2004a.

Wilcock, D.M., Rojiani, A., Rosenthal, A., Subbarao, S., Freeman, M.J., Gordon, M.N., Morgan, D. Passive immunotherapy against Abeta in aged APP-transgenic mice reverses cognitive deficits and depletes parenchymal amyloid deposits in spite of increased vascular amyloid and microhemorrhage. *J. Neuroinflammation* 1: 24, 2004b.

Wilcock, D.M., Alamed, J., Gottschall, P.E., Grimm, J., Rosenthal, A., Pons, J., Ronan, V., Symmonds, K., Gordon, M.N., Morgan, D. Deglycosylated anti-amyloid-beta antibodies eliminate cognitive deficits and reduce parenchymal amyloid with minimal vascular consequences in aged amyloid precursor protein transgenic mice. *J. Neurosci.* 26: 5340-5346, 2006.

Winklhofer, K.F., Tatzelt, J., Haass, C. The two faces of protein misfolding: gain- and loss-of-function in neurodegenerative diseases. *The EMBO journal* 27: 336-349, 2008.

Wisniewski, T., Konietzko, U. Amyloid-beta immunisation for Alzheimer's disease. *Lancet Neurol.* 7: 805-811, 2008.

Zou, J., Yao, Z., Zhang, G., Wang, H., Xu, J., Yew, D.T., Forster, E.L. Vaccination of Alzheimer's model mice with adenovirus vector containing quadrivalent foldable Abeta(1-15) reduces Abeta burden and behavioral impairment without Abeta-specific T cell response. *J. Neurol. Sci.* 272: 87-98, 2008.

In: Alzheimer's Disease and Dementia (Vol. 4)
Editor: Miao-Kun Sun
ISBN:978-1-60876-152-4

Chapter V

The Failure of the APP Transgenic Mouse Models to Predict Efficacy of Agents in Five Clinical Trials of Alzheimer's Disease Suggests that there is a Need for a New Paradigm for Drug Development

Jordan L. Holtzman*
Departments of Pharmacology and Medicine and Division of Environmental Health Sciences, University of Minnesota, Minneapolis, MN 55455, USA

Disclosures

The concepts outlined in the description of the new paradigm for the etiology of Alzheimer's disease are covered by both U.S. and International Patents and pending patents.

A. Introduction

The sporadic form of Alzheimer's disease as seen in the elderly is characterized by the development of dementia in association with the deposition in the extracellular space of the neocortex of a series of insoluble proteins, the β-amyloids. With the "graying" of the world's population this condition has become a major societal problem. For example, in the United States alone it is estimated that there are 4-5 million people suffering from Alzheimer's disease. This has not only placed a major burden on the families of these suffers, but has also

*Email: holtz003@umn.edu

led to an estimated expenditure of $100 130 billion per year for custodial care alone. As a result it is clear that there is currently a need for effective agents to reduce the impact of this devastating condition. To meet this need both public funding agencies and private foundations along with the pharmaceutical industry have invested massive sums of money in an effort to develop effective agents for controlling the cognitive decline characteristic of Alzheimer's disease. Yet, to date the results of these efforts have been disappointing. At the present time only cholinesterase and NMDA receptor inhibitors have been approved for the symptomatic relief of the cognitive symptoms. Yet their benefit is only modest and short term.

On the other hand, to date the efforts to develop disease modifying agents has have been unproductive. These efforts have been based on the currently accepted paradigm that the dementia associated with Alzheimer's disease is due to the toxicity of the β-amyloids. These peptides are the primary constituents of the plaques which are characteristic of this condition. They are produced during the normal processing of the Amyloid Precursor Protein (APP). It is thought that the deposition of plaque occurs because of an increase in the production with age of the more insoluble forms of the β-amyloids. Based on this concept a number of investigators have developed transgenic mouse models in which the animals have been tranfected with the gene for the human form of APP along with an active promoter. These animals exhibit the central characteristics of Alzheimer's disease, including an age related decline in cognitive function and the associated deposition in the neocortex of plaque containing the β-amyloids. As a result they have been extensively used for both the development of therapeutic agents and basic studies of the disease process. Yet, five drugs, which were effective in reversing the cognitive decline in APP transgenic mouse models, have proven to bewere ineffective in well designed, randomized, placebo controlled clinical trials in patients. I feel that the results of these trials seriously question whether the APP transgenic mice are valid models for the study of the sporadic form of the human disease.

In this review I shall expand on these concerns. I will first describe my perception of the β-amyloid paradigm and discuss its weaknesses. Next, I will outline in detail the five clinical trials in which agents which had been found to reverse the cognitive decline in APP transgenic mouse models were ineffective in patients. Next, I shall outline studies from my laboratory which suggest an alternative model based on recent advances in our understanding of the posttranslational processing of proteins in the endoplasmic reticulum (ER). Finally, I shall suggest how this new paradigm can lead to the development of possible cell and animal models for more reliable drug screening to treat this devastating condition.

B. A Brief Outline of the Currently Accepted Paradigm for the Etiology of the Dementia Associated with Alzheimer's Disease

Alzheimer's disease is characterized by the development of dementia and the deposition in the extracellular space of the neocortex of plaque formed from aggregates of a series of hydrophobic proteins, the ß-amyloids. In the early stages of the disease the dementia is not associated with evidence of cell death. On the other hand, even though there is only a loose correlation between the plaque burden and the degree of dementia, it is currently thought that the cognitive decline is secondary to the toxicity of either the plaque itself or oligomers of the β-amyloids. These proteins are a series of 40 to 43 amino acid peptides which are produced during the normal, posttranslational processing of APP. APP is a member of a family of pro-growth factors (Herzog *et al.* 2004). The other two are Amyloid Precursor Like Proteins 1 and 2 (APLP 1 and 2). These growth factors are highly conserved and homologues are found in *Caenorhabditis elegans*, *Drosophila*, and *Xenopus*. Furthermore, studies have indicated that they are necessary for normal development. Knocking out anyone of them leads to distinctive phenotypes. For example, the loss of APP is characterized by disorganized neuronal development (Dawson *et al.* 1999; Seabrook *et al.* 1999). The double knockout of both APP and APLP2 or all three leads to early neonatal death (von Koch *et al.* 1997; Heber *et al.* 2000). Clearly, these are important growth factors required for normal development and are produced throughout life in a large number of organs, including the brain and the liver (Herzog *et al.* 2004).

APP is synthesized in the ER as a single, type 1 transmembrane protein (Herzog *et al.* 2004) (Fig. 1). During its posttranslational processing, the active growth factor(s), soluble APP (sAPP), is cleaved off, and secreted into the extracellular space. APP can be cleaved at three sites by proteases designated as α-, β- and γ-secretase respectively (Fig. 1). B-secretase cleaves APP at the N-amino acid terminus of the β-amyloid peptide sequence; while the α-secretase cleaves it at a site producing αsAPP. Finally, the perimembrane portion of APP is cleaved by the γ-secretase. αsAPP is a 108 kDa glycoprotein which retains the first 16 N-terminus amino acids of β-amyloid (Turner *et al.* 2007). This portion of αsAPP has the epitopes that react with many of the anti-ß-amyloid antibodies, including the commonly used monoclonal antibody, 6E10.

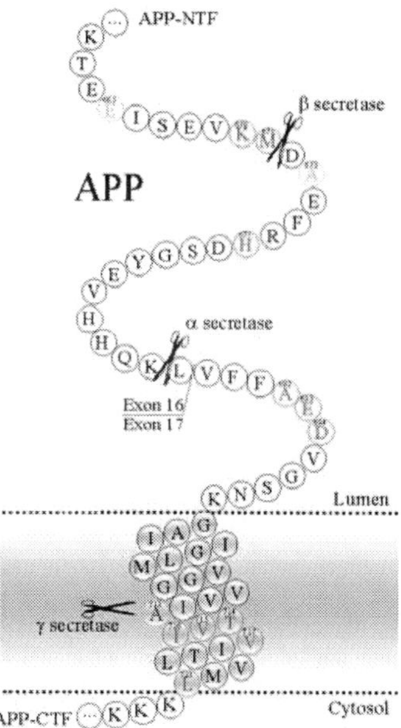

Figure 1. The Amino Acid Sequence of the Amyloid Precursor Protein

On the other hand, the combined cleavage by the β- and γ-secretases gives the ß-amyloids (Fig. 2). The cleavages produced by the α- and the β-secretases give active growth factors αsAPP and βsAPP respectively. Since the β-amyloids are partially derived from the membrane portion of APP, they are markedly hydrophobic and, on secretion into the aqueous, extracellular space, can precipitate to form the plaques characteristic of Alzheimer's disease. Aggregates of the synthetic peptides are also observed when they are dissolved in an aqueous buffer. This makes it difficult to establish standards to quantify the free β-amyloids by column chromatography or SDS-PAGE.

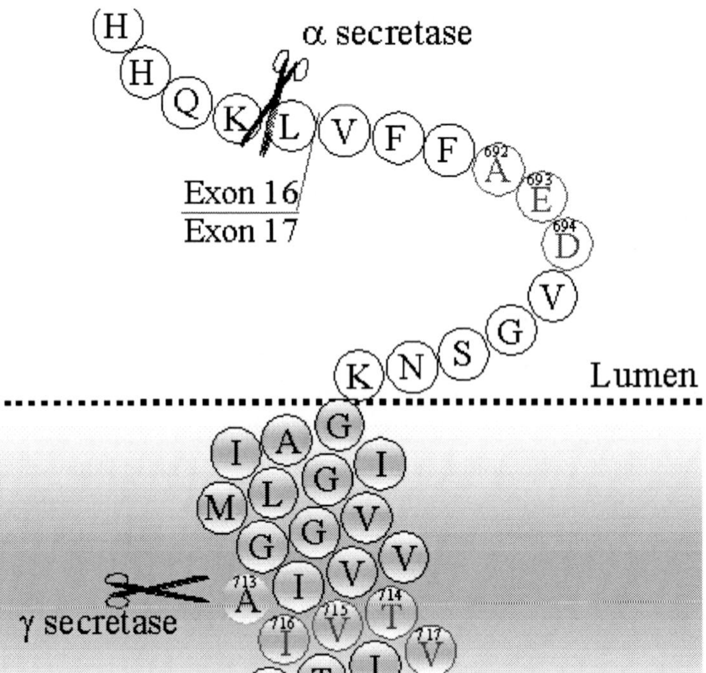

Figure 2. The sequence of the β-Amyloid portion of the APP

As the names for APP, APLP1 and APLP2 imply, most investigators have focused their attention on the β-amyloids, rather than on the biochemistry and cell biology of the synthesis and function of these proteins. Much of this focus has resulted from the discovery of several genetic forms of APP and two ancillary proteins, presenilin 1 and 2, which are associated with the early development of dementia (Selkoe 1999). Individuals with these mutations show significant cognitive decline in their 40's and 50's while symptoms of the sporadic form of the disease begin to appear in the seventh decade of life. Furthermore, individuals who reach the age of 85 years have a 50% chance of developing this form of the disease. Considering the frequency of this condition, it is not surprising that the sporadic form is not strongly associated with genetic variants of these or any other proteins. Similarly, patients with Down's syndrome show early signs of Alzheimer's disease. This condition is due to the duplication of chromosome 21 which contains the gene for APP. Finally individuals with either the genetic forms of the disease or Down's syndrome appear to over produce APP and the β-amyloids.

These findings in the genetic forms of the disease have led a number of workers to develop transgenic mouse models in which they have transfected the animals with a human form of the APP gene containing an active promoter leading to a markedly enhanced production of both APP and the β-amyloids. These animals demonstrate many of the characteristics of Alzheimer's disease, including the deposition of plaque containing the β-amyloids and an age related decline in cognitive function. They are currently the standard laboratory models for the study of Alzheimer's disease. Although they are possibly reasonable models for the genetic forms of the disease and the early cognitive decline seen in patients with Down's syndrome, there are several problems which raise the issue of whether they are valid models for the study of the sporadic form of the disease seen in the elderly.

The first is that these models are predicated on the unstated, concept assumption that there is an increase in APP production with age. Yet, this assumption flies in the face of one of the most profound attributes of the aging process: once we pass our prime, there is an overall decline in every metabolic pathway. This phenomenon is widely recognized by both researchers and the elderly themselves,

A second problem is that it is likely that normal growth and development is dependent upon a normal balance of the sAPP's and other growth factors. Hence, it is unclear whether the cognitive decline seen in the APP transgenic mice is due to the deposition of plaque or the secretion of excessive levels of the sAPP's. Such excessive levels are well recognized for other hormones and growth factors. This is exemplified by such metabolic syndromes as the Cushing syndrome with excessive cortisol, either due to endogenous secretion from a tumor or more commonly it occurs iatrogenically during therapy for a wide variety of conditions; hyperthyroidism and acromegaly from pituitary tumors. Besides metabolic abnormalities, excess growth factors can also cause structural defects. This has recently been found to be the case for Marfan's syndrome. This condition is due to a mutation in the matrix protein, fibrillin-1 (Ramirez and Dietz 2007). It was long thought that this mutation led directly to the structural defects characteristic of this syndrome. Yet, recent studies have suggested it is due to a more indirect effect. Fribillin-1 binds Transforming Growth Factor β (TGFβ) and is the major reservoir for this growth factor. Since the mutant form is less effective in binding the TGFβ, the levels of the free TGFβ are markedly elevated in patients with Marfan's syndrome. It is currently thought that it is these high levels that lead to the observed structural defects. Recognition of this possibility has led to the clinical use of losartan, an angiotensin receptor blocker, which also inhibits the TGFβ receptor and is thought to block the progression of Marfan's syndrome.

A similar role for APP has been suggested by the recent work of Nikolaev *et al.* (2009). During embryonic development an excess of neurons are produced and each of the embryonic neurons also has an excess of synaptic connections. For normal development it is important for the organism to prune both the number of neurons and the excessive number of synapses for the surviving neurons. These workers have found that APP regulates this pruning process by activating the Death Receptor 6 (DR6), a member of the TNFα superfamily. The question therefore arises in APP transgenic mice whether the excess of sAPP may lead to a continued pruning process even after the animals have reach maturity

(Nikolaev *et al.* 2009). If such is the case, then the various therapeutic agents which have been developed based on this model may be merely somehow decreasing the excessive levels of sAPP and not clearing the β-amyloids. These drugs would therefore be arresting the pruning process. Based on their results, it is of interest to speculate that the cognitive deficit characteristic of Down's syndrome may be due to the abnormal levels of sAPP leading to excessive pruning of both the neurons and synapses during development. As in the APP transgenic mice, this excessive pruning could occur both in the embryo and continue throughout life.

As will be discussed below, vaccine studies in these animal models have suggested that they may be effective in arresting the cognitive decline. This apparent benefit might suggest that the excess β-amyloids rather than an excess of APP could be the primary factor in the cognitive decline. Yet, an alternative interpretation could be that the vaccine may be reducing the free levels of αsAPP which retains one of the epitopes for the β-amyloids. Removal of this excess growth factor could serve to establish a normal, physiological balance for development.

A third problem, which will also be discussed in detail below, is that the excessive production of APP may overwhelm the posttranslational processing of proteins in the ER. This metabolic pathway is crucial for the synthesis of the synaptic membrane proteins which are necessary for memory and the myelin sheaths which speed the propagation of nerve impulses. Hence, decreases in the activity of this pathway could lead to the decreased cognitive skills seen in individuals with dementia due to a decreased capacity of the ER to produce and maintain those structures which are necessary for normal cognitive function.

In spite of these apparent problems, the APP transgenic mouse models have been the mainstay of those trying to understand the biochemistry and cell biology of this condition and to develop effective agents to treat it. In the next section I will discuss five clinical trials which examined agents that were effective in APP transgenic mouse models, but which failed to ameliorate this condition in patients. These failures would suggest that the transgenic animals are not a valid model for Alzheimer's disease and that we should consider other paradigms for the etiology of this condition so that we may have potentially more reliable drug screening procedures as well as a better understanding of the biochemistry and cell biology of Alzheimer's disease.

C. A Summary of Five Failed Clinical Trials of Agents Which had Been Found to be Effective in App APP Transgenic Mice

Recently, five clinical trials have served to reinforce the concern that the APP transgenic mouse models are not reliable for screening for potential therapeutic agents for the treatment of the sporadic form of Alzheimer's disease seen in the elderly. These five agents were ineffective in phase II or III clinical trials in humans. Not only do these failures imply that the cognitive decline seen in the sporadic form of Alzheimer's disease is not due to the toxicity of the β-amyloid (Erickson *et al.* 2005; Holtzman 2008; Holmes *et al.* 2008; Nicoll *et al.*

2008), but they also suggest that the heavy reliance on the APP transgenic mouse models for drug screening has led to several costly failures, and also may be impeding the search for effective agents. Since these failures raise serious concerns about the current approach to drug development, I should like to summarize each of them in detail.

C.1. The Failure of the B-Amyloid Vaccine from Elan to Either Halt or Reverse the Cognitive Decline Seen in Alzheimer's Patients

The most telling example of the failure of a clinical trial to lend support to the paradigm suggesting that the dementia of Alzheimer's disease is due to the toxicity of the β-amyloids was the follow-up study to the Elan vaccine trial. In the initial trial 372 patients with mild to moderate Alzheimer's disease received one or two injections of either a preparation of β-amyloid 1-42 containing an adjuvant or a placebo without adjuvant. The trial was stopped early because of the development of meningoencephalitis in18 of the patients, all of whom were in the treatment arm (Orgogozo *et al.* 2003). In a combined clinical/autopsy follow-up study of the patients who were in the initial trial, Holmes *et al.* (2008) reported that although at autopsy the patients who had received the vaccine had lower plaque burdens than those in the placebo group, there was no difference in the cognitive decline between the two groups. Yet, the vaccine did reduce the cognitive decline in an APP transgenic mouse model (Janus *et al.* 2000; Morgan *et al.* 2000). These data would suggest both that the mouse model does not replicate the human form of the disease and that the toxicity of the β-amyloids may not be the primary cause of the cognitive decline seen in the sporadic form of the human disease. I published these concerns in a letter to the *Lancet* (Holtzman 2008). In their reply, the authors of the report of the follow-up study indicated that they felt that I had raised a legitimate issue (Nicoll *et al.* 2008). Furthermore, in the last paragraph of their reply, they too suggested that the APP transgenic mouse may not be a valid model for the study of the sporadic form of Alzheimer's disease.

Because of the poor correlation between plaque burden and the obsserved cognitive decline (Katzman *et al.* 1988; Giannakopoulos *et al.* 1997; Wolf *et al.* 1999), over the years many investigators have expressed skepticism concerning the role of the β-amyloids in the development of the dementia characteristic of this disease. In response to this concern, Alzheimer's disease investigators have suggested that the actual toxic agent is not the plaque, but soluble aggregates of the β-amyloids (St. George-Hyslop and Morris 2008; Cleary *et al.* 2005). Furthermore, Petrushina *et al.* (2007) found that the administration of a vaccine reduced the plaque burden, but did not affect the levels of these aggregates in APP transgenic mice. Hence, one might conclude that the vaccine did not work because it cleared the plaque but not the soluble, toxic aggregates. Although it may be true that the soluble aggregates do impair cognitive function, this does not mean that they are the primary cause of the dementia seen in humans. Furthermore, the levels of the soluble aggregates are most likely determined by the solubility constants of the β-amyloids. Hence, as long as there is any plaque, there will be a constant level of the oligomers formed from the peptides which are in solution.

Furthermore, it is likely that the antibodies clear the plaque by binding to the soluble aggregates and delivering them through the normal flow of the CSF to the reticuloendothelial system where they are degraded. As an aside, it is of interest that antibodies to plaque are naturally found in both patients (45.1%) and age matched controls (41.2%) (Xu *et al.* 2008) suggesting that these antibodies should not have been thought to be an effective treatment for the prevention of the cognitive decline seen in humans.

As mentioned above there is an alternative explanation for the apparent efficacy of the vaccine in the APP transgenic mouse models. APP can be cleaved at two different sites on the lumenal portion of the protein by either the α- or the β-secretases to yield two different soluble forms of sAPP (Herzog *et al.* 2004). The form produced by cleavage by the α-secretase gives the growth factor, αsAPP. Many feel that this is the predominant form of the active growth factor, although we have never found it in the CSF or liver microsomes, both of which contain the β-amyloids. As noted above, αsAPP retains the first 16 amino acids of the β-amyloid sequence (Turner *et al.* 2007). This sequence contains an epitope reactive with many β-amyloid antibodies and hence the produced by the vaccine might clear the excess αsAPP. If such is the case, then the effect of the vaccine could be to reduce the excessive levels of this growth factor and thereby establish a more physiological balance of growth factors.

In spite of these concerns both Elan and several other pharmaceutical firms are still pursuing efforts to develop antibody mediated therapies (www.clinicaltrials.gov).

C2. The Failure of Mk-677 in Clinical Trials by Merck to Decrease the Cognitive Decline in Patients

MK-677 is an agent which enhances the secretion of the Insulin like Growth Factor 1 (IGF-1). The development of this agent resulted from observations from a number of groups showing that there is an inverse correlation between the levels of both insulin and IGF-1 and the development of Alzheimer's disease (Carro *et al* 2002). Furthermore, the β-amyloids appear to block the cellular response to IGF-1 (Carro *et al* 2002). Hence, it seemed logical to seek agents which enhanced the production of this hormone to overcome this inhibition. Finally, it was observed that MK-677 arrested the cognitive decline seen in an APP transgenic mouse model (Carro *et al* 2002). Yet, in a phase III clinical trial by Merck in which 416 patients were observed for 12 months, the agent was ineffective and the trial was ended early (Sevigny *et al* 2008).

C.3. The Failure of the γ-Secretase Inhibitor, R-Flurbiprophen, to Improve Cognitive Function in Patients in the Myriad/Lundbeck Phase Iii Clinical Trial

A third example of the failure of an APP transgenic mouse model to predict the efficacy of a therapeutic agent arose with a phase III clinical trial of a γ-secretase inhibitor, R-flurbiprophen. The trial was based on the concept that this agent would block the synthesis of the β-amyloids and thereby decrease the levels of these toxic peptides. This decrease would in turn reduce the cognitive decline attributed to their apparent toxicity. In both an APP transgenic mouse model (Kukar *et al* 2007) and in a phase II clinical trial (Wilcock *et al* 2008), the drug appeared to halt the progression of the cognitive decline. But in a larger phase III clinical trial it was found to be ineffective and the trial was terminated early (see www.FierceBiotech.com May 30, 2008). This was after an investment of $68 million. On accessing their web site, it would appear that the company running the trial, Myriad, for a Danish company, Lundbeck, has terminated its Alzheimer's program.

The structure of this agent was patterned after the widely used NSAID, ibuprofen. Observational studies had suggested that the use of this agent reduced the incidence of Alzheimer's disease. Like all observational studies, there may be many confounding factors which led to an erroneous conclusion. For example, individuals who routinely use these drugs may be less healthy than the nonusers and would therefore be more likely to fail to reach the age at which the cognitive decline begins. Furthermore, in a number of large randomized, placebo controlled, clinical trials in patients other NSAIDs, most recently naproxen and celecoxib, were not effective (ADAPT Research Group 2008).

The failure of R-flurbiprophen to block the cognitive decline might suggest that it is possible that it was ineffective in humans because it lacked sufficient inhibitory activity of the γ-secretase. Similarly, the agent may not have had sufficient lipid solubility to penetrate the blood brain barrier to give inhibitory concentrations to block the protease activity. Hence, it would seem reasonable to try to develop more potent agents which are also more lipid soluble. A major concern with this approach is that γ-secretase is involved is many important signal transduction systems. One of the more important is the receptor, notch-1 (D'Souza *et al.* 2008). This is a membrane bound receptor which is important both during development and in the normal function of adult cells. On activation a transcription factor is cleaved off the cytosolic tail of the receptor by γ-secretase. Potent inhibitors of this protease have been shown in *in vitro* systems to initiate cell death (Curry *et al.* 2005). In spite of these concerns and the failure of the R-flurbiprophen trial, Lilly is still seeking to develop a γ-secretase inhibitor, LY450139, as a possible therapeutic agent for the treatment of the sporadic form of Alzheimer's disease (www.clinicaltrials.gov NCT00762411). In early trials it has at least proven to be safe.

C.4. The Failure of Ginkgo Biloba in the Gem GEM Trial to Reduce the Cognitive Decline in Patients with Mild to Moderate Alzheimer's Disease

A fourth drug which has been claimed to be beneficial in the prevention and treatment of Alzheimer's disease is an extract of *Ginkgo biloba* leaves, EGb 761 (DeKosky *et al* 2008) This is a popular treatment which appears to act by decreasing the toxicity of the β-amyloids. It may also possibly act as an antioxidant. This property may be beneficial since oxidant stress is thought to enhance the toxicity of the β-amyloids. Furthermore, this extract was shown to limit the cognitive decline seen in an APP transgenic mouse model (Stackman *et al*

2003), but it had no effect on the plaque burden in these animals. Yet, it proved to be ineffective in a six year, phase III clinical trial with 523patients (DeKosky *et al* 2008). It should be noted that in 1999, when this trial was initially designed, the sales of this agent in the United States exceeded $249 million. This alone should give a clue as to the size of the Alzheimer's market and the desperation of the patients' families and of those who feel that they are likely to get the disease.

C.5. The Failure of Estrogen to Maintain Cognitive Function in the Elderly as Observed in the Women's Health Initiative (WhiWHI)

A fifth approach proposed to decrease the incidence of Alzheimer's disease in women is postmenopausal estrogen replacement. This proposal is based on the obvious correlation between menopause and the development of Alzheimer's disease. Furthermore, it has been found to have a significant beneficial effect on cognitive function in ovariectomized, female, APP transgenic mouse models as exemplified by the studies of Levin-Allerhand *et al.* (2002) and Carroll *et al.* (2007). Although in both of these studies there was an improvement in cognitive function, Levin-Allerhand *et al.* found that it had no effect on plaque burden while Carroll *et al.* reported that there was a significant decline in plaque as well as improved memory. On the other hand, when the effect of estrogen was examined in a substudy of a large, randomized, placebo-controlled, clinical trial in 2808 postmenopausal women in the WHI who had been followed for 5 to 7 years, those receiving hormone replacement therapy actually had slightly lower scores on tests of cognitive function than did the controls (Espeland *et al* 2004). Because of the size of this trial and the consistent minimal deficit, this finding was statistically significant.

Some investigators have argued that the WHI study should have examined a younger, perimenopausal population where there are suggestions that the drug might have been beneficial. This does not seem like a reasonable argument, since the study included women who are in the age group with the highest risk for the disease and would therefore have shown the greatest benefit. Furthermore, the main study was terminated early because there was a significant increase in the incidence of strokes in the treatment group (WHI 2004). Hence, it would not seem reasonable to treat women for 20 years to prevent a condition they may never get and at the same time expose them to a drug which could enhance their risk of death from strokes, a leading killer in the elderly.

The failure of estrogen might be a specific drug effect rather than a class effect, epecially since this agent appeared to increase vascular disease. Hence, it might seem reasonable to examine the effect of partial agonist/antagonists, such as tamoxafin and raloxifene, on cognitive function. Both of these agents have been used to treat breast cancer and may therefore be a safer alternative to estrogen. The former drug is not a good candidate because it does have some hepatic toxicity. On the other hand, raloxifene is a safer agent and is currently under investigation in a study sponsored by the National Institute of Aging (www.clinicaltrials.gov NCT00368459).

C.6. Drugs Which Have Shown Benefit in Preliminary Trials

For the sake of completeness I should like to discuss three agents that have recently received a great deal of publicity and which in preliminary trials have been claimed to be beneficial in the treatment of Alzheimer's disease. The first is resveratrol. This is an antioxidant found in red wine. It is commonly thought that the greater longevity of the French, in spite of a diet high in saturated fat and salt and a high cigarette consumption, is because of their high consumption of red wine. This benefit has been attributed to the presence of resveratrol. This agent has demonstrated efficacy in animal models for a wide variety of diseases, but the human dosages, which are equivalent to those used in the rodent studies, would require the consumption of 50 bottles of wine a day (Reagan-Shaw *et al.* 2007). Clearly, this agent is not the reason for the greater longevity of the French. In spite of this problem, this agent is currently under investigation in two phase III clinical trials (www.clinicaltrials.gov NCT00678431 and NCT00743743)

Another agent which has recently received a great deal of attention is dimebon. This is an old antihistamine which has been used clinically in Russia. It was reported to be a cholinesterase inhibitor and also was found to block the NMDA receptor (Bachurin *et al.* 2001). It does not appear to have been tested in any APP transgenic mouse models but has recently been reported to be effective in a small, randomized, placebo-controlled, clinical trial (Doody *et al.* 2008). This trial was performed in 11 centers in Russia and included 183 patients. In the initial report the patients had been followed for 26 weeks. Although an unpublished report of the experience at one year has been reported on the web where it appeared to exhibited a modest benefit. Yet, this benefit could have resulted from its cholinesterase or NMDA receptor inhibitory activity as seen with the currently clinically, available agents. It too is under clinical investigation in a phase III trial (www.clinicaltrials.gov NCT00829816).

The administration of another drug, methylene blue, has recently been reported to be beneficial in the treatment of Alzheimer's disease (see summary of T. Gura 2008). This agent is thought to serve as an antioxidant which presumably leads to the decline in tangles, another hallmark of severe Alzheimer's disease. Yet, there are no peer reviewed articles listed in PubMed for either pre-clinical or clinical investigations for its effect in Alzheimer's disease, but according to the news reports, the agent reduced the cognitive decline in patients. If this agent should prove to be effective, it would be a very sobering finding since it was first synthesized in 1876 and has been used as a treatment for malaria and is currently used clinically for the treatment of urinary tract infections. It has been available for the latter indication since the 1930's. Since urinary tract infections are common in the elderly, it would seem that years ago someone would have noted an improvement in cognitive function in their elderly patients. No clinical trials for the treatment of Alzheimer's disease are currently listed at www.clinicaltrials.gov.

D. An Alternative Paradigm for the Cognitive Decline Seen in the Sporadic Form of Alzheimer's Disease Based on the Known Biochemistry and Cell Biology of the Posttranslational Protein Processing System Found in the Endoplasmic Reticulum

These five failures of well designed, randomized, placebo-controlled, clinical trials which had both sufficient power and were performed for a long enough duration to the test the therapeutic potential of agents which were effective in the APP transgenic mouse models would suggest that these are not valid models for the discovery of drugs to treat patients with Alzheimer's disease (Holtzman 2008; Nicoll *et al.* 2008). A further problem with this animal model is that even within the mouse studies themselves, some drugs, such as estrogen (Levin-Allerhand *et al.* 2002; Carroll *et al.* 2007) and the Gingo extract, EGb 761 (Stackman *et al* 2003) reduced cognitive decline, but had no consistent effect on plaque burden. These observations provide further evidence that the dementia may not be due to the toxicity of the β-amyloids. Finally, the report by Nikolaev *et al.* (2009) raises a serious question concerning the cause of the cognitive deficiencies seen in the APP transgenic mice and that these declines nay bear no relationship to the disease seen in the elderly. These problems suggest that there is a need for a new model both for the basic study of the disease and for the development of new therapeutic agents.

In the next section I shall discuss an alternative paradigm which is based on the known biochemistry and cell biology of the posttranslational processing of membrane and secretory proteins in the ER. I feel that these concepts, which have been elucidated in this field over the past four decades, suggest an entirely different etiology for aging in general and Alzheimer's disease in particular (Holtzman 1997,1998; Erickson *et al.* 2005, 2006).

D.1. The Biochemistry and Cell Biology of the Posttranslational Processing of Proteins in the Endoplasmic Reticulum

In order to understand the significance of our findings, it is important to have at least some understanding of the biochemistry and cell biology of the posttranslational processing of newly synthesized proteins in the ER. But first I should like to give just a short history of how we became involved in a study of both this system and of Alzheimer's disease. My original interest was in the glutathione dependent enzymes which protect the cell against oxidant injury. During these studies we discovered a new member, ERp57, of a class of enzymes which are most properly termed thiol:protein disulfide oxidoreductases (Srivastrava *et al.* 1991,1993). These enzymes catalyze the oxidation and reduction of protein sulfurs groups. Whether they catalyze their oxidation or reduction depends upon the ratio of oxidized to reduced glutathione in the particular cell compartment. Hence, in the cytosol, where this ratio is 100:1, they reduce protein disulfides to their sulfhydro form. On the other hand, in the ER, where the ratio is only 2:1 they oxidize sulfhydro groups to form protein disulfides.[1] Shortly after we published our findings, I was asked to write a chapter reviewing the biochemistry of this newly characterized enzyme (Holtzman 1998). During my literature search I discovered that both ERp57 and its homologue, ERp55, more commonly known as protein disulphide isomerase (PDI)[2], were chaperones (Holtzman 1998). Chaperones are essential proteins found in all cellular organisms. They are involved in the posttranslational processing of most proteins and are critical for life. In fact knocking out most of them is a embryonic, lethal mutation. The field of posttranslational protein processing and the role of chaperones has been an area of intensive investigation over the past 40 years. As an aside, it is of interest that much of the information we have gained about these processes were originally derived from studies of yeast genetics. These findings have been readily extended to the homologous systems found in other families of eukaryotes, including humans. The high degree of conservation of these proteins clearly indicates their critical role in cell survival.

Briefly, as organisms have evolved they have developed mechanisms for faithfully translating the genetic code to give the correct amino acid sequence. It was originally thought that these nascent peptides would spontaneously fold into a configuration which has the lowest free energy (Holtzman 1997). But the problem that our ancient ancestors encountered was that proteins with molecular weights in excess of 20-30 kDa, could fold into any number of configurations with pseudo free energy minima (Holtzman 1997). In the absence of a process to direct these proteins into their active, native configurations, they aggregate to form something akin to cottage cheese or the proteins found in a hard boiled eggs. Our primitive ancestors evolved a set of proteins, the chaperones, to direct posttranslational folding to give a single active protein configuration. The homologues of the major family of these proteins, the Heat Shock Proteins (HSPs) are found in all cellular organisms, including the bacteria and the archae. The HSPs are the primary chaperones found in the posttranslational processing pathway associated with the cytoskeleton found in the cytosol of all eukaryotes. This pathway processes about 60% of the proteins synthesized in the cell. As the name HSP implies, they were initially identified because they are induced when cells are heated to modestly high temperatures, such as 43° C for mammalian cells (Holtzman 1997). This inductive capacity has been a retained feature of these proteins. Its benefit to the cell is that at elevated temperatures cellular proteins melt, i.e. lose their active configuration. The HSPs serve to reconfigure the melted proteins into their native state. This clearly reduces the energy demand on the cell since it no longer has to synthesize new proteins to replace the damaged ones. They also serve to clear aggregates which can interfere with normal cellular function. As a result they promote a survival benefit. Over the eons in eukaryotic cells the HSPs have also come to serve many other functions besides refolding denatured proteins.

---

[1]In the ER oxidized glutathione does not serve as the electron sink for the normal formation of protein disulfides. In fact in this system oxidized glutathione actually inhibits this reaction (Frand and Kaiser 1998). Hence, for the sake of clarity I have elected to skip over the details of this process, including the role of Ero1 in the transfer of electrons from the ERp57 to oxygen.

[2]For those interested in information concerning PDI, the search word on PubMed is PDI and not ERp55.

In eukaryotes the ER contains a second major system which catalyzes the posttranslational processing of proteins. This system is homologous to a posttranslational system found in the periplasmic space of bacteria and archae. The ER probably evolved as an invagination of this prokaryotic structure and is still associated with the plasma membrane (Zhang *et al.* 2006). It is involved in a number of other functions besides configuring nascent proteins. For example the nuclear membrane is a contiguous extension of the ER; the ER stores Ca^{++} which is released when cells are excited; it contains many of the cytochromes P450 which catalyze steroid hormone synthesis and the metabolism of xenobiotics; and it forms the autophagic vacuoles which remove both damaged organelles and cytosolic deposits of aggregated proteins. It is felt that it is defects in this latter function which lead to many of the neurodegenerative diseases of the elderly (Mizushima *et al.* 2008). But, like the periplasmic space of prokaryotes, a major function of the ER is to process all secretory and most membrane bound proteins. It contains a number of ER specific HSPs, such as BiP (GRp78) and GRp94, but it also contains several other families of proteins involved in posttranslational protein processing. Of particular interest for this discussion is that ERp57 appears to serve critical roles in the posttranslational processing of proteins and also acts as an ER chaperones (Holtzman 1998). Knocking out this protein is an embryonic lethal mutation (Garbi *et al.* 2006). Another family of eukaryotic ER chaperones are calreticulin and its membrane bound homologue, calnexin. Finally, a process unique to the ER is the modification of the lumenal portion of proteins by the N-glycosylation of asparagines. These N-glycosylation sites on the plasma membrane bound proteins are only observed on the extracellular portion of these proteins.

Proteins which undergo posttranslational processing in the ER have a hydrophobic peptide sequence, usually at the N-terminal end of the protein, termed the signal sequence. This is recognized by the "signal recognition particle" (SRP) which directs the polyribosomes to a pore in the ER membrane, called the translocon (Fig. 3). An homologous SRP is found in prokaryotes as well and binds the mRNA's of these proteins to an homologous pore on the periplasmic membrane. During the translation of the mRNA's, the nascent peptides are threaded into the lumen of the ER through the pore in the translocon where the protein is processed. On the other hand, the transmembrane portions of intrinsic membrane proteins move into the hydrophobic portions of the membrane while in the translocon. Once inside the lumen of the ER, the signal peptide is clipped off, the nascent proteins bind to the ER chaperones and most are N-glycosylated. Once the protein is configured and the appropriate posttranslational modifications are completed, it is packaged into trafficking vesicles and transported to the *golgi*. After further processing in the *golgi*, it is transported to the plasma membrane.

During the preparation of my chapter on ERp57, I discovered that it too was an ER chaperone. Of greater interest, there were reports that both ERp57 and ERp55 (PDI) are secreted from the cell bound to other proteins, such as the catalytic subunit of prolyl-4-hydroxylase (Holtzman 1998). At about this same time, I became aware of the current work in Alzheimer's disease. In light of the recent findings on the role of the ER in the processing of proteins, I felt that the current understanding of the etiology of this condition was not consistent with the result of the investigations of both the function of APP and the ER role in the catalysis of protein processing. I wondered whether the deposits of the β-amyloids could be due to a decline in ER chaperone function. I came to consider this question because of a major conundrum:

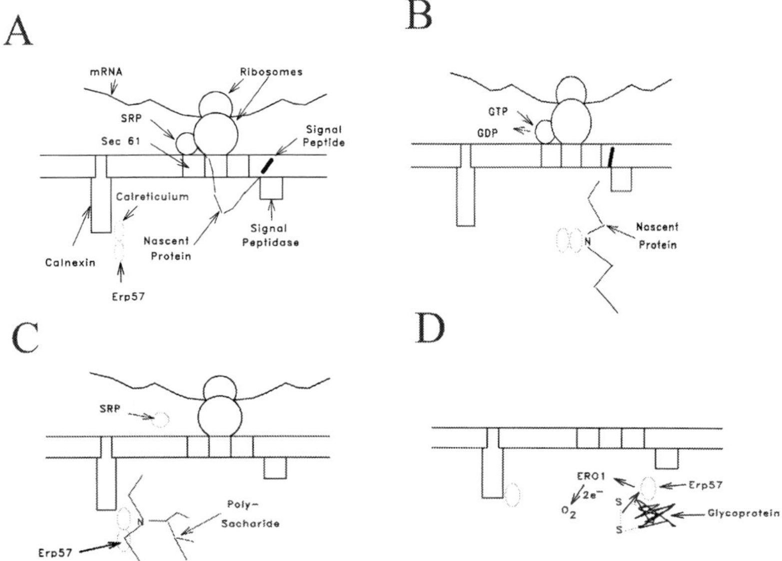

Figure 3a. Scheme of the Posttranslational Processing in the ER of Secretory Proteins

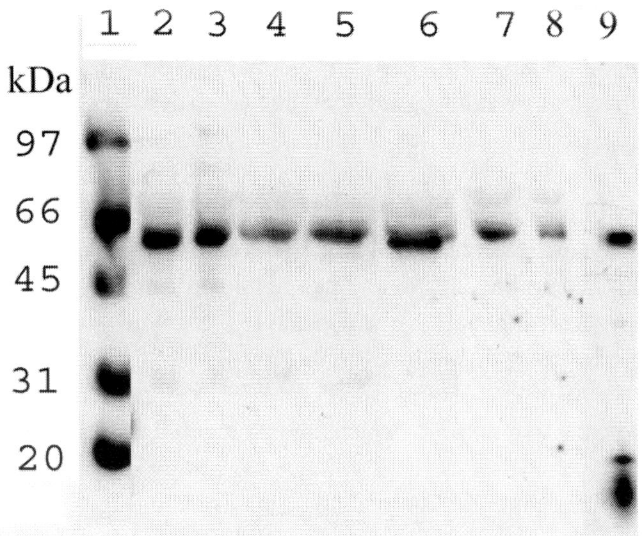

Figure 3b. ECL, immunoblots with rabbit polyclonal antibodies to β-amyloid (1282) of normal human CSF after treatments to dissociate the β-amyloid-ERp57 complex. Channel 1 - molecular weight markers; channel 2 - untreated CSF; channel 3 - CSF treated with 70% formic acid; channel 4 - CSF treated with 80% trifluoroacetic acid; channel 5 - CSF treated with 6 M guanidine isothiocyante; channel 6 - CSF treated with 6 M urea; Channel 7 - CSF proteins which did not bind to a boronate column; Channel 8 - CSF proteins which bound to a boronate column; channel 9 - treatment of the complex with glycine buffer, pH 9.0. (Data taken from Erickson *et al.* 2005).D.2. The Possible Role of Declines in the Activity of the Er ER to Catalyze Protein Processing in the Cognitive Decline Seen in Alzheimer's Disease

Since the β-amyloids are produced in everyone as a result of sAPP synthesis, why is plaque formation only observed in the brains of the elderly?

Currently, the standard reply to this question is that as individuals age there is a shift from the secretion of the more soluble β-amyloid 1-40 to the less soluble 1-42 peptide. Yet, clinical trials have not reported such a shift (Mehta *et al.* 2000). Furthermore, it would seem strange that the same protease, the γ-secretase, would change its mode of action with age. The fact that both the 1-40 and 1-42 are observed in CSf CSF would suggest that the β-amyloids are normally produced as the 1-42 or 1-43 peptide. These are then cleaved by an extracellular peptidase to give the 1-40 peptide.

We elected to examine an alternative mechanism. Based on the observation that some proteins are secreted from the cell bound to chaperones, we reasoned that in normals the β-amyloids do not precipitate after secretion into the extracellular aqueous space because they are bound to one or more ER chaperones. These could then serve to keep these hydrophobic peptides in solution. This would further imply that as we age, there is a decline in the formation of these complexes with the resultant excretion of the naked, hydrophobic peptides found in plaque.

D.3. The Observed Binding of □-Amyloids to Er ER Chaperones in the CsfCSF

If the β-amyloids are secreted as a complex with one or more chaperones, then these soluble proteins could serve to keep the normally insoluble β-amyloids in solution. Furthermore, this paradigm would suggest that the plaque deposits are merely a biomarker for a decline in the capacity of the ER to form such complexes. This would further imply that with age there is a decline in thc capacity of the ER to catalyze the posttranslational processing of many of the proteins necessary for normal cognitive function.

And indeed when we examined CSF for the presence of chaperones, we found that it contained two ER chaperones, ERp57 and calreticulin (Erickson *et al.* 2005). Furthermore, our western blots indicated that all of the detectable β-amyloids in straight CSF and in liver microsomes were covalently bound to ERp57 (Fig. 4) (Erickson *et al.* 2005). This complex was stable under reducing conditions on SDS-PAGE. It was unaffected by neat formic or trifluoroacetic acids, the two reagents which are commonly used to solubilize the β-amyloids from plaque (Fig. 4; channels 3 & 4). Similarly, the complex was stable in the presence of chaotropic agents, such as urea and guinadine isothiocyanate (Fig. 4; channels 5 & 6). But it was sensitive to hydrolysis by base (Fig. 4; channel 9). Furthermore, it could be pulled out of solution by boronate beads (Fig. 4; channels 7 & 8). These beads are used to bind protein bound carbohydrates, such as those found in hemoglobin A_{1c}. This suggested that the β-amyloids are N-glycosylated at asparagine 27. When we ran the PAGE on a native gel, that is without detergent or dithiothreotol, we observed that the complex contained a second ER chaperone, calreticulin (Fig. 5). This chaperone appeared to be reversibly bound to the ERp57 (Erickson *et al.* 2005). Such complexes between ERp57 and calreticulin were initially reported by High's group (Elliot *et al* 1997; Oliver *et al.* 1997) and confirmed by numerous other investigators. These complexes have been primarily observed in models of the synthesis of soluble N-glycosylated proteins in the ER. In these models the calreticulin is thought to be a lectin which binds to the oligosaccharide bound to the N-glycosylation site. The ERp57 then binds to the calreticulin.

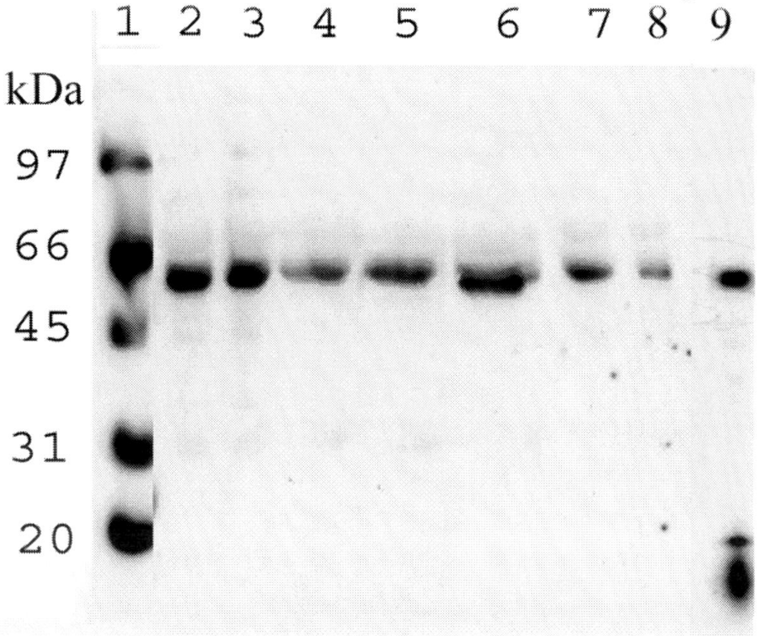

Figure 4. ECL, immunoblots with rabbit polyclonal antibodies to β-amyloid (1282) of normal human CSF after treatments to dissociate the β-amyloid-ERp57 complex. Channel 1 - molecular weight markers; channel 2 - untreated CSF; channel 3 - CSF treated with 70% formic acid; channel 4 - CSF treated with 80% trifluoroacetic acid; channel 5 - CSF treated with 6 M guanidine isothiocyante; channel 6 - CSF treated with 6 M urea; Channel 7 - CSF proteins which did not bind to a boronate column; Channel 8 - CSF proteins which bound to a boronate column; channel 9 - treatment of the complex with glycine buffer, pH 9.0. (Data taken from Erickson *et al.* 2005).

In line with the possible N-glycosylation of asparagine 27, we found that of the five anti-β-amyloid antibodies we employed, only the monoclonal antibody 4G8 failed to react (Erickson *et al.* 2005). This antibody is directed to an epitope of amino acids 17 -24. The binding of a bulky oligosaccharide to asparagine 27 would be expected to sterically hinder the binding of this antibody. This observation is consistent with the posttranslational modification of this amino acid.

We were also able to purify the ERp57-β-amyloid complex from CSF by immunoprecipitation with anti-ERp57 and anti-β-amyloid antibodies (Fig. 6). Of note in this study, although we did not observe the soluble aggregates in the straight CSF, we did observe them when we concentrated them by immunoprecipitation with an anti-β-amyloid antibody. The antibody used in this study was prepared against the synthetic 1-42 peptide and served to concentrate the naked peptides that were not N-glycosylated. When taken together our data indicate that the bulk of the β-amyloids in the CSF are present as a complex with ERp57. We have observed and partially purified this same complex from preparations of human CSF and hepatic microsomes for proteomic studies.

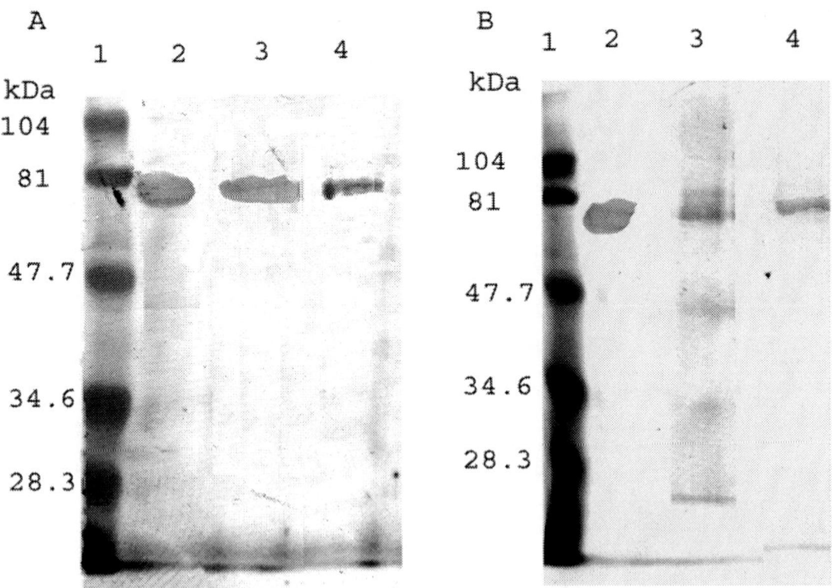

Figure 5a. Immunoblots with A) polyclonal antibodies to ERp57 and B) to bamyloid. Channel 1 - prestained standards; channels 2 - CSF; channel 3 - CSF Separated by affinity chromatography with anti-β-amyloid antibodies; channel 4 - CSF separated by affinity chromatography with anti-ERp57 antibodies. The bands were detected with the alkaline phosphatase reaction.

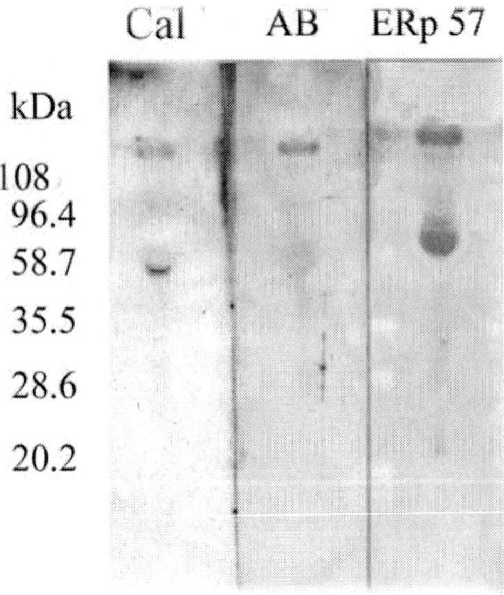

Figure 5b. Immunoblot of CSF run on a native Gel. Channel 1 - anti-calreticulin; channel 2 - anti-β-amyloid; channel 3 - anti-ERp57. (Data taken from Erickson *et al.* 2005).

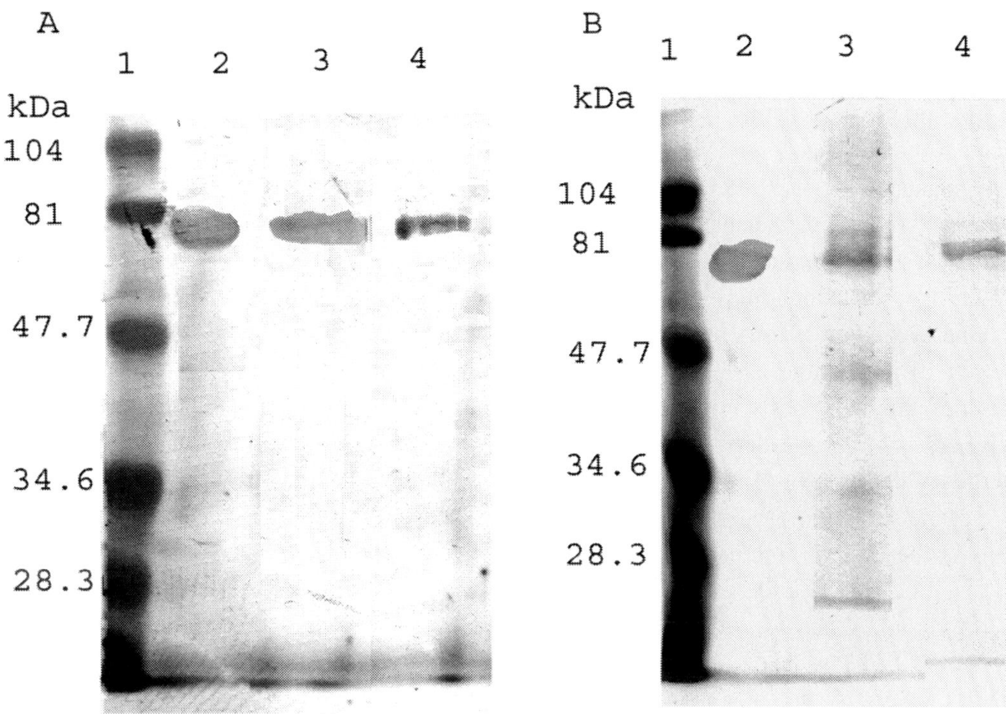

Figure 6a. Immunoblots with A) polyclonal antibodies to ERp57 and B) to bamyloid. Channel 1 - prestained standards; channels 2 - CSF; channel 3 - CSF Separated by affinity chromatography with anti-β-amyloid antibodies; channel 4 - CSF separated by affinity chromatography with anti-ERp57 antibodies. The bands were detected with the alkaline phosphatase reaction. (Data taken from Erickson *et al,* 2005)

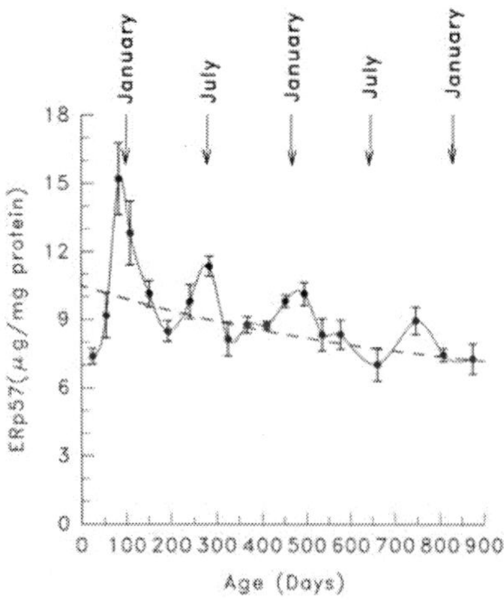

Figure 6b. The Effect of Age on Hepatic, ER D.4. The Correlation of the Presence of Plaque in the Brain to the Level of Erp57 ERp57 in the CsfCSF

Other workers have also observed on SDS-PAGE of CSF a β-amyloid band at around 60 kDa (Koudinov *et al.* 1996). Similarly, Cleary *et al.* (2005) observed this band in fractions obtained from transfected CHO and 7PA2 cells; while Shankar *et al.* (2007) observed it in homogenates of brains from patients with Alzheimer's disease. This latter observation suggests that even though patients with this condition secrete the naked peptide, they are still able to produce some of the complex.

One problem with this model is that it is generally held that the N-glycosylation only occurs at the consensus sequence N-X-S, while in the β-amyloids the asparagines are present in the sequence S-N-K (See Fig. 2). Furthermore, it is also thought that this step only occurs after about 15 amino acids have been translocated through the translocon pore while in the β-amyloids the asparagine is separated from the membrane by a single lysine. A possible resolution of this conundrum will be discussed below.

One prediction of this new paradigm is that there should be a correlation between the level of ERp57 in the CSF and the presence of plaque in the brain. In a pilot study we examined this hypothesis in samples of CSF obtained at autopsy from subjects in the Nun study. As controls we determined the levels of this chaperone in CSF obtained from the emergency department of a local hospital and from individuals undergoing spinal anesthesia for prostate surgery. Based on these determinations we found that the normal range of ERp57 levels in the CSF in both samples from the young individuals in the emergency department and from the elderly undergoing prostate surgery were the same. The normal range was 18.4 to 38.9 ng/ml. When we analyzed the autopsy samples we observed that about half of the individuals had low levels of ERP57 ERp57 in their CSF, i.e. less than 18.4 ng/ml. These subjects, invariably had plaque in the brain (Table 1).

These data lend support to the concept that the deposition of plaque is due to a failure of the ER to catalyze the formation of the complex between the β-amyloids and ERp57. Unfortunately, we were unable to obtain reliable cognitive scores on these subjects, as a result we could not determine whether there is a correlation between cognitive function and the levels of ERp57 in the CSF.

TABLE 1. The Correlation Between the CSF Levels of ERp57 and the Number of Participants in the Nun Study with Plaque Deposits.

CSF ERp57Levels (ng/mL)	< 18.4	>18.4
No Plaque	0	5
Significant Plaque	9	7

$\chi^2 = 4.922$, $p < 0.03$

D.5. The Effect of Age on the Levels of the Er ER Chaperones and the Activity of the N-Glycosylation Pathway

A major implication of our observations and the vast body of information on the biochemistry and cell biology of the ER posttranslational protein processing is that the deposition of the β-amyloids and any increases in the soluble aggregates are not the cause of the dementia, but are merely biomarkers of a decline with age in the capacity of the ER to catalyze posttranslational protein processing suggesting that there is a decline in the levels of the ER chaperones with age. And indeed in a separate study we found that in hepatic microsomes there was a significant decline in the content of several ER chaperones (Erickson *et al.* 2006) (Table 2). In particular, we observed a significant age related decline in ERp57 in the liver, a relatively well conserved organ (Fig. 7)[3]. On the basis of these observations, we suggested that this decline in chaperone content could decrease the capacity of the ER to catalyze the posttranslational processing of membrane and secretory proteins and in turn reduce the capacity of the neurons to form the new synapses necessary to initiate, consolidate and retrieve memory (Erickson *et al.* 2005).

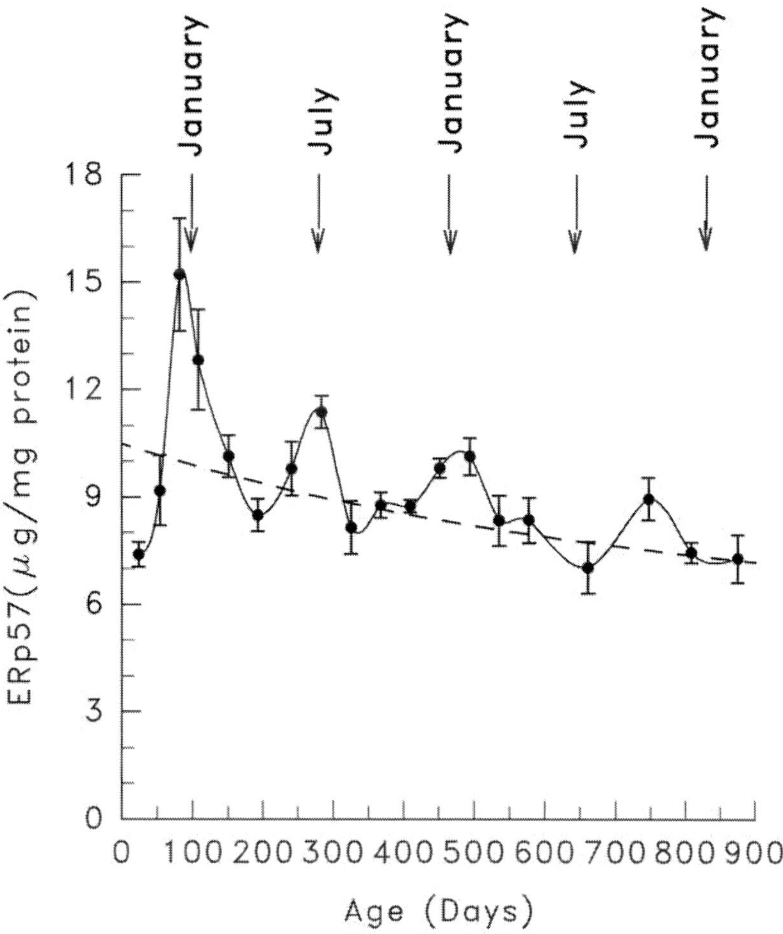

Figure 7 The Effect of Age on Hepatic, ER ERp57 (Data taken from Erickson *et al.* 2006).

[3]One enigma of this plot is that there were semiannual peaks in the content of the ERp57. There were similar cyclic variations in the contents of ERp55 (PDI) and BiP (GRp78) (Table 2). Yet, these animals were maintained in a state-of-the art facility from weaning until death with a constant temperature of 68° C and a constant 12 hour light-dark cycle. Hence, there was no obvious environmental reason for this cyclic pattern. Furthermore, other chaperones, such as ERp72 and calnexin, did showed only a steady decline with age.

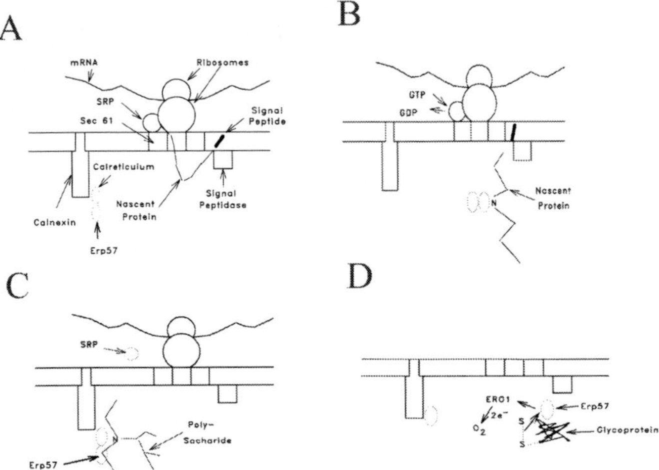

Figure 7 (Continued). Scheme of the Posttranslational Processing in the ER of Secretory Proteins

TABLE 2. Effect of Age and Cyclic Variation on The Concentrations of the Various ER Chaperones.

Chaperone	Peak Concentration μg/mg Protein	Concentration @ 874 Days μg/mg Protein	Constitutive Decline %	Show Cyclic Variation	Cyclic Variation % Decline
BiP	80.0	48.5	39	Yes	50
Calnexin	57.4	40.5	29	No	---
Calreticulin	7.6	4.8	8	No	---
ERp55	34.8	13.1	51	Yes	73
ERp57	15.4	8.2	32	Yes	71
ERp72	141	100	30	No	---
Total	336.2	215.1	37		

(Data taken from Erickson *et al.* 2006)

Similarly, a number of studies have suggested that there is also a decrease in the N-glcosylation pathway with age. The initial step in this pathway is the synthesis of dolichol (Yan and Lennarz 1999; Kelleher and Gilmore 2006), a large terpine which serves as a cofactor for the cytosolic synthesis of a 15 sugar oligosaccharide. Once the complex is fully synthesized, it is transferred to the lumen of the ER and bound to an asparagine by a oligosaccharide transferase (OST) (Helenius and Aebi 2002). The addition of the individual sugars to the carbohydrate complex is catalyzed by a family of specific monosaccharide transferases (MST) (Yan and Lennarz 1999; Helenius and Aebi 2002; Kelleher and Gilmore 2006). The first sugars added to the dolichol phosphate are a pair of N-acetyl glucosamines, followed by nine mannoses and three glucoses. A large number of studies have shown that as animals age there is a marked increase in the cellular content of both dolichol and dolichol phosphate (for example see Marino *et al.* 1997,1998). Since there is no increase in the synthesis of dolichol. this finding would suggest that there is a decline in the activity of the first MST that binds the first N-acetyl glucosamine to the dolichol phosphate, thus blocking N-glycosylation.

As noted above a major conundrum of our observation that the β-amyloids are N-glycosylated at asparagines 27 is that it is too close to the membrane and has the wrong consensus sequence for this reaction. This problem may be resolved by the recent studies of Ruiz-Canada *et al.* (2009). They found that there is a second form of the catalytic component of the terminal OST, STT3B, that could catalyze the transfer of the carbohydrate complex to asparagines. It is possible that this newly identified OST isoform catalyzes this step with the β-amyloids. Completion of on going purification studies and planned knock down studies may help to resolve this issue.

In conclusion the combined loss of the chaperones and decreases in the activity of the N-glycosylation pathway could have profound effects on the capacity of the cell to produce the membrane proteins which are necessary for normal cellular function. In the case of the neuron, it could lead to decreases in the capacity of the cell to produce the membrane proteins necessary to form the synapses that initiate, consolidate and retrieve membranememory. Similarly, it could explain the frequently observed loss of white matter in the brains of the elderly. The myelin sheaths which encase the axons are an onion-like structure formed from the plasma membranes of Schwann cells and the brain microglia (Fig. 8).

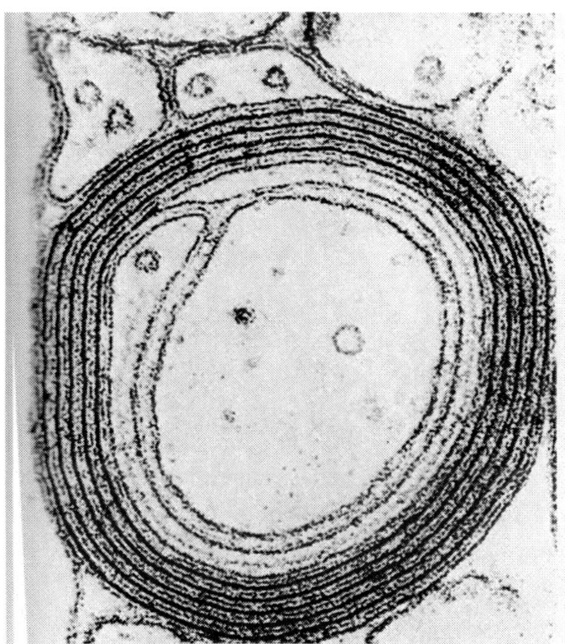

Figure 8. Electron Micrograph of a Schwann Cell.

As the organism ages if there is a decrease in the capacity of the these cells to produce the plasma membrane proteins forming these structures, there will be a decline in the size of the myelin sheaths. This would reduce the velocity of nerve conduction and could be the etiology of the well known "Senior Moments" which afflict the elderly in which there is an increased delay in retrieving specific memories. The decrease in synthesis of synapses and myelin membranes could also explain the well known clinical observation that there is a decrease in brain size seen on CT or MRI brain scans of the elderly.

D.6. Studies Suggesting that Erp57 ERp57 Binds to Other Proteins Processed in the ErR

The binding of ERp57 to β-amyloid is not unique, but has also been observed in or suggested by studies of a number of plasma membrane receptor proteins. Hence, our suggestion that it is bound to the lumenal portion of APP is merely an extension of studies of other membrane bound proteins. The first such study was an investigation by Aiyar *et al.* (1989) of the vasopressin receptor. These workers had initially cloned and sequenced ERp57 from hamster ovary cells (Bennett *et al.* 1988), but mistakenly identified it as a phospholipase C form 1a (Srivastrava *et al.* 1991; 1993). This error was due to contamination with a phospholipase of their preparation of ERp57 since when we (Srivastrava *et al.* 1993) and Bourdi *et al.* (1995) expressed the plasmid, the resulting protein had no phospholipase c activity. Based on their erroneous identification of the enzymatic activity of this protein, they went on to perform a very elegant study in which they sought to examine a possible association of ERp57 with the vasopressin receptor (Aiyar *et al* 1989). The vasopressin response is mediated by the second messenger, inositol triphosphate (IP3). On binding of vasopressin the receptor activates a G-protein dependent phospholipase c. The activated enzyme cleaves off IP3 from membrane bound phosphatidyl inositol. Hence, the vasopressin receptor should have an associated G-proteins and a phospholipase c. To test this hypothesis, they designed a study in which they affinity-labeled hepatocyte, plasma membranes with ^{14}C-vasopressin. They treated the membranes with a cross linking reagent, solubilized them and then ran the preparation over an ion-exchange column. They reported that the radioactivity eluded from the column in a fraction which also reacted with antibodies to both ERp57 and a G-protein suggesting that the ERp57 was bound to this receptor.

Similarly, Nime (2005) examined the structure of the 1,25-dihydroxyvitamin D_3 receptor on the plasma membrane of chick, embryo enterocytes. This receptor is not to be confused with the cytosolic receptor which is involved in the nuclear activity of the vitamin. But rather it stimulates the uptake of Ca^{++} into intestinal cells. She was able to isolate the receptor and found that it contained ERp57. Furthermore, she produced antibodies to the carboxy terminus of ERp57 and found that these antibodies blocked the uptake of Ca^{++} into the enterocytes. These data strongly support the concept that the ERp57 is bound to yet another plasma membrane receptor.

Finally, we have examined the effect of two agents on glutathione oxidation in *in vitro* models (McConkey *et al.* 1987; Holtzman, unpublished data). These studies were predicated on the observation that ERp57 is an oxidoreductase (TPDO). As noted above, these enzymes are members of the gluterdoxin/thioredoxin/protein disulfide isomerase superfamily (Holtzman 1998) which catalyze both the oxidation and reduction of protein sulfur groups. In our studies we found that in an anaerobic, *in vitro* assay, both glucagon (McConkey *et al.* 1987) and morphine (unpublished studies) increased the oxidation of glutathione at physiological and pharmacologically relevant concentrations. These findings suggests that the activation of these receptors leads to the stimulation of TPDO activity. Based on the studies by Aiyar *et al.* and Nime, this enzyme may well be ERp57.

This body of evidence suggests that the binding of ERp57 to membrane proteins is not unique to APP as indicated by its binding to β-amyloid, but rather is a generalized phenomenon observed in several plasma membrane receptors which are also type 1 transmembrane proteins. The combined observations that ERp57 may serve some role in receptor function and the decline in the capacity of the cell to form the ERp57-β-amyloid complex would suggest that the decreased functional capacity of receptors with age could be due to a failure of the ER to form this complex with plasma membrane receptors. For example, it is well known that the elderly have a muted β-adrenergic response without a significant loss of total number of receptors or G-proteins. This loss could be due to the failure of the ER to add the ERp57 to this receptor.

E. New Cell and Animals Models for Drug Discovery

The failure of the clinical trials outlined in this review suggests that there is a need for a new approach to seeking disease modifying treatments for Alzheimer's disease. Our new paradigm suggests both new cell and animal models for the screening of potential therapeutic agents. If as our studies suggest this condition is due to a decline in the components of the posttranslational protein processing system, it would seem reasonable to seek agents which increase their content in the ER. In line with this we have found that the insecticide, methoxychlor, does increase the ERp57 in rat liver suggesting that this could be a potential agent to examine. (Morrell *et al.* 2000). Yet, the methodology we employed in this study is not applicable for massive drug screening. It is clear that it would be necessary to develop cell based systems to facilitate this crucial step in drug development.

The standard approach would be to knock down the mRNA's with either antisense DNA's or RNAi's. These reagents would decrease the translation of the specific components of the ER posttranslational protein processing pathway. An initial test of the new paradigm, would be to knock down the ERp57 and the early MST's involved in the N-glycosylation pathway and determine whether there is an accumulation of the β-amyloids. These could be detected with anti-β-amyloid antibodies which have been tagged with a fluorescent dye. Alternatively, they could also be directly detected with a fluorescent dye, such as thioflavin-T. This dye binds to the β-amyloids. With this established cell culture model it would be possible to screen whole panels of drugs in microtiter plates. Alternatively, it would be possible to monitor the effects of various agents in cells or animals by transfecting them with the promoters for each of the components attached to a classical reporter gene, such as green, red or yellow fluorescent proteins (GFP, GRP, or GYP). A similar approach can be taken with whole animals in which they are transfected with the appropriate promoter and a reporter such as luciferase. In the latter case it would be possible to monitor the effect by imaging the whole animal. A wide variety of cell systems could be employed for these studies, such as primary neuron cultures or a variety of cell lines.

Finally, similar procedures based on this paradigm can be used to test the effect of agents on cognitive function. If our model is correct, then the chronic administration of either antisense DNA's or RNAi's to intact animals should lead to a decline in cognitive function. In such a model probably the best agents would be antisense morpholino DNA's. These agents have long half lives, do not require metabolic activation and are not degraded through the same pathways as the RNAi's. Hence, any effects of drugs which might be observed would not be due to interference with the metabolic processes, such as dicer activation of the RNAi's or P-protein degradation. Hence, the antisense morpholino DNA's for the one or more of the components of the ER system can be chronically administered either by injection or by some form of infusion pump, such as an osmotic pump. After the optimal dose and pretreatment times have been established, then the drugs, such as methoxychlor, which show promise during the screening studies, can be administered. The cognitive function of the animals can be tested by any number of well established procedures, such as the swimming pool test, before and after the administration of the test drug.

F. Summary

I feel that the body of evidence to date indicates that the dementia characteristic of Alzheimer's disease is not due to the toxicity of the β-amyloids. Even if their toxicity is a factor in the development of the dementia, it is not clear that the APP transgenic mice are valid models to study this toxicity. In fact, many agents which arrested cognitive decline did so without significantly altering the plaque burden (Levin-Allerhand *et al.* (2002; Stackman *et al* 2003; Carroll *et al.* (2007). These data argue that this decline is not due to the presence of toxic levels of the β-amyloids. Furthermore, the work of Nikolaev *et al.* (2009) suggests rather that the cognitive decline may be due to the continued pruning of neurons and synapses in the adult animal due to the excessive levels of sAPP. If this is correct, then the apparent therapeutic benefit observed in these models for many of the proposed agents may be due to an inhibition of the APP pathway rather altering the basic disease as seen in the elderly. Finally, the poor track record of this model to identify potential disease modifying therapeutic agents would suggest that consideration should be given to alternative paradigms and test systems, such as those that I have outlined in this review.

References

ADAPT Research Goup Cognitive function over time in the Alzheimer's disease anti-inflammatory Prevention Trial (ADAPT) *Arch. Neurol.* 2008;65: 896-905

Aiyar, N., Bennett, C.F., Namei, P. Valinsky, W., Angoli, M., Minnich, M. and Crooke, S.T. Solubilization of rat liver vasopresin receptors as a complex with a guanine-nucleotide-binding protein and a phophoinositide-specific phospholipase C. *Biochem. J.* 1988;261:63-70

Bachurin, S., Bukatina, E., Lermontova, N., Tkachenko, S., Afanasiev, A., Grigoriev, V., Grigorieva, I., Ivanov, Y.U., Sablin, S. and Zefirov, N. Antihistamine agent dimebon as a novel neuroprotector and a cognitive enhancer. *Ann. NY Acad. Sci.* 2001;939:425-436

Bennett, C.F., Balcarek, J.M., Varrichio, A., and Crooke, S.T. Molecular cloning and complete amino-acid sequence of form-I phosphoinositide-specific phopholipase C. *Nature* 1988;334:268-270

Bourdi, M., Demady, D., Martin, J.L., Jabbour, S.K., Martin, B.M., George, J.W. and Pohl, L.R. cDNA cloning and baculovirus expression of the human liver endoplasmic reticulum P58: Characterization as a protein disulfide isomerase isoform, but not as a protease or a carnitine acetyltransferase. *Arch. Biochem. Biophys.* 1995;323:397-403

Carro, E., Trejo, J.L., Gomez-Isla, T., LeRoth, D. and Torres-Aleman, L. Serum insulin-like growth 1 regulates brain amyloid-β levels. *Nature Med.* 2002;12:1390-1397

Carroll, J.C., Rosario, E.R., Chang, L., Stanczyk, F.Z., Oddo, S., LaFerla, F.M. and Pike, C.J. Progesterone and estrogen regulate Alzheimer-like neuropathology in female 3xTg-AD mice. *J. Neurosci.* 2007;27:13357-13365

Cleary, J.P., Walsh, D.M., Hofmeister, J.J., Shankar, G.M., Koskowski, M.A., Selkoe, D.J. and Ashe, K.H. Natural oligomers of the amyloid-β protein specifically disrupt cognitive function. *Nature Neuroscience* 2005;8:79-84

Curry, C.L., Reed, L.L., Golde, T.E., Miele, L., Nickoloff, B.J. and Foreman, K.E., Gamma secretase inhibitor blocks Notch activation and induces apoptosis in Kaposi's sarcoma tumor cells. *Ongene* 2005;24:633-644

Dawson, G.R., Seabrook, G.R., Zheng, H., Smith, D.W., Graham, S., O'Dowd, G., Bowery, B.J., Boyce, S., Trumbauer, M.E., Chen, H.Y., Van der Ploeg, L.H. and Sirinathsinghji, D.J. Age-related cognitive deficits, impaired long-term potentiation and reduction in synaptic marker density in mice lacking the beta-amyloid precursor protein. *Neuroscience* 1999;90:1-13

DeKosky, S.T., Williamson, J.D., Fitzpatrick, A.L., Kronmal, R.A., Ives, D.G., Saxton, J.A., Lopez, O.L., Burke, G., Carlson, M.C., Fried, L.P., Kuller, L.H., Robbins, J.A., Tracy, R.P., Woolard, N.F., Dunn, L., Snitz, B.E., Nahin, R.L., Furberg, C.D. and Ginkgo Evaluation of Memory (GEM) Study Investigators. *Ginkgo biloba* for revention of dementia: A randomized controlled trial. *JAMA*. 2008;300:2253-2262

Doody, R.S., Govrilova, S., Sano, M., Thomas, R,G., Aisen, P.S.. Bachirun, S.O., Seely, L. and Hung, D. Effect of dimebon on cognition, activities of daily living, behaviour, and global function in patients with mild-to-moderate Alzheimer's disease: a randomised double-blind, placebo-controlled study. *Lancet* 2008;372:207-215

D'Souza, B., Miyamoto, A. and Weinmaster, G. The many facets of notch ligands. *Oncogene* 2008;27:5148-5167

Elliott, J.G., Oliver, J.D. and High, S. The thiol-dependent reductase ERp57 interacts specifically with N-glycosylated integral membrane proteins. *J. Biol. Chem.* 1997;272: 13849-13855

Erickson, R.R., Dunning, L.M., Olson, D.A., Cohen, D.A., Davis, A.T., Wood, W.G., Kratzke' R.A. and Holtzman, J.L. In Cerebrospinal Fluid ER Chaperones ERp57 and Calreticulin Bind β-Amyloid. *Biochem. Biophys. Res. Commun.* 2005;332: 50-57

Erickson, R.R., Dunning, L.M. and Holtzman, J.L. The Effect of Aging on the Chaperone Concentrations in the Hepatic, EndoplasmicReticulum of Male Rats: The Possible Role of Protein Misfolding Due to the Loss of Chaperones in the Decline in Physiological Function Seen with Age. *J. Gerontol. Biol. Med.* 2006;61A:435-443

Espeland, M.A., Rapp, S.R., Shumaker, S.A., Brunner, R., Manson, J.E., Sherwin, B.B., Hsia, J., Margolis, K.L., Hogan, P.E., Wallace, R., Dailey, M., Freeman, R., Hays, J., for Women's Health Initiative Memory Study. Conjugated equine estrogens and global cognitive function in postmenopausal women: Women's Health Initiative Memory Study. *JAMA.* 2004;291:2959-2968

FierceBiotech June 30, 2008

Frand, A.R. and Kaiser, C.A. The ERO1 gene of yeast is required for the oxidation of protein thiols in the endoplasmic reticulum. Mol. *Cell* 1998;1:161-170

Gura, T. Hope in Alzheimer's fight emerges from unexpected places. *Nature Med.* 2008;14:894 2008

Garbi, N., Tanaka, S., Momburg, F. and Hämmerling, G.J. Impaired assembly of the major histocompatibility complex class 1 peptide-loading complex in mice deficient in the oxidoreductase ERp57. *Nat. Immunol.* 2006;7:93-102

Giannakopoulos, P., Hof, P.R., Michel, J.P., Guimon, J. and Bouras, C. Cerebral cortex pathology in aging and Alzheimer's disease: a quantitative survey of large hospital-based geriatric and psychiatric cohorts. *Brain Res. Brain Res. Rev.* 1997;25: 217-245

Heber, S., Herms, J., Gajic, V., Hainfellner, J., Aguzzi, A., Rulicke, T., von Kretzschmar, H., von Koch, C., Sisodia, S., Tremml, P., Lipp, H.P., Wolfer, D.P. and Muller, U. Mice with combined gene knock-outs reveal essential and partially redundant functions of amyloid precursor protein family members. *J.Neurosci.* 2000;20:7951-7963

Helenius, J. and Aebi, M. Transmembrane movement of dolichol linked carbohydrates during N-glycoprotein biosynthesis in the endoplasmic reticulum. *Seminars in Cell & Developmental Biology.* 2002;13:171-178

Herzog, V., Kirfel, G., Siemes, C. and Schmitz, A. Biological roles of APP in the epidermis. *Eur. J. Cell Biol.* 2004;83:613-624

Holmes, C., Bache, D., Wilkinson, D., Yadegarfar, G., Hopkins, V., Bayer, A., Jones, R.W., Bullock, R., Love, S., Neal, J.W., Zotova, E. and Nicoll, J.A.R. Long-term effects of $A\beta_{42}$ immunisation in Alzheimer's disease: follow-up of a randomized, placebo-controlled phase 1 trial. *Lancet* 2008;372:216-223

Holtzman, J.L. : The Roles of the Thiol:Protein Disulfide Oxidoreductases in Membrane and Secretory Protein Synthesis Within the Lumen of the Endoplasmic Reticulum. *J. Invest. Med.* 1997;45:28-34

Holtzman, J.L. The Physiological Roles of the Thiol:Protein Disulfide Oxidoreductases. In: Prolyl-4-hydroxylase, protein disulfide isomerase and other structurally related proteins (Ed. Guzman, N.) *Marcel Deker*, New York pp. 173-236, 1998

Holtzman, J.L. Amyloid-β vaccination for Alzheimer's dementia. Lancet 2008;372:216

Janus, C., Pearson, J., McLaurin, J., Mathews, P.M., Jiang, Y., Schmidt, S.D., Chishti, M.A., Horne, P., Heslin, D., French, J., Mount, H.T.J., Nixon, R.A., Mercken, M., Bergeron, C., Fraser, P.E., St. George-Hyslop, P. and Westaway, D. Aβ peptide immunization reduces behavioural impairment and plaques in a model of Alzheimer's disease. *Nature* 2000;408:979-982

Katzman, R., Terry, R., DeTeresa, R., Brown, T., Davies, P., Fuld, P., Renbing, X. and Peck, A. Clinical, pathological, and neurochemical changes in dementia: a subgroup with preserved mental status and numerous neocortical plaques. *Ann. Neurol.* 1988;23: 138-144

Kelleher,D.J. and Gilmore, R. An evolving view of the eukaryotic oligosaccharyltransferase. *Glycobiology* 2006;16:47R-62R

Koudinov, A.R., Koudinova, N.V., Kumar, A., Beavis, R.C. and Ghiso, J. Biochemical characterization of Alzheimer's soluble amyloid beta protein in human cerebrospinal fluid: association with high density lipoproteins. *Biochem. Biophys. Res. Commun.* 1996;223: 592-597

Kukar, T., Prescott, S., Eriksen, J., Holloway, V., Murphy, M.P., Koo, E.H., Golde, T.E. and Nicolle, M. Chronic administration of R-flurbiprofen attenuates learning impairments in transgenic amyloid precursor protein mice. *BMC Neuroscience* 2007;8:54-66

Levin-Allerhand, J.A., Lominska, C.E., Wang, J. and Smith, J.D. 17Alpha-estradiol and 17beta-estradiol treatments are effective in lowering cerebral amyloid-beta levels in AbetaPPSWE transgenic mice. *J. Alzheimer's Dis.* 2002;4:449-457

Marino, M., Dolfi, C., Paradiso, C., Cavallini, G., Gori, Z., Innocenti, B., Maccheroni, M., Masini, M., Pollera, M., Trentalance, A. and Bergamini, E. Accumulation of dolichol and impaired signal transduction in aging. *Aging* 1997;9: 433-434

Marino, M., Dolfi, C., Paradiso, C., Cavallini, G., Masini, M., Gori, Z., Pollera, M., Trentalance, A. and Bergamini, E. Age-dependent accumulation of dolichol in rat liver: is tissue dolichol a biomarker of aging?. *J. Gerontol. A Biol. Sci. Med. Sci.* 1998;53: B87-B93

Mehta, P.D., Pirttila, T., Mehta, S.P., Sersen, E.A., Aisen, P.S. and Wisniewski, H.M. Plasma and cerebrospinal fluid levels of amyloid beta proteins 1-40 and 1-42 in Alzheimer disease. *Arch. Neurol.* 2000;57:100-105

Mizushima, N., Levine, B., Cuervo, A.M. and Klionsky, D.J. Autophagy fights disease through cellular self-digestion. *Nature* 2008;451:1069-1075

Morrell, S.L., Fuchs, J.A. and Holtzman, J.L. The Effect of Methoxychlor Administration to Male Rats on the Hepatic, Microsomal Iodothyronine 5'-Deiodinase, Form I. *J. Pharmacol. Expertl. Therap.* 2000;294: 308-312

Morgan, D., Diamond, D.M., Gottschall, P.E., Ugen, K.E., Dickey, C., Hardy, J., Duff, K., Jantzen, P., DiCarlo, G., Wilcock, D., Connor, K., Hatcher, J., Hope, C., Gordon M. and Arendash, G.W. Aβ peptide vaccination prevents memory loss in an animal model of Alzheimer's disease. *Nature* 2000;*408*:982-985

Nicoll, J.A.R., Bache, D. and Holmes, C. Authors' reply. Lancet 2008;372:216-217

Nikolaev, A., McLauglin, T., O'Oleary, D.D.M. and Tessier-Lavigne, M. APP binds DR6 to trigger axon pruning and neuron death via distinct caspases. *Nature* 2009;457:981-989

Nime, I. The 1,253-MARRS protein: Contribution to steroid stimulated calcium uptake in chicks and rats. *Steroids* 2005;70:455-457

Oliver, J.D., van der Wal, F.J., Bulleid, N.J. and High, S. Interaction of the thiol dependent reductase ERp57 with nascent glycoproteins. *Science* 1997;275: 86-88

Orgogozo, J.-M., Gilman, S., Dartigues, J.-F., Laurent, B., Puel, M., Kirby, L.C., Jouanny, P., Dubois, B., Eisner, L., Flitman, S., Michel, B.F., Boada, M., Frank, A. and Hock, C. Subacute meningoencaphalitis in a subset of patients with AD after Aβ42 immunization. *Neurology* 2003;61:46-54

Petrushina I., Ghochikyan, A., Mktrichyan, M., Mamikonyan, G., Movsesyan, N., Davtyan, H., Patel, A., Head, E., Cribbs, D.H. and Agadjanyan, M.G. Alzheimer's disease peptide epitope vaccine reduces insoluble but not soluble/oligomeric Abeta species in amyloid precursor protein transgenic mice. *J.Neurosci.* 2007;27:12721-12731

Reagan-Shaw, S., Nihal, M. and Ahmad, N. Dose translation from animal to human studies revisited. *FASEB J.* 2007;22:629-661

Ruiz-Canada, C., Kelleher, D.J. and Gilmore, R. Cotranslational and posttranslational N-glycosylation of polypeptides by distinct mammalian OST isoforms. *Cell* 2009;136:272-283

Seabrook, G.R., Smith, D.W., Bowery, B.J., Easter, A., Reynolds, T., Fitzjohn, S.M.. Morton, R. A., Zheng, H. Dawson, G.R. Sirinathsinghji, D.J., Davies, C.H., Collingridge, G.L. and Hill, R.G. Mechanisms contributing to the deficits in hippocampal synaptic plasticity in mice lacking amyloid precursor protein. *Neuropharmacology* 1999;38:349-359

Selkoe, D.J. Translating cell biology into therapeutic advances in Alzheimer's disease. *Nature* 1999;399 (Supp. 24): A23-A31

Sevigny, J.J., Ryan, J.M., van Dyek, C.H., Peng, Y., Lines, C.R. and Nessly, M.I. Growth hormone secretagogue MK-677; No clinical effect on AD progression in a randomized trial. *Neurology* 2008;71:1702-1708

Shankar, G.M., Li, S., Mehta, T.H., Garcia-Munoz, A., Shepardson, N.E., Smith, I., Brett, F.M., Farrell, M.A., Rowan, M.J., Lemere, C.A., Regan, C.M., Walsh, D.M., Sabatini, B.L. and Selkoe, D.J. Amyloid-beta protein dimers isolated directly from Alzheimer's brains impair synaptic plasticity and memory. *Nature Medicine* 2008;14:837-842

Srivastava, S.P., Chen, N.-Q., Liu, Y.-X. and Holtzman, J.L.: Purification and characterization of a new isozyme of thiol:protein disulfide oxidoreductase from rat hepatic microsomes: Relationship of this isozyme to cytosolic, phosphatidylinositol specific phospholipase C form 1A. *J. Biol. Chem.* 1991;266:20337-20344

Srivastava, S.P., Fuchs, J.A. and Holtzman, J.L.: The reported cDNA sequence for phospholipase Ca encodes protein disulfide isomerase, isozyme Q-2 and not phospholipase C. *Biochem. Biophys. Res. Commun.* 1993;193: 971-979

St George-Hyslop, P.H. and Morris, J.C. Will anti-amyloid therapies work for Alzheimer's disease? *Lancet* 2008;372:80-182

Stackman, R.W., Eckenstein, F., Frei, B., Kulhanek, D., Nowlin, J. and Quinn, J.F. Prevention of age-related spatial memory deficits in a transgenic mouse model of Alzheimer's disease by chronic Ginkgo biloba treatment. *Exp. Neurol.* 2003;184:510-520

Turner, P.R., Bourne, K., Garama, D., Carne, A., Abraham, W.C. and Tate, W.P. Production, purification and functional validation of human secreted amyoloid precursor proteins for use as neuropharmacological reagents. *J. Neurosci. Methods* 2007;134:68-74

von Koch, C.S., Zheng, H., Chen, H., Trumbauer, M., Thinakaran, G., van der Ploeg, L. H., Price, D.L. and Sisodia, S. S. Generation of APLP2 KO mice and early postnatal lethality in APLP2/APP double KO mice. *Neurobiology of Aging* 1997;18:661-669, 1997

WHI Effects of conjugated equine estrogen in postmenopausal women with hysterectomy: The Women's Health Initiative Randomized Controlled Trial. *J.Amer. Med. Soc.* 2004;291:1701-1712

Wolf, D.S., Gearing, M., Snowdon, D.A., Mori, H., Markesbery, W.R. and Mirra, S.S. Progression of regional neuropathology in Alzheimer disease and normalelderly: findings from the Nun study. *Alzheimer Dis. Assoc. Disord.* 1999;13: 226-231

Wilcock, G.K., Black, S.E., Hendrix, S.B., Zavitz, K.H., Swabb, E.A., Laughlin, M.A. Efficacy and safety of tarenflurbil in mild to moderate Alzheimer's disease: a randomized phase II trial. *Lancet Neurol.* 2008;7:483-493

Yan, Q. and Lennarz, W.J. Oligosaccharyltransferase: a complex multisubunit enzyme of the endoplasmic reticulum. *Biochem. Biophys. Res. Commun.* 1999;266:684-689

Xu, W., Kawarabayashi, T., Matsubara, E., Deguchi, K., Murakami, T., Harigaya, Y., Ikeda, M., Amari, M., Kuwano, R., Abe, K. and Shoji, M. Plasma antibodies to Aβ40 and Aβ42 in patients with Alzheimer's disease and normal controls. *Brain Res.* 2008;1219:169-179

Zhang, S.L., Yeromin, A.V., Zhang, X.H.-F., Yu, Y., Safrina, O., Penna, A., Roos, J., Stauderman, K.A. and Cahalan, M.D. Genome-wide RNAi screen of Ca^{2+} influx identifies genes that regulate Ca^{2+} release-activated $Ca2^{+}$ channel activity *Proc. Nat. Acad. Sci. USA* 2006;103:9357-9362

In: Alzheimer's Disease and Dementia (Vol. 4)
Editor: Miao-Kun Sun
ISBN:978-1-60876-152-4

Chapter VI

Apolipoprotein E and Alzheimer's Disease: An Update on Allele-Specific Effects of Disease Etiology

Ann M. Saunders

Genetics Research, GlaxoSmithKline R&D, Five Moore Drive, MAI.A1259, Research Triangle Park, North Carolina 27709-3398, USA, Tele: 919-483-9349

Abstract

Alzheimer disease (AD) has multiple etiologies, including genetic mutations, susceptibility genes and environmental factors. Apolipoprotein E (*APOE*=gene; apoE=protein) is a suceptiblity gene involved in the development of late-onset AD that accounts for approximately 50% of late onset AD. Remarkable progress has been made in understanding the susceptibility genetics of *APOE* and AD and the influence of a common polymorphism on recovery from acute brain stresses. While the role of apoE as a peripheral plasma lipid-transport molecule has been well documented, the normal functions of apoE in the brain and its role in the etiology of AD have not been solidly identified. Research suggests critical functions in the central nervous system that include metabolism, lipid transport, repair, toxicity, signaling, and cholinergic dysfunction. Furthermore, there are increasing epidemiological data supporting an interaction of *APOE* with diabetes and in the development of dementia in the elderly, suggesting that AD may represent a "type 3 diabetes" in the central nervous system.

Abbreviations

AD, Alzheimer's disease
APOE, apolipoprotein E gene
apoE, apolipoprotein E protein

APP,	amyloid β-protein precursor
Aβ,	amyloid β-protein
Arg,	arginine
CNS,	central nervous system
Cys,	cysteine
ε2,	epsilon 2 genetic variant of apolipoprotein E
ε3,	epsilon 3 genetic variant of apolipoprotein E
ε4,	epsilon 4 genetic variant of apolipoprotein E
HDL,	high-density lipoprotein
HIV-1,	human immunodeficiency virus, subtype 1
ICH,	intracerebral hemorrhage
kDa,	kilodalton
LDL	low-density lipoprotein
PPARγ,	peroxisomes proliferative-activated receptor, gamma
PS,	presenilin
TAT	trans-activator of transcription
VLDL	very low-density lipoprotein

Introduction

Alzheimer disease (AD) has multiple etiologies, including genetic mutations, susceptibility genes and environmental factors. Mutations in three genes, the amyloid precursor protein (APP) and presenilin (PS) 1 and 2 genes, nearly always cause the disease [7]. Study of these mutations is important for basic neurobiological research in understanding mechanisms involving these protein mutations. However, from the perspective of the more common form of AD seen in clinical practice, the autosomal dominant forms represent less the 2% of the incidence or prevalence. Apolipoprotein E (*APOE*=gene; apoE=protein) is a fourth genetic factor involved in the development of AD. Unlike the three deterministic gene mutations, *APOE* is a genetic risk factor that accounts for approximately 50% of late onset AD [72]. Remarkable progress has been made in understanding the susceptibility genetics of *APOE* and AD and the influence of a common polymorphism on recovery from acute brain stresses. While the role of apoE as a peripheral plasma lipid-transport molecule has been well documented, the normal functions of apoE in the brain and its role in the etiology of AD have not been solidly identified. Research over the past 15 years suggests critical functions in the central nervous system that include energy metabolism, lipid transport and synaptic repair, neurotoxicity, signaling, and cholinergic dysfunction. Furthermore, there are increasing epidemiological data supporting an interaction of a common *APOE* polymorphism with diabetes and in the development of dementia in the elderly, suggesting that AD may represent a “type 3 diabetes” in the CNS.

Genetic and Biochemical Background

The *APOE* gene is located on chromosome 19 within an apolipoprotein gene family and encodes three common alleles, designated *ε2*, *ε3* and *ε4*. *APOE ε3* is the most common variant (allele frequency in populations; 60-70%), followed by *APOE ε4* (15-20%) and *APOE ε2* (5-10%). ApoE is a polymorphic 299 amino acid protein, and the protein isoforms differ only at residues 112 and 158 (Figure 1). ApoE3 has Cys-112 and Arg-158, whereas apoE4 has arginine at both sites and apoE2 has cysteines [96]. The apoE protein has two structural domains that allow the protein to bind lipids and deliver them to cells. The 22-kDa N-terminal domain contains the low-density lipoprotein (LDL) receptor binding site, through which apoE mediates the cellular uptake of lipid complexes via the LDL-receptor and other related receptors. The 10-kDa C-terminal domain contains the major lipid binding site. Via this domain, plasma apoE is a component of both very low-density lipoprotein (VLDL), a subclass of high-density lipoprotein (HDL), and chylomicrons, which transport dietary cholesterol and triglycerides. The apoE2 protein is defective in LDL-receptor binding, and inheritance of two *ε2* alleles is associated with type III hyperlipoproteinemia [55, 96].

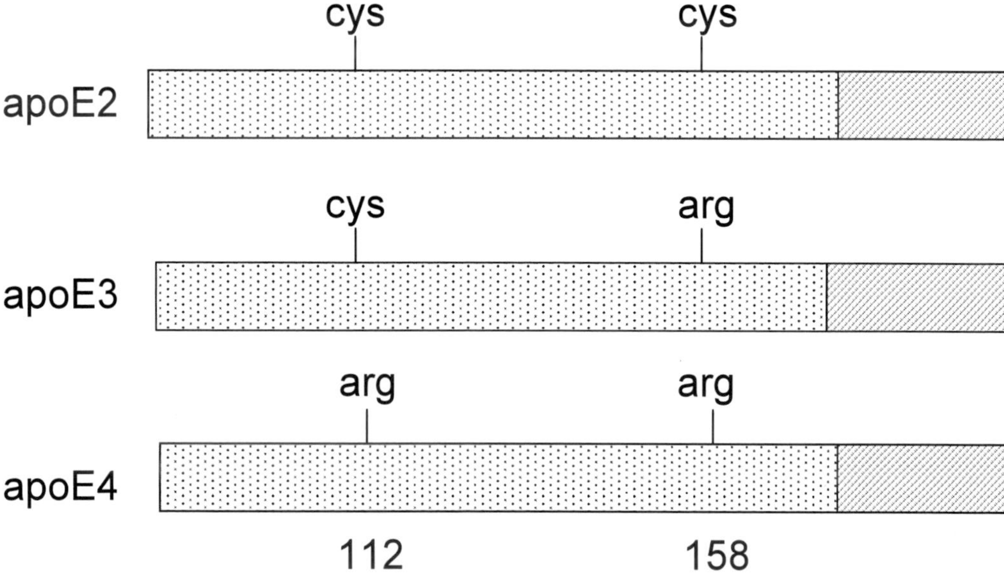

Figure 1. A schematic of the three common apoE protein isoforms, illustration the seemingly minor differences between the ancesteral apoE4 form with two arginines and the more recently evolved apoE3 (one arginine and one cysteines) and apoE2 (two cysteines). The stippled N-terminal domain is the LDL-receptor binding site and the hatched C-terminal domain is the major lipid binding site.

ApoE is abundant in the brain, second only to liver in synthesis of apoE [20]. Brain apoE is synthesized locally, as shown in liver transplant cases [48], and is the major apolipoprotein in the cerebrospinal fluid [97]. While astrocytes are the primary cell type that produces apoE, low levels of neuronal expression in the CNS has also been documented in cortical and hippocampal neurons in humans [99] and in transgenic mice expressing human apoE under the control of the human apoE promoter [100]. It is not known whether nascent apoE in the CNS preferentially associates with lipids and lipoprotein particles or if it complexes with other proteins. Biochemical analyses of apoE-containing lipoproteins in human cerebrospinal fluid have shown that apoE isl a constituent of HDL-like particles or phospholipids discs [67]. In contrast, nascent apoE-containing lipoprotein secreted by cultured rat astrocytes contain very little core lipid and are smaller [43]. ApoE-containing lipoproteins can deliver lipids, including cholesterol, to injury sites for cellular repair. ApoE3 and apoE2 are more effective than apoE4 in the repair and maintenance of cells, and apoE4 may even be harmful in the process [63].

APOE as a Genetic Risk Factor for AD

Polymorphic variations at the *APOE* locus, acting as inherited risk factors, affect genetic susceptibility to AD [77, 84]. Despite seemingly slight coding variations among the three common alleles, the different genotypes (combinations of inherited alleles) have a significant effect on both the risk and the age-at-onset distribution of AD. The *APOE ε4* allele is associated with an earlier age at onset of the common form of AD [13], while the rarer *ε2* allele confers a decreased risk and an older age at of onset [11, 22]. Each person inherits 2 alleles, and the risk and onset distribution of AD varies among the six common genotypes. *APOE ε4/4* homozygotes, approximately 2% of the general population, have the greatest risk of developing the disease. Statistically, AD will commence in 50% of *ε4/4* individuals before they reach 70 years of age. *APOE ε2/3* heterozygotes, represented in 12-14% of the population, have a median age of onset well over 90 years. The age-at-onset distribution of the *APOE ε3/3* population, bearing the most common genotype, falls in between. On the basis of *APOE* genotype alone, there is more than a twenty year difference in the median age-at-onset distributions.

The prevalence of each genotype varies among ethnic and racial groups [22]. In Japan, where the *APOE ε4* allele frequency is about half that of Caucasian populations, most of the *ε4*-positive AD patients have the *APOE ε3/4* genotype. Consequently, there are fewer Japanese patients with disease onset before 70 years of age. Finland provides a second example, where the *ε4* allele frequency in the general population is on the high end of the spectrum at 22%. However, age-matched controls for AD cases in the Finnish population had a lower allele frequency of 16.5%. The attrition of many *APOE ε4*-positive individuals before the age of risk for AD may be influenced by the high incidence of fatal myocardial infarction in Finland, which the *ε4* allele also serves as a risk factor. The presence of *APOE ε4* has clear effects on risk and age at onset in Caribbean Hispanics and African Americans; however, other genetic factors are likely involved [12, 35, 44, 93]. Any association appears to be absent in both east and west African communities [9, 10, 66, 78].

The influence of *APOE ε4* on accelerating progression of cognitive decline and modifying disease duration has been examined by a number of investigators. The majority of studies have shown no effect of *APOE* genotype on rate of cognitive decline [2, 4, 5, 16, 16, 21, 28, 29, 37, 39, 41, 42, 45, 61, 62, 80]. However, some investigators have reported that the presence of one *ε4* allele may increase [15, 36, 61] or even decrease [25, 83] the rate of cognitive decline. Likewise, disease duration does not appear to be influenced by *APOE ε4* but rather the age of onset [12]. Since the *ε4/4* genotype is associated with earlier ages at onset, these patients generally have a longer disease course. However, comparison of patients with onsets in the same age range (e.g. *APOE ε4/4* and *APOE ε3/3* with onsets between 65 and 69 years of age), the disease duration is similar and independent of *APOE* risk.

APOE Allele-Specific Effects on Brain Injury Repair

The effects of *APOE ε4* are not limited to AD, and have been implicated in recovery from several types of acute brain and chronic stress. The first suggestion that *ε4* played a role in the recovery of brain injury appeared within a study of amyloid load in head trauma patients who were comatose and died within a 30 day period after trauma [64]. Their interpretation was that there was a much higher *ε4* allele frequency in patients who died with increased amyloid deposits in their brains than in patients who died without increased amyloid deposition. Further examination of the Nicoll et al. data noted that the average age of the amyloid-bearing patients was over 50 years old, more than two decades older than the non-amyloid bearing patients. A proposed alternative interpretation was that head trauma patients lacking an *APOE ε4* allele did not qualify for inclusion in the neuropathological study because they did not die [73]. This second hypothesis suggested that head injury patients without a *ε4* allele had more efficient recovery from their injury. The younger patient group may have reflected the general population with more severe head injuries. Similar *APOE ε4* allele-specific effects on recovery from post-traumatic coma have also been reported [81].

The head trauma hypothesis led to the initiation numerous investigations on the influence of *APOE ε4* on recovery from brain insults; and soon thereafter, the findings that the *ε4* allele is a risk factor for poor outcome after moderate to severe closed head injury began to emerge in the literature [24, 58, 59, 68, 90, 91]. Further, a consecutive series of intracerebral hemorrhage (ICH) patients demonstrated a significant difference in mortality between *APOE ε4*-positive and -negative subjects [3]. There are also intriguing data suggesting that *ε4*-positive cardiopulmonary bypass patients do not recover some neuropsychological parameters as well as *APOE ε4*-negative patients [88]. Nearly all patients in the study exhibited cognitive deficits immediately following surgery; however, cognition remained significantly impaired in *APOE ε4*-beraring patients several months following the procedure.

Inheritance of *APOE ε4* also appears to influence cognitive function decades following traumatic brain injury. Mayeux and colleagues extended observations on the relationship between *APOE ε4* and recovery from brain injury by examining the association between *APOE*, head trauma and AD, basing their study on an earlier suggestion that head injury was a risk factor for AD [58, 59]. There was a relatively striking 10-fold increase in the risk of AD when an *ε4* allele bearing subject had a history of traumatic brain injury, compared with a 2-fold increase in risk with the *ε4* alone. Head injury in the absence of an *APOE ε4* allele did not increase the risk for the disease. These risk factors appear to act synergistically, whereby *APOE ε4*-positive individuals are even more likely to develop AD if they sustain a closed head injury earlier in life. Several later case-control studies confirmed that *APOE ε4* together with head injury increases the risk of developing AD later in life [46, 50, 58, 59, 68, 87]. Given the similarities between AD and dementia pugilistica, the relationship between *APOE* alleles and chronic traumatic brain injury in boxers was evaluated a few years later [40]. Their finding suggested that possession of a *ε4* allele was associated with increased severity of chronic neurological deficits in boxers with high exposure (number of boxing bouts). Somewhat contrary to what one would predict, a recent study of demographic, structural and genetic predictors of long-term cognitive outcome in Vietnam veterans more than thirty years after suffering penetrating head injury did not find an association between *APOE ε4* and cognitive decline in later life [69].

It is not known whether the same mechanism that leads to an increased risk and earlier onset of AD is involved in poorer recovery from brain stresses. There is some evidence suggesting that both *APOE ε4* and closed head injury may influence to risk of AD via interactions with amyloid-β (Aβ). Diffuse Aβ deposits can be found in approximately one third of the subjects who either have undergone surgical treatment within hours of traumatic brain injury [38] or who die shortly after closed head injury [71]. A significant percentage of these patients are *APOE ε4*-positve [18, 47, 64, 65, 91]

Apoe and the Etiology of AD

The genetics of *APOE* as a major risk for AD and its role in neuropathology have been well documented over the past 16 years. However, neither the normal nor pathological functions of apoE in the CNS are solidly known and accepted. Prior to the discovery of the association of *APOE* with susceptibility to AD, there were only a handful of studies on apoE in the CNS. Accumulating data suggest that CNS apoE has multiple functions, and so far, it is the only protein that has been associated with both the pathological and metabolic disturbances of the disease, including amyloid plaque deposition, neurofibillary tangle formation, glucose utilization, synaptic loss, cholinergic dysfunction, oxidative stress, and lipid homeostasis deregulation [8, 53].

Apoe and Neuropathology

Amyloid plaques and neurofibrillary tangles are the two pathological hallmarks of AD. The extracellular role of apoE in amyloid plaque formation and Aβ peptide clearance has generated much experimental activity. ApoE is present in amyloid plaques and Aβ levels are increased in brains of AD patients bearing an *APOE ε4* allele [79]. Similar findings have been reported in transgenic mice expressing human apoE isoforms [19, 34]. Several studies have shown apoE isoform-specific binding to Aβ; however, it remains to be determined whether apoE4 has an active, detrimental role in facilitating amyloid deposition or if apoE2 and apoE3 have a protective role in enhanced Aβ clearance. Both in vitro and in vivo studies demonstrate that apoE4 both stimulates Aβ depositon and inhibits Aβ clearance resulting in amyloid plaques. [51, 76, 84, 98]

ApoE may also have an isoform-specific influence on the abnormal phosphorylation of tau, leading to the formation of neurofibrillary tangles. In vitro studies have demonstrated that apoE3, but not apoE4, forms a detergent stable complex with nonphorphorylated tau. ApoE3 does not interact with phosphorylated tau, suggesting that apoE3 may be able to inhibit abnormal tau hyperphosphorylation [85]. A neuronal effect of apoE4 on tau phosphorylation has been indicated in transgenic mice studies. Increased tau phosphorylation was observed in mice expressing human apoE4 in neurons, but not in mice with apoE expression limited to astrocytes [6, 92]. The N-terminal domain of apoE3 irreversibly binds to the tau protein's microtubule-binding repeat regions [85], and C-terminal truncated apoE stimulates tau phorphorylation and neuronal neurofibrlillary tangle-like inclusion formation [33]. Over the years, there has been skepticism that apoE, a normally secreted protein, could interact with tau in the cytoplasm. Recent research has identified several membrane penetrating proteins, including HIV-1 TAT which are taken up by cells and ultimately enter the cytosol. As reviewed by Mahley et al [57], apoE closely resembles these cell-penetrating peptides, and domain mapping has identified that the positively charged receptor binding region and the hydrophobic lipid binding regions are required for apoE translocation into the cytosol. Furthermore, ultrastructural evidence of cytoplasmic apoE has been noted human neurons [31] and liver [30]. The apoE immunoreactivity associates with the outer membranes of mitochondria and peroxisomes.

Apoe and Neuronal Repair

Neurons are repaired and remodeled throughout life to maintain connectivity. ApoE, as a lipid transporter, has an important function in these processes. ApoE2 and apoE3 are effective in maintaining and repairing neuronal cells while apoE4 is less efficient [56]. This is likely due to the impaired ability of apoE4 in promoting cholesterol efflux from both neurons and astrocytes [60]. An interesting observation in an olfactory nerve repair study in *APOE* knockout mice was markedly delayed regeneration of the olfactory nerve in the absence of apoE [86]. The study's end point of regeneration was not different between wild type and *APOE* knockout mice which suggested that apoE affected the rate of repair but not the endpoint of recovery. The authors speculate that the delay in olfactory nerve regeneration in the knock out mouse represents inefficient lipid utilization. In the absence of apoE protein, lipid would require less efficient methods of delivery.

Apoe and Neurotoxicity

Relatively recent research on apoE structure and function from the Gladstone Institute has cumulated in new hypotheses for AD-related neurodegeneration that are independent of amyloid (for detailed reviews, see [54, 57]). They have proposed that neuron-specific cleavage of apoE results in neurotoxic fragments. Further, the differing conformational stability of the three apoE isoforms leads to differing susceptibility to enzymatic cleavage, with apoE4 being the least stable isoform and most vunerable to proteolysis by the neuron-specific enzyme. The conformation of apoE3 is more stable, and the isoforms is cleaved to a lesser degree.

Protein instability is a major component of several neurodegenerative disorders, including Alzheimer's disease, Parkinson's disease, Huntington's disease, frontotemporal lobe dementia, prion diseases, and motor neuron disease [89]. With regard to apoE and AD, the Gladstone researchers propose that neuronal expression of apoE is induced to promote neuronal repair or protection. However, apoE4 is less effective in these processes and becomes detrimental to the health of a neuron because of its susceptibility to neuronal proteolysis.

C-terminal truncated apoE fragments are present in the brains of AD patients and transgenic mice expressing neuronal apoE. The cleaving enzyme is neuron-specific, and apoE4 is highly susceptible to proteolysis. ApoE3 is less so. The truncated apoE is translocated into the cytosol and has several effects, including neurotoxicity and accumulation of the fragments with mitochondria and neurofibrillary tangle-like structures. Mitochondrial dysfunction has been described in AD patients, particularly those with an *APOE ε4* allele [27]. There are supporting data that the localization of toxic apoE fragments to the mitochondria could have the deleterious consequences of induction of the mitochondrial apoptosis pathway, disruption of mitochondrial regulation of glucose metabolism, decreased synaptogenesis, and disruption of mitochondrial trafficking [57].

Apoe and Mitochondrial Dysfunction

Several independent discoveries over the past 16 years resulted in the formulation of a new hypothesis supporting the role of mitochondrial metabolic dysfunction in the pathogenesis of AD [74]. In the proposal, apoE4>apoE3 toxic degradation products alter mitochondrial function, metabolism and axonal transport. These events result in a chronic decreased rate of glucose utilization and a subsequent impairment of mitochondrial transport to maintain dendritic plasticity, and precede the secondary formation of amyloid plaques, neurofibrillary tangles and atrophy. The discoveries include 1) the association of *APOE* genotypes with age of onset distributions for late-onset AD and subsequent studies in *APOE* knockout and humanized transgenic mice demonstrating alteration in protein levels of key glucose metabolic enzymes 2) the influence of *APOE ε4* on lower glucose utilization in AD patients and normal, healthy subjects two decades before the onset of disease 3) the finding that neuronal apoE4>apoE3>apoE2 degradation products are toxic to mitochondrial function; 4) demonstration of increased mitogenesis and associated increased gene expression of subunits of glucose metabolizing enzymes with PPARγ agonists treatment; and 5) Phase IIA clinical trial data with rosiglitazone maleate, a PPARγ agonist marketed to treat type 2 diabetes, suggesting better efficacy in subjects lacking a *ε4* allele.

As noted by Sager and Johnson [75], this hypothesis joins others in the opinion that there is an important role for abnormal glucose utilization in the development of the disease [14, 82]. Elevated plasma insulin and reduced insulin sensitivity have been demonstrated in AD patients, and both of these factors have been linked to the development of dementia later in life [23, 49]. Likewise, diabetes has been identified as a risk factor for later cognitive decline and dementia [17, 52].

The suggestive influence of *APOE* alleles on treatment with rosiglitazone is interesting. The first hint was in a small preliminary phase IIA study of AD patients that was initiated in 2001. Efficacy results hinted at the possibility of increased responsiveness in a few patients lacking an *APOE ε4* allele [94, 95]. These clinical trial data helped support the rationale for a strategic decision to move forward with a larger dose-ranging phase IIB study with a new, un-marketed formulation of rosiglitazone. Prospectively defined exploratory analyses of the Phase IIB data raised the possibility of an interaction between treatment efficacy and the absence or presence of the *ε4* allele. *APOE ε4*-negative subjects showed significant clinical improvement [70]. Phase III studies are underway to confirm efficacy and to determine whether there is a gradient of benefit that is observed in all subjects depending on their specific *APOE* genotypes, or whether there are some subjects who receive no benefit.

There are also hints that *APOE ε4*-negative AD patients have better efficacy on cognition and function taking Ketasyn, a ketogenic shake in clinical development by Accera[1]. Like the investigations of rosiglitazone to ameliorate CNS glucose hypometabolism, the ketones generated by the liver following ingestion of the shake offer an alternate food source to the brain. Two small pilot studies of another PPARγ agonist, pioglitazone, have noted small benefits in cognition; *APOE* effects were not noted [26, 32].

Conclusion

Since the discovery of the robust genetic association of *APOE* with AD in 1993, remarkable advances have been made in defining the susceptibility genetics of *APOE* in AD and the detrimental influence of the *ε4* variant on recovery from acute brain stresses. While the peripheral role of apoE as plasma lipid-transport molecule has been well documented over the past few decades, delineation of the normal functions of apoE in the central nervous system and the protein's role in the etiology of AD has lagged behind. Unfortunately, both purified ApoE and the APOE mouse models can be temperamental in the laboratory, hampering experimental efforts. Research over the past 15 years suggests apoE is a protein that is involved in several distinct biological responses, with critical functions in the central nervous system that include energy metabolism, lipid transport and synaptic repair, neurotoxicity, signaling, and cholinergic dysfunction. Perhaps the most intriguing developments over the past few years are the AD as a "type 3 diabetes" and mitochondrial dysfunction hypotheses. These views are independent of the favored amyloid and tau strategies of drug development, and open the door to exploration of new therapeutic interventions for the disease based on manipulation of apoE fragment neurotoxicity and CNS glucose metabolism.

References

[1] Accera. Experimental Drug Ketasyn (AC-1202) treats Alzheimer's as Diabetes of the Brain. *http://www.accerapharma.com/2007/news21.html* . 2009.

[2] Aerssens,J. *et al.* APOE genotype: No influence on galantamine treatment efficacy nor on rate of decline in Alzheimer's disease. *Dementia and Geriatric Cognitive Disorders* 12, 69-77 (2001).

[3] Alberts,M.J. *et al.* ApoE genotype and survival from intracerebral haemorrhage [7]. *Lancet* 346, 575 (1995).

[4] Asada,T., Kariya,T., Yamagata,Z., Kinoshita,T., & Asaka,A. ApoE ε4 allele and cognitive decline in patients with Alzheimer's disease. *Neurology* 47, 603 (1996).

[5] Basun,H., Grut,M., Winblad,B., & Lannfelt,L. Apolipoprotein e4 allele and disease progression in patients with late-onset Alzheimer's disease. *Neuroscience Letters* 183, 32-34 (1995).

[6] Brecht,W.J. *et al.* Neuron-Specific Apolipoprotein E4 Proteolysis Is Associated with Increased Tau Phosphorylation in Brains of Transgenic Mice. *Journal of Neuroscience* 24, 2527-2534 (2004).

[7] Brouwers,N., Sleegers,K., & Van Broeckhoven,C. Molecular genetics of Alzheimer's disease: An update. *Annals of Medicine* 40, 562-583 (2008).

[8] Cedazo-Mínguez,A. Apolipoprotein e and Alzheimer's disease: Molecular mechanisms and therapeutic opportunities: Alzheimer Review Series. *Journal of Cellular and Molecular Medicine* 11, 1227-1238 (2007).

[9] Chen,C.H. *et al.* A comparative study to screen dementia and APOE genotypes in an ageing East African population. *Neurobiology of Aging . Ref Type:* In Press

[10] Chen,C.H. *et al.* A comparative study to screen dementia and APOE genotypes in an ageing East African population. *Neurobiology of Aging* In Press, Corrected Proof.

[11] Corder,E.H. *et al.* Protective effect of apolipoprotein E type 2 allele for late onset Alzheimer disease. *Nature Genetics* 7, 180-184 (1994).

[12] Corder,E.H. *et al.* Apolipoprotein E, survival in Alzheimer's disease patients, and the competing risks of death and Alzheimer's disease. *Neurology* 45, 1323-1328 (1995).

[13] Corder,E.H. *et al.* Gene dose of apolipoprotein E type 4 allele and the risk of Alzheimer's disease in late onset families. *Science* 261, 921-923 (1993).

[14] Craft,S. *et al.* Memory improvement following induced hyperinsulinemia in Alzheimer's disease. *Neurobiology of Aging* 17, 123-130 (1996).

[15] Craft,S. *et al.* Accelerated decline in apolipoprotein E-4 homozygotes with Alzheimer's disease. *Neurology* 51, 149-153 (1998).

[16] Dal Forno,G. *et al.* Apolipoprotein E genotype and rate of decline in probable Alzheimer's disease. *Archives of Neurology* 53, 345-350 (1996).

[17] Dash,S.K. Cognitive impairment and diabetes. *Recent Patents on Endocrine, Metabolic and Immune Drug Discovery* 2, 218-223 (2008).

[18] DeKosky,S.T. *et al.* Association of increased cortical soluble $A\beta_{42}$ levels with diffuse plaques after severe brain injury in humans. *Archives of Neurology* 64, 541-544 (2007).

[19] Dolev,I. & Michaelson,D.M. A nontransgenic mouse model shows inducible amyloid-β (Aβ) peptide deposition and elucidates the role of apolipoprotein E in the amyloid

cascade. *Proceedings Of The National Academy Of Sciences Of The United States Of America* 101, 13909-13914 (2004).

[20] Elshourbagy,N.A., Liao,W.S., Mahley,R.W., & Taylor,J.M. Apolipoprotein E mRNA is abundant in the brain and adrenals, as well as in the liver, and is present in other peripheral tissues of rats and marmosets. *Proceedings Of The National Academy Of Sciences Of The United States Of America* 82, 203-207 (1985).

[21] Farlow,M.R. *et al.* Metrifonate treatment of AD influence of APOE genotype. *Neurology* 53, 2010-2016 (1999).

[22] Farrer,L.A. *et al.* Effects of age, sex, and ethnicity on the association between apolipoprotein E genotype and Alzheimer disease: A meta-analysis. *Journal of the American Medical Association* 278, 1349-1356 (1997).

[23] Fishel,M.A. *et al.* Hyperinsulinemia provokes synchronous increases in central inflammation and β-amyloid in normal adults. *Archives of Neurology* 62, 1539-1544 (2005).

[24] Friedman,G. *et al.* Apolipoprotein E-ε4 genotype predicts a poor outcome in survivors of traumatic brain injury. *Neurology* 52, 244-248 (1999).

[25] Frisoni,G.B. *et al.* Gene dose of the ε4 allele of apolipoprotein E and disease progression in sporadic late-onset Alzheimer's disease. *Annals of Neurology* 37, 596-604 (1995).

[26] Geldmacher D, Fritsch T, & McClendon M A pilot study of pioglitazone in Alzheimer's disease. *Int Conf Alz Dis Rel Dementias Madrid*(2006).

[27] Gibson,G.E. *et al.* Mitochondrial damage in Alzheimer's disease varies with apolipoprotein E genotype. *Annals of Neurology* 48, 297-303 (2000).

[28] Gomez-Isla,T. *et al.* Clinical and pathological correlates of apolipoprotein ε4 in Alzheimer's disease. *Annals of Neurology* 39, 62-70 (1996).

[29] Growdon,J.H., Locascio,J.J., Corkin,S., Gomez-Isla,T., & Hyman,B.T. Apolipoprotein E genotype does not influence rates of cognitive decline in Alzheimer's disease. *Neurology* 47, 444-448 (1996).

[30] Hamilton,R.L., Wong,J.S., Guo,L.S.S., Krisans,S., & Havel,R.J. Apolipoprotein E localization in rat hepatocytes by immunogold labeling of cryothin sections. *Journal of Lipid Research* 31, 1589-1603 (1990).

[31] Han,S.H. *et al.* Apolipoprotein E is localized to the cytoplasm of human cortical neurons: A light and electron microscopic study. *Journal of Neuropathology and Experimental Neurology* 53, 535-544 (1994).

[32] Hanyu,H., Sato,T., Kiuchi,A., Sakurai,H., & Iwamoto,T. Pioglitazone improved cognition in a pilot study on patients with alzheimer's disease and mild cognitive impairment with diabetes mellitus. *Journal of the American Geriatrics Society* 57, 177-179 (2009).

[33] Harris,F.M. *et al.* Carboxyl-terminal-truncated apolipoprotein E4 causes Alzheimer's disease-like neurodegeneration and behavioral deficits in transgenic mice. *Proceedings Of The National Academy Of Sciences Of The United States Of America* 100, 10966-10971 (2003).

[34] Hartman,R.E. *et al.* Apolipoprotein E4 influences amyloid deposition but not cell loss after traumatic brain injury in a mouse model of Alzheimer's disease. *Journal of Neuroscience* 22, 10083-10087 (2002).

[35] Harwood,D.G., Barker,W.W., Ownby,R.L., Mullan,M., & Duara,R. Apolipoprotein E polymorphism and cognitive impairment in a bi-ethnic community-dwelling elderly sample. *Alzheimer Disease and Associated Disorders* 16, 8-14 (2002).

[36] Hirono,N., Hashimoto,M., Yasuda,M., Kazui,H., & Mori,E. Accelerated memory decline in Alzheimer's disease with apolipoprotein ε4 allele. *Journal of Neuropsychiatry and Clinical Neurosciences* 15, 354-358 (2003).

[37] Holmes,C., Levy,R., McLoughlin,D.M., Powell,J.F., & Lovestone,S. Apolipoprotein E: Non-cognitive symptoms and cognitive decline in late onset Alzheimer's disease. *Journal of Neurology Neurosurgery and Psychiatry* 61, 580-583 (1996).

[38] Ikonomovic,M.D. *et al.* Alzheimer's pathology in human temporal cortex surgically excised after severe brain injury. *Experimental Neurology* 190, 192-203 (2004).

[39] Jonker,C., Schmand,B., Lindeboom,J., Havekes,L.M., & Launer,L.J. Association between apolipoprotein E ε4 and the rate of cognitive decline in community-dwelling elderly individuals with and without dementia. *Archives of Neurology* 55, 1065-1069 (1998).

[40] Jordan,B.D. *et al.* Apolipoprotein E ε4 associated with chronic traumatic brain injury in boxing. *Journal of the American Medical Association* 278, 136-140 (1997).

[41] Kleiman,T. *et al.* Apolipoprotein E ε4 allele is unrelated to cognitive or functional decline in Alzheimer's disease: Retrospective and prospective analysis. *Dementia and Geriatric Cognitive Disorders* 22, 73-82 (2006).

[42] Kurz,A. *et al.* Apolipoprotein E ε4 allele, cognitive decline, and deterioration of everyday performance in Alzheimer's disease. *Neurology* 47, 440-443 (1996).

[43] LaDu,M.J. *et al.* Nascent astrocyte particles differ from lipoproteins in CSF. *Journal of Neurochemistry* 70, 2070-2081 (1998).

[44] Lee,J.H. *et al.* Age-at-onset linkage analysis in Caribbean Hispanics with familial late-onset Alzheimer's disease. *Neurogenetics* 9, 51-60 (2008).

[45] Lehtovirta,M. *et al.* Longitudinal SPECT study in Alzheimer's disease: Relation to apolipoprotein E polymorphism. *Journal of Neurology Neurosurgery and Psychiatry* 64, 742-746 (1998).

[46] Lendon,C.L. *et al.* Genetic variation of the APOE promoter and outcome after head injury. *Neurology* 61, 683-685 (2003).

[47] Lichtman,S.W., Seliger,G., Tycko,B., & Marder,K. Apolipoprotein E and functional recovery from brain injury following postacute rehabilitation. *Neurology* 55, 1536-1539 (2000).

[48] Linton,M.F. *et al.* Phenotypes of apolipoprotein B and apolipoprotein E after liver transplantation. *Journal of Clinical Investigation* 88, 270-281 (1991).

[49] Luchsinger,J.A., Tang,M.X., Shea,S., & Mayeux,R. Hyperinsulinemia and risk of Alzheimer disease. *Neurology* 63, 1187-1192 (2004).

[50] Luukinen,H. *et al.* Risk of dementia associated with the ApoE ε4 allele and falls causing head injury without explicit traumatic brain injury. *Acta Neurologica Scandinavica* 118, 153-158 (2008).

[51] Ma,J., Yee,A., Brewer,J., Das,S., & Potter,H. Amyloid-associated proteins α1-antichymotrypsin and apolipoprotein E promote assembly of Alzheimer β-protein into filaments. *Nature* 372, 92-94 (1994).

[52] Maggi,S. *et al.* Diabetes as a risk factor for cognitive decline in older patients. *Dementia and Geriatric Cognitive Disorders* 27, 24-33 (2009).

[53] Mahley,R.W. & Huang,Y. Apolipoprotein E: From atherosclerosis to Alzheimer's disease and beyond. *Current Opinion in Lipidology* 10, 207-217 (1999).

[54] Mahley,R.W., Huang,Y., & Weisgraber,K.H. Detrimental effects of apolipoprotein E4: Potential therapeutic targets in Alzheimer's disease. *Current Alzheimer Research* 4, 537-540 (2007).

[55] Mahley,R.W. & Rall,J. Apolipoprotein E: Far more than a lipid transport protein. *Annual Review of Genomics and Human Genetics* 1, 507-537 (2000).

[56] Mahley,R.W. & Rall,J. Apolipoprotein E: Far more than a lipid transport protein. *Annual Review of Genomics and Human Genetics* 1, 507-537 (2000).

[57] Mahley,R.W., Weisgraber,K.H., & Huang,Y. Apolipoprotein E4: A causative factor and therapeutic target in neuropathology, including Alzheimer's disease. *Proceedings Of The National Academy Of Sciences Of The United States Of America* 103, 5644-5651 (2006).

[58] Mayeux,R. *et al.* Synergistic effects of traumatic head injury and apolipoprotein-ε4 in patients with Alzheimer's disease. *Neurology* 45, 555-557 (1995).

[59] Mayeux,R. *et al.* Genetic susceptibility and head injury as risk factors for Alzheimer's disease among community-dwelling elderly persons and their first-degree relatives. *Annals of Neurology* 33, 494-501 (1993).

[60] Michikawa,M., Fan,Q.W., Isobe,I., & Yanagisawa,K. Apolipoprotein E exhibits isoform-specific promotion of lipid efflux from astrocytes and neurons in culture. *Journal of Neurochemistry* 74, 1008-1016 (2000).

[61] Mori,E. *et al.* Accelerated hippocampal atrophy in Alzheimer's disease with apolipoprotein E ε4 allele. *Annals of Neurology* 51, 209-214 (2002).

[62] Murphy,J., Taylor,J., Kraemer,H.C., Yesavage,J., & Tinklenberg,J.R. No association between Apolipoprotein E ε4 allele and rate of decline in Alzheimer's disease. *American Journal of Psychiatry* 154, 603-608 (1997).

[63] Neely,M.D. & Montine,T.J. CSF lipoproteins and Alzheimer's disease. *Journal of Nutrition, Health and Aging* 6, 383-391 (2002).

[64] Nicoll,J.A.R., Roberts,G.W., & Graham,D.I. Apolipoprotein E ε4 allele is associated with deposition of amyloid β- protein following head injury. *Nature Medicine* 1, 135-137 (1995).

[65] Nicoll,J.A.R., Roberts,G.W., & Graham,D.I. Amyloid +¦-protein, APOE genotype and head injury. 777, 271-275. 1996. Ref Type: Serial (Book,Monograph)

[66] Osuntokun,B.O. *et al.* Lack of an association between apolipoprotein E ε and Alzheimer's disease in elderly Nigerians. *Annals of Neurology* 38, 463-465 (1995).

[67] Pitas,R.E., Boyles,J.K., Lee,S.H., Hui,D., & Weisgraber,K.H. Lipoproteins and their receptors in the central nervous system. Characterization of the lipoproteins in cerebrospinal fluid and identification of apolipoprotein B,E(LDL) receptors in the brain. *Journal of Biological Chemistry* 262, 14352-14360 (1987).

[68] Plassman,B.L. *et al.* Documented head injury in early adulthood and risk of Alzheimer's disease and other dementias. *Neurology* 55, 1158-1166 (2000).

[69] Raymont,V. *et al.* Demographic, structural and genetic predictors of late cognitive decline after penetrating head injury. *Brain* 131, 543-558 (2008).

[70] Risner,M.E. *et al.* Efficacy of rosiglitazone in a genetically defined population with mild-to-moderate Alzheimer's disease. *Pharmacogenomics Journal* 6, 246-254 (2006).

[71] Roberts,G.W., Gentleman,S.M., Lynch,A., & Graham,D.I. βA4 amyloid protein deposition in brain after head trauma. *Lancet* 338, 1422-1423 (1991).

[72] Roses,A.D., Devlin,B., & Conneally,P.M. Measuring the genetic contribution of APOE in late-onset Alzheimer disease (AD). *Am J Hum Genet* 57, (1995).

[73] Roses,A.D., Saunders,A., Nicoll,J.A.R., Graham,D.I., & Roberts,G.W. Head injury, amyloid β and Alzheimer's disease [2]. *Nature Medicine* 1, 603-604 (1995).

[74] Roses,A.D. & Saunders,A.M. Perspective on a pathogenesis and treatment of Alzheimer's disease. *Alzheimer's and Dementia* 2, 59-70 (2006).

[75] Sager,M.A. & Johnson,S.C. Commentary on "Perspective on a pathogenesis and treatment of Alzheimer's disease." Comment on the mitochondrial metabolism hypothesis. *Alzheimer's and Dementia* 2, 74-75 (2006).

[76] Sanan,D.A. *et al.* Apolipoprotein E associates with β amyloid peptide of Alzheimer's disease to form novel monofibrils. Isoform ApoE4 associates more efficiently than ApoE3. *Journal of Clinical Investigation* 94, 860-869 (1994).

[77] Saunders,A.M. *et al.* Association of apolipoprotein E allele ε4 with late-onset familial and sporadic Alzheimer's disease. *Neurology* 43, 1467-1472 (1993).

[78] Sayi,J.G. *et al.* Apolipoprotein e polymorphism in elderly East Africans. *East African Medical Journal* 74, 668-670 (1997).

[79] Schmechel,D.E. *et al.* Increased amyloid β-peptide deposition in cerebral cortex as a consequence of apolipoprotein E genotype in late-onset Alzheimer disease. *Proceedings Of The National Academy Of Sciences Of The United States Of America* 90, 9649-9653 (1993).

[80] Slooter,A.J.C. *et al.* Apolipoprotein E genotype and progression of Alzheimer's disease: The Rotterdam Study. *Journal of Neurology* 246, 304-308 (1999).

[81] Sorbi,S., Nacmius B., & Piacentini S. Apolipoprotein E genotypes and outcome after post-traumatic coma. Neurology 46, A307. 1996. Ref Type: Generic

[82] Steen,E. *et al.* Impaired insulin and insulin-like growth factor expression and signaling mechanisms in Alzheimer's disease - Is this type 3 diabetes? *Journal of Alzheimer's Disease* 7, 63-80 (2005).

[83] Stern,Y. *et al.* The absence of an apolipoprotem ε4 allele is associated with a more aggressive form of Alzheimer's disease. *Annals of Neurology* 41, 615-620 (1997).

[84] Strittmatter,W.J. *et al.* Apolipoprotein E: High-avidity binding to β-amyloid and increased frequency of type 4 allele in late-onset familial Alzheimer disease. *Proceedings Of The National Academy Of Sciences Of The United States Of America* 90, 1977-1981 (1993).

[85] Strittmatter,W.J. *et al.* Hypothesis: Microtubule instability and paired helical filament formation in the Alzheimer disease brain are related to apolipoprotein E genotype. *Experimental Neurology* 125, 163-171 (1994).

[86] Struble,R.G., Cady,C., Nathan,B.P., & McAsey,M. Apolipoprotein E may be a critical factor in hormone therapy neuroprotection. *Frontiers in bioscience : a journal and virtual library* 13, 5387-5405 (2008).

[87] Sundström,A. *et al.* Increased risk of dementia following mild head injury for carriers but not for non-carriers of the APOE ε4 allele. *International Psychogeriatrics* 19, 159-165 (2007).

[88] Tardiff,B.E. *et al.* Preliminary report of a genetic basis for cognitive decline after cardiac operations. *Annals of Thoracic Surgery* 64, 715-720 (1997).

[89] Taylor,J.P., Hardy,J., & Fischbeck,K.H. Toxic proteins in neurodegenerative disease. *Science* 296, 1991-1995 (2002).

[90] Teasdale,G.M., Murray,G.D., & Nicoll,J.A.R. The association between APOE ε4, age and outcome after head injury: A prospective cohort study. *Brain* 128, 2556-2561 (2005).

[91] Teasdale,G.M., Nicoll,J.A.R., Murray,G., & Fiddes,M. Association of apolipoprotein E polymorphism with outcome after head injury. *Lancet* 350, 1069-1071 (1997).

[92] Tesseur,I. *et al.* Expression of human apolipoprotein E4 in neurons causes hyperphosphorylation of protein tau in the brains of transgenic mice. *American Journal of Pathology* 156, 951-964 (2000).

[93] Tycko,B. *et al.* APOE and APOC1 promoter polymorphisms and the risk of Alzheimer disease in African American and Caribbean Hispanic individuals. *Archives of Neurology* 61, 1434-1439 (2004).

[94] Watson,G.S. *et al.* Preserved cognition in patients with early Alzheimer disease and amnestic mild cognitive impairment during treatment with rosiglitazone: A preliminary study. *American Journal of Geriatric Psychiatry* 13, 950-958 (2005).

[95] Watson,G.S. & Craft,S. The role of insulin resistance in the pathogenesis of Alzheimer's disease: Implications for treatment. *CNS Drugs* 17, 27-45 (2003).

[96] Weisgraber,K.H. Apolipoprotein E: Structure-function relationships. *Advances in Protein Chemistry* 45, 249-302 (1994).

[97] Wiederkehr,F., Ogilvie,A., & Vonderschmitt,D.J. Cerebrospinal fluid proteins studied by two-dimensional gel electrophoresis and immunoblotting technique. *Journal of Neurochemistry* 49, 363-372 (1987).

[98] Wisniewski,T., Castan?o,E.M., Golabek,A., Vogel,T., & Frangione,B. Acceleration of Alzheimer's fibril formation by apolipoprotein E in vitro. *American Journal of Pathology* 145, 1030-1035 (1994).

[99] Xu,P.T. *et al.* Specific regional transcription of apolipoprotein E in human neurons. *Am. J. Pathol.* 154, 601-611 (1999).

[100] Xu,P.T. *et al.* Human apolipoprotein E2, E3, and E4 isoform-specific transgenic mice: Human-like pattern of glial and neuronal immunoreactivity in central nervous system not observed in wild-type mice. *Neurobiology of Disease* 3, 229-245 (1996).

In: Alzheimer's Disease and Dementia (Vol. 4)
Editor: Miao-Kun Sun
ISBN:978-1-60876-152-4

Chapter VII

Chronic Inflammation and Alzheimer's Disease

Douglas G. Walker*[*], *Jason Yuan and Lih-Fen Lue
Laboratory of Neuroinflammation, Sun Health Research Institute, Sun City, Arizona, U.S.A.

Abstract

More than 20 years ago, pathological studies of postmortem Alzheimer's disease (AD) affected brains identified the significant presence of activated microglia in association with senile amyloid beta peptide containing plaques and neurofibrillary tangles, the hallmark pathological features of the disease. These studies, along with the identification of activated complement in association with these structures, led to the hypothesis that a form of chronic inflammation was ongoing in AD brains, likely contributing to degenerative processes. The apparent absence of neutrophil and lymphocyte infiltrations in AD brains indicated that a chronic, rather than acute, inflammatory response was ongoing, likely fueled by the persistence of the plaques and tangles. Since then a large number of different studies, including gene expression profiling and proteomic analyses of AD brains or biofluids, have identified many inflammatory components to be upregulated in association with AD pathology. Also, a number of retrospective epidemiology studies have demonstrated that anti-inflammatory drugs appear protective for AD. Despite these data, the failure of prospective clinical trials of anti-inflammatories to show effectiveness in treating AD, and the effectiveness of the Aβ vaccine strategy, at least in mice models of AD, caused interest in "*inflammation and AD*" to diminish. Although neuroinflammation is a prominent feature in most neurodegenerative diseases, abandoning control of inflammation as a therapeutic strategy has only been proposed in AD; this seems an unreasonable shift in paradigm, and is based mainly on studies with AD mice models, which do not completely represent

[*]Correspondence: Dr. Douglas G. Walker, Sun Health Research Institute, 10515 West Santa Fe Drive, Sun City, AZ, 85351, U.S.A., Tel no: (623)-876-5623, Email: Douglas.walker@bannerhealth.com

the human AD brain. In this article, we will examine recent evidence that a type of chronic inflammation is ongoing in AD brains. Neuroinflammation in AD brains can be considered a breakdown of existing inflammatory control mechanisms, a feature of aging that is exacerbated in AD. We suggest new approaches are needed to effectively treat this chronic inflammation so as to reduce the neuronal damage that leads to memory symptoms in AD patients.

Introduction

With the aging of the population, and as a result of more effective treatments for heart disease, cancer, cerebrovascular disease and infectious diseases, the incidence of death due to Alzheimer's disease (AD) can expect to climb. The impending epidemic of AD in the aged is becoming apparent, but at present is underrepresented in official death records. Current mortality statistics for 2005 in the United States show AD as the 7th overall certified cause of death in the whole population (Kung *et al.* 2008). Of a total of 2,448,017 certified deaths in 2005, 71,599 were listed as being due to AD; this compares to 652,091 due to heart disease, 559,312 due to cancer, and 143,579 due to stroke/cerebrovascular disease. It is widely appreciated that AD patients can die due to pneumonia, if institutionalized, or from cerebrovascular or cardiac disease, so it is understood that AD as a certified cause of death is under reported. This is apparent in the fact that there has been a 1,200% increase from 1970 to 1998 in AD as a reported cause of death (Kung *et al.* 2008). This is believed due to increasing consciousness of physicians of AD as a disease entity; previous generations of doctors had likely simply diagnosed AD as senility of the aged. However, these same statistics clearly show that AD is a disease that only affects the aged (Kung *et al.* 2008). Of those 71,599 certified to have died from AD, 67,045 were 75 years or older. Basing the incidence of AD on death certification is likely to make the disease incidence to be highly underrepresented; a study of death certificates of Canadians over 65 years of age with a clinical diagnosis of AD showed that 85.2% had other causes of death listed (Chamandy and Wolfson 2005;Koutsavlis and Wolfson 2000). These studies of elderly Canadians showed firstly that dementia was associated with pneumonia as an increased cause of death, and secondly that most dementia subjects had cardiovascular or cerebrovascular diseases listed as the primary cause of death (Chamandy and Wolfson 2005;Koutsavlis and Wolfson 2000).

The Alzheimer's Association estimates that there are 4.5 million people in the U.S. with AD; a number that is expected to rise to 12 million by 2050. At present, it is estimated that 1 in 10 over 65 years of age have AD, and up to half for those over 85 years. The incidence rates and prevalence of AD in developed Western nations are similar to the U.S. The annual cost of caring for an AD patient is currently estimated at \$ 35,000 - 75,000 (depending on the level of care) and the total can be expected to rise proportionally with the expected higher incidence of cases. The major reason for outlining these statistics is to highlight that AD is becoming a silent epidemic in developed nations as the population ages, and also to put inflammatory causes for this disease back into perspective along with the other major causes of death in the elderly (heart disease, stroke, cancer), all of which have chronic inflammation as significant pathological features.

There have been a number of excellent reviews of AD and inflammation in recent years that address whole aspects of the field [Examples (Dheen *et al.* 2007;Heneka and O'Banion 2007;Simi *et al.* 2007;Wyss-Coray 2006)]. Many of these articles reference the large numbers of transgenic mice models to draw conclusions for AD; however all of these models still have to be considered as incomplete representations of human AD (Duyckaerts *et al.* 2008;Schwab *et al.* 2004). Significant work has demonstrated that the deposited Aβ in different transgenic mice has key biochemical differences (molecular sizes, modifications and solubility) compared to AD brain-derived plaques (Kalback *et al.* 2002;Kuo *et al.* 1997;Kuo *et al.* 2000;Kuo *et al.* 2001); as Aβ is the key feature for developing therapeutic treatments by most researchers, these differences in Aβ structure need to be considered when interpreting the effectiveness of Aβ lowering treatments from results with these mice models. Although we do not intend to downplay transgenic studies, and will discuss their key findings about inflammation in following sections, the focus of this article will be to assess what can be learnt from studies with human AD brains or human microglia about inflammatory processes *in vivo*. These studies include recent gene expression profiling or proteomics studies of human disease-affected tissues or biological fluids (blood or CSF) that have identified novel inflammation-related biomarkers of early disease diagnosis/mechanisms.

Features of Chronic Inflammation: Lessons from the Periphery

In the periphery, inflammation is the biological response to injurious stimuli, such as microbial pathogens, damaged cells, or irritants. It involves a complex coordinated response involving a large number of potentially damaging bioactive compounds (cytokines) which are produced by specialized cells (macrophages, neutrophils), and is an essential part of the protective attempt by the organism to remove the injurious stimuli and start the reparative process for the affected tissue. In situations where inflammatory responses are deficient, wounds and infections can not heal, which can compromise the survival of the infected host. However, uncontrolled (chronic) inflammation can lead to a host of diseases; one only needs to look at the examples of atherosclerosis, cancer and rheumatoid arthritis to understand what lessons from these disease mechanisms can be applied to AD (Douglas *et al.* 2007;Gomez-Mejiba *et al.* 2009;Langheinrich and Bohle 2005).

Acute inflammation is a well-regulated and time-limiting response to harmful stimuli, and characterized by trafficking of plasma and leukocytes from the blood into the affected tissues. A cascade of biochemical events, involving the local vascular system, the immune system, and various cells within the injured tissue, propagates and evolves the inflammatory response to completion. Prolonged inflammation, known as chronic inflammation, leads to a progressive shift in the types of cells that are present at the site of inflammation, and is characterized by simultaneous destruction and healing of the tissue from the inflammatory process. A common feature of chronic inflammation is that there is a persistence of the stimuli. This can be as a non-degradable pathogen (tuberculosis bacteria), a non-degradable foreign agent (asbestos), or an autoimmune response to a natural component that is repaired and damaged persistently due to an autoimmune response (involving lymphocytes). In AD, there is a lack of trafficking of plasma or leukocytes into the brain, but there are persistent and non-degradable cellular components, namely Aβ peptide, which is aggregated and chemically modified into neuritic plaques, or neurofibrillary tangles, which represent the aggregated skeletons of dead neurons, to fuel the inflammatory response (Mott and Hulette 2005;Small and Cappai 2006).

Inflammation and Alzheimer's Disease

Despite over 20 years of intense study of inflammation and AD, it has still not been resolved whether inflammation is an initiating factor, a progressing factor, a bystander, or is even beneficial (Wyss-Coray 2006). AD is characterized clinically by a progressive decline in cognitive function; pathologically the hallmark features of the disease are the presence of extracellular Aβ peptide containing plaques, and neurofibrillary tangles. The cause of AD remains unknown; a small percentage of cases have a solely genetic component with mutations in the amyloid precursor protein (APP) gene, the protein from which the 40 or 42 amino acid Aβ is derived by proteolytic cleavage, or in presenilin (PS)-1 or PS-2, which are components of the gamma secretase enzyme complex involved in APP cleavage at the C-terminal of the Aβ peptide (Bertram and Tanzi 2008). These rare genetic mutations, which are autosomal dominant for AD, have provided the strongest evidence for the amyloid hypothesis for AD. As chronic neuroinflammation is still considered by many to be a propagating and progressing factor for tissue loss and cognitive decline in AD (Parachikova *et al.* 2007;Sokolova *et al.* 2008;Venneti *et al.* 2008), the goal of this article is to consider firstly the role of chronic inflammation (both cerebral and vascular) in AD pathology and, secondly to justify why inflammation is still a significant pathogenic process in AD despite arguments to the contrary (Boche and Nicoll 2008). When one considers the inflammatory pathology observed in neurodegenerative conditions besides AD, including Parkinson's disease (PD), multiple sclerosis, amyotrophic lateral sclerosis (ALS), human immunodeficiency virus (HIV) dementia, and also acute conditions such as stroke (Esiri 2007;Jander *et al.* 2007;Sawada *et al.* 2006;Simi *et al.* 2007;Steinman 2008), significant roles for inflammation are apparent. Only in AD, because of the use of immune therapy, is there now a downplaying of the significance of inflammation in pathological processes (Foster *et al.* 2009;Holtzman 2008;McGeer 2008). This can be considered short sighted for several reasons; firstly chronic inflammatory processes are invariably damaging irrespective of the disease or tissue and offer a range of therapeutic targets; secondly there have been significant autoimmune side-effects in humans in the clinical trials of the Aβ vaccine or humanized antibodies to Aβ (Foster *et al.* 2009;Holtzman 2008;McGeer 2008).

The role of Aβ is generally considered central to the etiology of AD. Aβ peptide in different forms can cause direct neurotoxicity with recent emphasis on the role of soluble Aβ oligomers as the driving force for neurotoxicity (De Felice *et al.* 2009;Di 2009;Hung *et al.* 2008). In addition, Aβ can activate a number of inflammatory processes in microglia by binding to cell-surface receptors such as the Receptor for Advanced Glycation Endproducts (RAGE) (Lue *et al.* 2001b;Yan *et al.* 1997) or Toll-like receptor 2 (Jana *et al.* 2008), or directly interact with complement C1q and initiate the classical complement cascade (Rogers *et al.* 1992). However, other components are involved in the disease progression, including the apolipoprotein E ε4 allele, oxidative stress, high cholesterol, blood-brain barrier peripheral vascular changes and cerebral inflammatory changes (Cagnin *et al.* 2007;Cankurtaran *et al.* 2008;Coon *et al.* 2007;Deane *et al.* 2003;DeLegge and Smoke 2008;Hirsch-Reinshagen and Wellington 2007;Panza *et al.* 2007).

With the availability of suitable immunological reagents, pioneering studies were carried out using autopsy derived brain tissues from AD and control cases that demonstrated the distinct presence of activated microglia, the brain resident macrophages, in AD brains associated with the plaque and tangle structures (Dickson and Mattiace 1989;Itagaki *et al.* 1989;Luber-Narod and Rogers 1988;McGeer *et al.* 1987;McGeer *et al.* 1988). These studies, which primarily utilized antibodies to the major histocompatibility complex class II protein HLA-DR, identified stronger staining in microglia that were in close association with AD pathological structures. There was generally observed to be increased numbers of cells immunoreactive for these antigens that had a hypertrophic morphology compared to resting microglia. This increase in staining of tissue microglia showed that the innate immune system was activated in the AD brain. Further studies at that time demonstrated complement activation was also ongoing in the AD brain; it was demonstrated that activated complement fragments C3, C4 and C9 were attached to Aβ plaques, dystrophic neurites and neurofibrillary tangles (Akiyama *et al.* 1991;McGeer *et al.* 1989;Webster *et al.* 1997). Complement C1q, the initiating protein of the classical complement pathway, was also deposited on plaques and tangles (Akiyama *et al.* 1991;McGeer *et al.* 1989;Rogers *et al.* 1992). Although it has been possible to demonstrate the presence of some infiltrating lymphocytes into AD brains (Fiala *et al.* 2002;Itagaki *et al.* 1988;Togo *et al.* 2002), these cells were not a prominent feature in comparison to the infiltration observed in multiple sclerosis. A recent study even suggested that there were decreased numbers of T cells in AD frontal cortex and hippocampus (Parachikova *et al.* 2007). These data suggested that a type of chronic inflammation was ongoing in AD brains with some of the components of an acute antigen-specific adaptive immune response being missing.

Inflammation Studies in Vitro

The inflammatory hypothesis of AD has been extensively studied in experimental models since these earlier pathological studies. Experimental *in vitro* studies using microglia derived from animal sources or from human postmortem brains showed that aggregated (fibrillar and oligomeric) Aβ could activate these cells leading to increased production of many different cytokines, chemokines, reactive oxygen species and proinflammatory enzymes, including interleukin (IL)-1β, IL-6, tumor necrosis factor (TNF)-α and monocyte chemoattractant protein (MCP)-1 [examples (Bianca *et al.* 1999;Lue *et al.* 2001a;Qin *et al.* 2002;Walker *et al.* 2006)]. A fundamental difference exists between rodent and human microglia in that the latter cell type does not have the capacity to produce significant amounts of nitric oxide (Lee *et al.* 1993). Aβ treatment of rodent microglia induces high levels of NO, which can be neurotoxic, while human microglia produce little or none (Roy *et al.* 2008;Tan *et al.* 2000;Walker *et al.* 1995).

Animal Models of AD Inflammation

In the different transgenic mice models of AD, constructed with copies of the human APP gene containing various of the identified mutations, microglial responses to Aβ plaques could be detected (Apelt and Schliebs 2001;Benzing *et al.* 1999;Bornemann *et al.* 2001), but these responses appear less well developed compared to what was observed in AD brains (Schwab *et al.* 2004). It has been suggested that the transgenic mice models of AD are poor representations of human AD as the Aβ deposits are more easily dissolved than human AD plaque amyloid (Kalback *et al.* 2002), and also complement activation by C1q binding to Aβ in mice is a less efficient procedure than human complement activation (Webster *et al.* 1999). For example, as mouse C1q does not interact directly with Aβ peptide with the same efficiency as human C1q; it has been suggested that this reduced level of complement activation in these mice models leads to less inflammatory pathology. C1q can still be considered to have a significant role in AD as demonstrated by one study showing that Aβ plaque developing transgenic mice deficient in C1q had significantly less neuropathology than Aβ mice expressing normal levels of C1q (Fonseca *et al.* 2004).

Other mechanistic studies of inflammation and AD have been carried out by developing double transgenic mice that express mutant APP, and also overexpress or have gene deletions for inflammatory-associated proteins. The overall aim of these studies was to determine the consequences of overexpressing or removing inflammatory-associated proteins on Aβ plaque development and neuropathology in these model systems. Mice that overexpressed cyclooxygenase-2 (COX-2) under control of a neuron specific promoter produced enhanced prostaglandin E2 and had enhanced Aβ accumulation (Xiang *et al.* 2002); however mice deficient in PGE2 receptor (EP2) had reduced Aβ accumulation (Liang *et al.* 2005). Culture studies with microglia lacking EP2 showed that they were significantly more effective at phagocytosing Aβ than wild type microglia (Shie *et al.* 2005). These data suggest that increased COX activity, resulting in increased levels of PGE2, reduced microglia Aβ clearance. Similarly, mice deficient in CD40L, the activating ligand for CD40, showed reduced Aβ accumulation and reduced microglia activation (Tan *et al.* 2002). Mutant APP mice overexpressing α-1 antichymotrypsin (α1-ACT) or MCP-1 under the control of the astrocyte glial fibrillary acidic protein (GFAP) promoter both resulted in enhanced Aβ accumulation and enhanced glial activation (Nilsson *et al.* 2001;Yamamoto *et al.* 2005). By comparison, mice overexpressing the anti-inflammatory protein TGF-β1 under the GFAP promoter had reduced Aβ cerebral accumulation, enhanced accumulation of vascular Aβ, but increased microglial and astrocytic activation (Wyss-Coray *et al.* 2001). From these representative results, it can be seen that enhancement of inflammatory proteins can have effects on Aβ accumulation; two possible mechanisms could be enhancement of microglial phagocytosis of Aβ, or enhancement of microglial mediated neurotoxicity resulting in increased production of Aβ by damaged neurons.

What Does Aβ Immune Therapy and Anti-Inflammatories Say About AD Inflammatory Mechanisms

Due to the apparent failure of anti-inflammatory drug trials for AD in recent years, the inflammatory hypothesis for AD has fallen out of favor as a therapeutic target (Boche and Nicoll 2008). Most efforts at developing new therapies have focused on mechanisms for reducing the formation and aggregation of the amyloid beta (Aβ) peptide, even using immune activation to stimulate microglial phagocytosis to remove Aβ from the brain (Boche and Nicoll 2008). Initial studies showed that PDAPP mice immunized with Aβ peptide developed a circulating antibody titer to the peptide, and these animals developed significantly fewer plaques. Immunization of older animals with established plaques resulted in significant reduction in plaque load. Initial data suggested that the microglia were being stimulated to enhanced phagocytosis of antibody opsonized Aβ plaques (Schenk *et al.* 1999). A subsequent study by this group suggested that human microglia could remove Aβ from tissue slices of AD brains by the same mechanism. This study used an *ex vivo* tissue and microglia culture model, where tissue sections pretreated with Aβ antibody showed enhanced Aβ removal while those treated with control antibodies did not (Bard *et al.* 2000). A large number of subsequent studies in transgenic mice replicating these findings have been published [examples (Jensen *et al.* 2005;Morgan 2006;Wilcock *et al.* 2004b)]; these data indicated that mechanisms that enhanced inflammation in mice could aid in the clearance of Aβ and improve cognitive function, however human trials of the Aβ vaccine resulted in inflammatory-associated side effects such as meningoencephalitis, and had to be terminated (Schenk *et al.* 2005).

Dismissing inflammation as a factor in AD is premature, as is the suggestion that anti-inflammatory drug trials have failed; the drugs tested, primarily non steroidal anti-inflammatory drugs (NSAIDS), which are mainly cyclooxygenase (COX) inhibitors, did not show effectiveness in prospective clinical trials of AD patients [example (Aisen *et al.* 2003)]. A number of these drugs also have anti-inflammatory properties for activating the peroxisome proliferator-activated receptors (PPARs), a group of nuclear receptor proteins that function as transcription factors (Bright *et al.* 2008). These drugs are functional against very few of the multiple targets associated with inflammation in the brain. Anti-inflammatory drug discovery has progressed in recent years, and many new agents against a range of targets are now available; in addition, established agents such as statins have been shown to have significant anti-inflammatory effects through non-COX or -PPAR mechanisms (Paraskevas *et al.* 2007). It can also be suggested (and has been) that many clinical trials of effective drugs are likely to fail as they are being tested in patients whose disease has progressed extensively before being diagnosed as AD. Unfortunately the ADAPT trial, a preventive trial of two anti-inflammatory drugs, was stopped prematurely due to cerebrovascular side effects (ADAPT research group 2006).

Inflammation and Aging

A range of animal studies have demonstrated that increased chronic inflammation was a feature of aging and accompanied by a decrease in endogenous anti-inflammatory proteins (Morgan *et al.* 2007). Microglia cultured *in vitro* from aged rats showed higher levels of spontaneous proliferation and activation marker expression compared to microglia isolated from younger rats (Rozovsky *et al.* 1998). In addition, aged rats had increased numbers of activated microglia and astrocytes and increased expression of GFAP, APOE, clusterin, complement receptor 3 and TGFβ-1 compared to younger animals (Morgan *et al.* 1999). In this study, spontaneous glial activation was downregulated in animals fed a diet restricted in calories. Other studies have shown increased levels of IL-1β with increasing age, along with decrease in the expression of genes for anti-inflammatory proteins IL-4 and CD200 (Griffin *et al.* 2006;Lyons *et al.* 2007a;Maher *et al.* 2004;Nolan *et al.* 2005). A similar feature has been observed in humans; this has lead to the term "inflammaging" that describes increased markers of inflammation and oxidative stress with increasing age (Salvioli *et al.* 2006). From this concept, it is suggested that inflammation could be further enhanced by the presence of initiating AD pathology, which exacerbates this age-related enhanced inflammation (Giunta *et al.* 2008). The interaction of these two events is not unreasonable; since Aβ is produced by neurons as a byproduct of APP metabolism, but does not start to become deposited until late in life, it can be expected that microglia in the younger healthy brain are contributing to the removal of Aβ. Later in life, this phagocytic processes became replaced by activation processes, leading to microglial activation, production of damaging inflammatory products resulting in neurotoxicity and enhanced Aβ deposition. One group has suggested from model studies with aging rats that age-related loss of the anti-inflammatory cytokine IL-4 could be a central coordinator of this change from phagocytosis to activation by microglia (Lyons *et al.* 2007b).

Chronic Vascular Inflammation Compared to Chronic Cerebral Inflammation

The term plaque has different meaning when considering vascular atherosclerosis and AD pathology, though there is now a blurring in distinction between vascular dementia, AD and atherosclerosis. Atherosclerotic plaques develop as a chronic inflammatory response in the walls of arteries, mainly due to the accumulation of macrophages and other white blood cells and are promoted by low density lipoproteins; the plaques accumulate due to lack of adequate removal of fats and cholesterol from the macrophages by functional high density lipoproteins (Viles-Gonzalez *et al.* 2006). By comparison, since the identification of the amyloid precursor protein (APP) as the protein from which the 4kD Aβ peptide is derived from, and basic studies have shown that APP is most abundantly expressed in brain compared to other tissues, the basic amyloid hypothesis for AD has focused on the disease starting and progressing in the brain without influence of peripheral factors. However, a competing vascular hypothesis of AD has also emerged that hypothesizes that peripheral vascular components, including chronic vascular inflammation, could influence Aβ formation and deposition in the brain. How this can occur is still controversial, but Roher and colleagues measured the degree of atherosclerosis occlusion in a large series of Circle of Willis arteries collected at autopsy from AD and non-demented donors (Beach *et al.* 2007;Roher *et al.* 2003). In these two separate studies, it was shown that the degree of occlusion, an index of severity of atherosclerosis, correlated positively with the diagnosis of AD and the degree of AD plaque and tangle pathology. The mechanism of how these two events are connected can be suggested; the degree of occlusion of this crucial vascular structure leads to hypoperfusion of blood, glucose and oxygen throughout the brain resulting in enhanced oxidative stress, which causes neurotoxicity and inflammation (Beach *et al.* 2007;de la Torre 2000;de la Torre 2002;de la Torre 2004;Roher *et al.* 2003). In addition, severe atherosclerosis results in significantly increased peripheral chronic inflammation that could have consequences on the cerebrovasculature. This chronic process could set up a positive feedback cycle as the degree of occlusion, hypoperfusion and inflammation becomes progressively more severe.

Immunohistochemical studies of human postmortem brains demonstrated that the degree of cerebral vascular inflammation, as shown by increased expression of vascular inflammatory markers such as ICAM-1 and CD40, in cerebral endothelial cells, correlated with the degree of peripheral inflammation, as shown by levels of C-reactive protein (CRP) (Uchikado *et al.* 2004). The correlation was stronger in cases with no parenchymal brain lesions, but this was due to a few cases showing strong parenchymal inflammation (activated microglia) without vascular inflammation; most of the AD cases in this study also showed strong peripheral inflammation.

How do Peripheral Vascular Events Affect Inflammation and Plaque Development in the Brain ?

As mentioned in the previous section, there is evidence that peripheral vascular events, including endothelial activation, can contribute to Aβ plaque development and inflammation in the brain. Many studies have documented significant levels of Aβ in the blood; activated platelets are an abundant source of Aβ in the periphery (Davies *et al.* 2000;Johnston *et al.* 2008). Transport of Aβ into and out of the brain has been characterized in various models. In the brain, Aβ is primarily produced and released by neurons. It has been shown that low-density lipoprotein receptor-related protein (LRP)-1 is the major endothelial protein responsible for transport of Aβ from brain to blood, while RAGE is the major protein responsible for transport of Aβ from blood to brain (Deane *et al.* 2004;Deane *et al.* 2003;Zlokovic 2005). Blockade of RAGE reduced Aβ accumulation and inflammation in the brains of treated transgenic mice (Deane *et al.* 2003). In cerebral vessels in AD brains, it has been seen that RAGE levels are enhanced while LRP-1 levels are reduced (Donahue *et al.* 2006;Miller *et al.* 2008). The consequence of this could be to reduce Aβ transport out of the brain and increase Aβ transport into the brain.

Many Aβ immunotherapy studies have been characterized in transgenic AD mice models (examples (Jensen *et al.* 2005;Lemere *et al.* 2006;Morgan 2005;Wilcock *et al.* 2004a;Wilcock *et al.* 2006); although the promising results from these studies have not translated into effective therapy for AD patients (Boche and Nicoll 2008;Schenk *et al.* 2005), they have indicated some interesting disease mechanisms. In the transgenic mouse models, enhanced expression of mutated APP predominantly occurs in neurons due to the neuron-specific promoters attached to the various transgenes, but even in these models, there is significant trafficking of Aβ into the blood. Immunization of mice with Aβ peptide produced an anti-Aβ antibody titer resulting in inhibition of Aβ plaque formation in younger immunized mice, and significant reduction in plaque load in older mice with established plaques (Schenk *et al.* 2004). Although a subject of controversy, since most of the antibody does not penetrate into the brain, it has been suggested that the effect of immunization was to sequester/neutralize the Aβ **in the blood** and prevent it from entering or reentering the brain. One study using passive injection into mice of an Aβ antibody that did not cross into the brain showed significant effectiveness in reducing cerebral Aβ plaque load (DeMattos *et al.* 2002;DeMattos *et al.* 2001). Other researchers have concluded that the small percentage of antibody to Aβ that does cross into the brain and binds to plaques is responsible for enhancing the phagocytosis of plaque material by microglia through Fcg immunoglobulin receptor mechanism. In some of the human subjects that had received Aβ vaccination, there appeared to be significant plaque clearance by microglia (Nicoll *et al.* 2006;Patton *et al.* 2006). While immunization was effective in reducing plaque load, it was not effective at clearing vascular amyloid (Patton *et al.* 2006).

Inflammatory Gene Expression Profiling of AD

Defining chronic inflammation in AD brains is dependent on the criteria being used, but we are considering any increase in levels of inflammatory cytokines/chemokines in the absence of interferon-gamma as an indication of this feature. The development of global gene expression profiling or proteomics techniques to examine brain or biofluids has identified different groups of molecules associated with disease; many of these molecules are inflammatory-related. Gene expression profiling of carefully selected AD brain tissues, when compared to matched control samples, allows an unbiased measurement of gene expression to identify differential expression due to disease. Various approaches to investigating AD through gene expression profiling have been attempted, and data have identified changes in many classes of genes involved in cellular metabolism, synapse formation, cellular stress and inflammation. A number of these studies have identified increased or decreased expression of inflammatory markers in AD brains; however, the lack of consistency in results has still not allowed the identification of key inflammatory mediators. An earlier study using pooled RNA samples from CA1 region of hippocampus, a region affected early in AD degeneration, from 6 AD and 6 control cases identified 19 genes upregulated more than 3-fold and 19 genes downregulated by the same amount (Colangelo *et al.* 2002). Of the 19 upregulated genes, 13 were inflammatory genes; these genes were cytosolic phospholipase-2 (cPLA2), the inflammatory transcription factors NFκB-p52, NFκB-p100 and NF-IL 6, dipeptidylpeptidase-1 precursor (DPP1), IL-1α and IL-1β, interferon-gamma (IFN-γ) inducible protein (IFIND), B94, a tumor necrosis factor inducible protein, COX-2, chemokine exodus protein (CEX1), and human JE cytokine-like glycoprotein. This study used a gene chip with approximately 12,000 genes, but since then whole genome profiling has become possible. Subsequent studies have identified inflammatory changes ongoing in AD brains, but there has been a lack of consistency between studies, probably due to differences in experimental design, methodology and quality of human brain tissues. A recent study on whole genome arrays utilizing RNA from inferior parietal lobe of AD and ND cases, along with validation using a series of tissue samples from AD, ND and non-AD cases with neurological diseases, identified a range of immunological/inflammatory-associated genes and genes involved in nervous system development. Of the inflammatory-associated genes that were significantly upregulated, there were 14 genes involved in B-Cell receptor signaling, 9 involved in chemokine signaling, 13 involved in the ERK/MAPK signaling pathways, 8 involved in insulin growth factor-1 signaling, 8 involved in T-cell receptor signaling, 6 involved in JAK/STAT signaling, 5 involved in IL-2 signaling and 19 involved in NFκB signaling (Weeraratna *et al.* 2007). This study identified IL-28A for the first time to be increased in AD brains by 179 fold (validated by real time PCR techniques), as was CCL27 by 5-fold (also known as T-cell attracting chemokine). IL-28A is a type III interferon cytokine with identified roles in anti-viral activity and T cell function, as is CCL27; their involvement in AD pathology is unclear. Significant upregulation of CXCR2 (interleukin-8 receptor β) and CXCR4 (receptor for CXCL12 – stromal cell derived factor-1) and CCR3 (receptor for the following chemokines: CCL5 (RANTES), CCL7 (MCP-3), CCL11 (eotaxin), CCL13 (MCP-4), CCL15 (MIP5), CCL26 (MIP4a)) was validated by real time PCR. A similar study employing RNA derived from frontal cortex and hippocampus of ND and mild to moderate AD cases, using Affymetrix whole genome arrays, showed that there was an increase in expression of inflammatory markers, which positively correlated with early changes in cognitive function (Parachikova *et al.* 2007). These changes were more marked in frontal cortex than hippocampus; 39 inflammatory-associated genes were significantly upregulated in frontal cortex, ranging from IL-15R at a mean value of 4.8 fold to ICAM-2 at 1.44 fold. As genes for the immunoglobulin IgG Fc receptors CD16 and CD64 and for different components of the major histocompability complex (MHC) were upregulated, these data suggested that increased activation of microglia was occurring with early changes of cognitive function. Interestingly, this study also showed, contrary to others, that there were reduced numbers of T cells in AD brains compared to control samples. Another study using AD and control frontal cortex samples identified interferon induced transmembrane protein-3 (IFITM-3) as the only upregulated inflammatory-associated protein (Ricciarelli *et al.* 2004). This study used samples from more advanced AD cases compared to the previous mentioned study (Parachikova *et al.* 2007), with controls showing significant AD pathology. These discrepancies between reports illustrate the problems with obtaining a definitive picture of AD inflammation based on gene expression profiling. Gene expression profiling datasets are complex and large in nature; many different ways have been developed to analyze this data. It was recently shown that a technique called Fast independent component analysis (ICA) was superior than principal component analysis (PCA) for identifying significantly altered genes. Using a deposited data set of hippocampal gene expression from 8 controls and 5 severe AD cases, ICA identified 50 genes that were significantly upregulated, including the following inflammatory genes AMIGO2, BTG1, CD24, CD44, CDC42EP4, IFITM1, IFITM2, IRF7, FI44L, IL4R, IRAK1, NFKBIA, by comparison, PCA identified only 2 inflammatory related genes (BCL-6 and CD24) (Kong *et al.* 2009). There are large numbers of gene expression datasets of AD and ND microarray experiments that have been deposited, and could be reanalyzed using these enhanced methods.

AD Inflammatory Gene Expression Changes in the Blood

Gene expression profiling of blood mononuclear cells from clinically diagnosed AD patients is being used to produce a transcription signature for possible changes in the periphery reflective of pathological changes in the AD brain [for example (Maes *et al.* 2007)]. This approach has produced some interesting results; there was down-regulation of genes concerned with cytoskeletal maintenance, cellular trafficking, cellular stress, redox homeostasis and DNA repair (Maes *et al.* 2007). There was a significant difference in profile between samples from females compared to males in this study. Changes in expression of inflammatory-associated genes was not prominent, with only vascular cell adhesion molecule -1 (VCAM-1) and Coagulation factor II receptor-like 1 being significantly upregulated in both the female and male samples.

An interesting use of peripheral blood mononuclear cells for a AD biomarker study was to examine those patients that participated in the Aβ vaccine study. This approach to treating AD in humans was abandoned due to a percentage of patients developing meningoencephalitis. Gene expression profiling of blood samples from those participants showed that a proinflammatory and apoptosis profile, especially high levels of expression of the inflammatory transcription factors STAT1 and STAT5a, as well as IL-9, IL-19, IL-25, IL-27R, and CD80, predicted a high risk of developing meningoencephalitis, while those blood samples with a profile of expression of protein synthesis and trafficking genes had a significantly greater immunoglobulin production response to Aβ vaccination (O'Toole *et al.* 2005). Using this method, which appears to identify a group of individuals predisposed to inflammatory activation and therefore not suitable candidates for vaccination, might be useful if Aβ vaccination can be reconsidered as an AD therapy.

A significant study of levels of 120 proteins in plasma samples of a large series of diagnosed AD cases, matched controls or those with other diagnoses identified a panel of 18 inflammatory or growth factor-associated proteins whose changes in levels in the plasma might be used as a predictor for clinical diagnosis of AD (Britschgi and Wyss-Coray 2009;Ray *et al.* 2007). These proteins were CCL5 (RANTES), CCL7 (monocyte chemoattractant protein-3), CCL15 (macrophage inflammatory protein (MIP)-5, CCL18 (macrophage inflammatory protein 4), ANG-2 (angiopoietin-2), TNF-α, GCSF (granulocyte colony stimulating factor), macrophage colony stimulating factor (MCSF), IL 1α, IL-3, IL-11, ICAM-1, CXCL8 (also known as IL-8), PDGF-BB (platelet derived growth factor), GDNF (glial cell line derived neurotrophic factor, EGF (endothelial growth factor), TRAIL-R4 and IGFBP-6. All of these molecules have multiple modes of action, and also have functional roles as inflammatory mediators. This study has provided evidence for peripheral inflammation as a feature, and therefore a potential mechanism, for AD, but requires replication by other investigators.

Gene Expression Profiling in Transgenic Mouse Models

It has also been possible to compare gene expression profiles between wild type and Aβ plaque-developing animals, or other transgenic mice, in a more defined manner than if using human tissues; the following studies have produced interesting results of potential significance to AD. Comparing the profiles of 2 month-old transgenic and non-transgenic mice demonstrated upregulation of a number of genes related to mitochondrial metabolism and apoptosis (Reddy *et al.* 2004); abnormal expression of these genes can lead to enhanced oxidative stress resulting in inflammatory changes. Another study investigated the effect of the apoE4 isoform on the inflammatory response to administration of lipopolysaccharide (LPS) as inflammatory activating agent in apoE3 and apoE4 transgenic mice. Genome-wide gene expression profiling was used to assess the effects of the apoE genotype on inflammatory activation in hippocampus. From the data, it was possible to conclude that the neuroinflammatory response to acute LPS treatment is more prolonged and up-regulated in apoE4 mice; this response was linked to enhanced NF-κB signaling (Ophir *et al.* 2005). Specifically, the genes for TNFα, MCP-1 (CCL2), MIP-1α (CCL3), α-2 macroglobulin (α2-MG), and BIRC3 responded more robustly to LPS treatment in apoE4 mice than in apoE3 mice at 10 hours, while IL-6, IL-1β, interferon-induced protein-10 (CXCL10), ICAM-1 and NFκB2 transcripts were higher in apoE3 mice than in apoE4 mice at 5 h, but higher in apoE4 mice at 10 hours. These data show that apoE4 causes an enhanced inflammatory response to stimuli. In a similar study, it was shown that microglia derived from apoE4 mice had enhanced production of TNF-α, IL-6 and IL-12 in response to LPS compared to microglia from apoE3 mice (Vitek *et al.* 2007). Sera from AD patients that had one or two apoE 4 alleles caused enhanced activation of microglia (Lombardi *et al.* 1998).

MCP-1 as a Key Chemokine in AD Chronic Inflammation

Gene expression profiling studies of AD brains have shown increased expression of MCP-1, and additional data have suggested that this abundant chemokine might have a significant role in the progression of AD pathology. Measurement of cerebrospinal fluid (CSF) levels of IP-10, MCP-1 and IL-8 concentrations showed that they were significantly increased in patients with mild cognitive impairment (MCI) and mild AD; in severe AD patients, MCP-1 and IL-8 levels continued to increase, while IP-10 decreased. There was a significant positive correlation between Mini-Mental State Examination score and CSF IP-10 or MCP-1 concentrations in patients with AD (Galimberti *et al.* 2006b). The same researchers showed that serum levels of MCP-1 were significantly increased in MCI and early AD, but declined as the disease progressed (Galimberti *et al.* 2006a). From these studies, it can be concluded that MCP-1 increased prior to the development of AD pathology. However, another study using CSF samples from control, AD, alcoholic dementia, frontal temporal dementia and depression cases showed that MCP-1 increased with age and did not distinguish between control and AD cases (Blasko *et al.* 2006). Using a multi-analyte approach to simultaneously measure protein levels of 18 cytokines in tissue extracts of AD brains, the results suggested that significantly increased levels of MCP-1, along with IL-6 and IL-8 were responsible for maintaining chronic neuroinflammation in AD. Although technically well done with state of the art methodology, these findings need to be confirmed by others as this study combined young and aged controls in one group and compared their cytokine values with a group comprising young AD cases due to PS-1 mutations and aged sporadic AD cases (Sokolova *et al.* 2008).

Summary

Although accumulated data from different sources have indicated that chronic inflammation must be involved in AD pathological processes, these findings have not turned into effective therapies. Findings from neuropathology identified increased numbers of activated microglia and astrocytes associated with AD amyloid plaques and neurofibrillary tangles have been replicated in many different studies with a range of different markers. The detailed studies on IL-4, its loss in aging and how if supplemented by pharmacological treatments can reduce inflammation are promising new therapeutic avenues. These studies in aging rats, and our findings that IL-4 is deficient in aging brain resulting in reduced levels of the anti-inflammatory molecules CD200 and CD200 receptor (Walker *et al.* 2009), support this suggestion. Finally, the retrospective epidemiological studies showing that taking NSAIDS for an extended period of time can protect from AD needs to be considered before inflammation and AD is rejected as a disease mechanism. In 1996, a meta-analysis of 17 previous studies demonstrated significant protective properties for NSAIDS (McGeer *et al.* 1996); since then further large studies have again confirmed these findings [example (Vlad *et al.* 2008)]. This last study examined records from a total of 246,199 subjects. Interestingly, data on the mechanisms of action of statins in neurological disease suggest that they might be effective due to anti-inflammatory properties, not due to their well-known cholesterol lowering properties (Orr 2008). Further promising agents with anti-inflammatory properties, along with other functions (like inhibiting Aβ aggregation, anti-oxidants, signal transduction inhibitors) need to be tested in AD. Promising preliminary data from transgenic mouse studies with curcumin or omega-3 fatty acids have been published (Cole *et al.* 2005; Cole *et al.* 2007). As clinical trials with AD or MCI patients are expensive and time-consuming to conduct, but if backed up by rigorous and balanced scientific studies, further attempts to treat AD or pre-AD with anti-inflammatories are justified and needed.

References

ADAPT research group. Cardiovascular and Cerebrovascular Events in the Randomized, Controlled Alzheimer's Disease Anti-Inflammatory Prevention Trial (ADAPT). *PLoS Clin Trials*. 1: e33, 2006.

Aisen, P. S., Schafer, K. A., Grundman, M., Pfeiffer, E., Sano, M., Davis, K. L., Farlow, M. R., Jin, S., Thomas, R. G., Thal, L. J. Effects of rofecoxib or naproxen vs placebo on Alzheimer disease progression: a randomized controlled trial. *JAMA*. 289: 2819-2826, 2003.

Akiyama, H., Yamada, T., Kawamata, T., McGeer, P. L. Association of amyloid P component with complement proteins in neurologically diseased brain tissue. *Brain Res*. 548: 349-352, 1991.

Apelt, J., Schliebs, R. beta-Amyloid-induced glial expression of both pro- and anti-inflammatory cytokines in cerebral cortex of aged transgenic Tg2576 mice with Alzheimer plaque pathology. *Brain Res*. 894: 21-30, 2001.

Bard, F., Cannon, C., Barbour, R., Burke, R. L., Games, D., Grajeda, H., Guido, T., Hu, K., Huang, J., Johnson-Wood, K., Khan, K., Kholodenko, D., Lee, M., Lieberburg, I., Motter, R., Nguyen, M., Soriano, F., Vasquez, N., Weiss, K., Welch, B., Seubert, P., Schenk, D., Yednock, T. Peripherally administered antibodies against amyloid beta-peptide enter the central nervous system and reduce pathology in a mouse model of Alzheimer disease. *Nat Med*. 6: 916-919, 2000.

Beach, T. G., Wilson, J. R., Sue, L. I., Newell, A., Poston, M., Cisneros, R., Pandya, Y., Esh, C., Connor, D. J., Sabbagh, M., Walker, D. G., Roher, A. E. Circle of Willis atherosclerosis: association with Alzheimer's disease, neuritic plaques and neurofibrillary tangles. *Acta Neuropathol* (Berl). 113: 13-21, 2007.

Benzing, W. C., Wujek, J. R., Ward, E. K., Shaffer, D., Ashe, K. H., Younkin, S. G., Brunden, K. R. Evidence for glial-mediated inflammation in aged APP(SW) transgenic mice. *Neurobiol Aging*. 20: 581-589, 1999.

Bertram, L., Tanzi, R. E. Thirty years of Alzheimer's disease genetics: the implications of systematic meta-analyses. *Nat Rev Neurosci*. 9: 768-778, 2008.

Bianca, V. D., Dusi, S., Bianchini, E., Dal, P., I, Rossi, F. beta-amyloid activates the O-2 forming NADPH oxidase in microglia, monocytes, and neutrophils. A possible inflammatory mechanism of neuronal damage in Alzheimer's disease. *J Biol Chem*. 274: 15493-15499, 1999.

Blasko, I., Lederer, W., Oberbauer, H., Walch, T., Kemmler, G., Hinterhuber, H., Marksteiner, J., Humpel, C. Measurement of thirteen biological markers in CSF of patients with Alzheimer's disease and other dementias. *Dement Geriatr Cogn Disord*. 21: 9-15, 2006.

Boche, D., Nicoll, J. A. The role of the immune system in clearance of Abeta from the brain. *Brain Pathol*. 18: 267-278, 2008.

Bornemann, K. D., Wiederhold, K. H., Pauli, C., Ermini, F., Stalder, M., Schnell, L., Sommer, B., Jucker, M., Staufenbiel, M. Ab-Induced Inflammatory Processes in Microglia Cells of APP23 Transgenic Mice. *Am J Pathol*. 158: 63-73, 2001.

Bright, J. J., Kanakasabai, S., Chearwae, W., Chakraborty, S. PPAR Regulation of Inflammatory Signaling in CNS Diseases. *PPAR Res*. 2008:658520.: 658520, 2008.

Britschgi, M., Wyss-Coray, T. Blood protein signature for the early diagnosis of Alzheimer disease. *Arch Neurol*. 66: 161-165, 2009.

Cagnin, A., Zambon, A., Zarantonello, G., Vianello, D., Marchiori, M., Mercurio, D., Micciche, F., Ermani, M., Leon, A., Battistin, L. Serum lipoprotein profile and APOE genotype in Alzheimer's disease. *J Neural Transm Suppl*. 175-179, 2007.

Cankurtaran, M., Yavuz, B. B., Cankurtaran, E. S., Halil, M., Ulger, Z., Ariogul, S. Risk factors and type of dementia: vascular or Alzheimer? *Arch Gerontol Geriatr*. 47: 25-34, 2008.

Chamandy, N., Wolfson, C. Underlying cause of death in demented and non-demented elderly Canadians. *Neuroepidemiology*. 25: 75-84, 2005.

Colangelo, V., Schurr, J., Ball, M. J., Pelaez, R. P., Bazan, N. G., Lukiw, W. J. Gene expression profiling of 12633 genes in Alzheimer hippocampal CA1: transcription and neurotrophic factor down-regulation and up-regulation of apoptotic and pro-inflammatory signaling. *J Neurosci Res*. 70: 462-473, 2002.

Cole, G.M., Lim, G.P., Yang, F., Teter, B., Begum, A., Ma, Q., Harris-White, M.E., Frautschy, S.A. Prevention of Alzheimer's disease: Omega-3 fatty acid and phenolic anti-oxidant interventions. Neurobiol Aging. 26: Suppl 1:133-6, 2005.

Cole, G.M., Teter, B., Frautschy, SA. Neuroprotective effects of curcumin. *Adv Exp Med Biol.* 595:197-212, 2007

Coon, K. D., Myers, A. J., Craig, D. W., Webster, J. A., Pearson, J. V., Lince, D. H., Zismann, V. L., Beach, T. G., Leung, D., Bryden, L., Halperin, R. F., Marlowe, L., Kaleem, M., Walker, D. G., Ravid, R., Heward, C. B., Rogers, J., Papassotiropoulos, A., Reiman, E. M., Hardy, J., Stephan, D. A. A high-density whole-genome association study reveals that APOE is the major susceptibility gene for sporadic late-onset Alzheimer's disease. *J Clin Psychiatry*. 68: 613-618, 2007.

Davies, T. A., Long, H. J., Eisenhauer, P. B., Hastey, R., Cribbs, D. H., Fine, R. E., Simons, E. R. Beta amyloid fragments derived from activated platelets deposit in cerebrovascular endothelium: usage of a novel blood brain barrier endothelial cell model system. *Amyloid*. 7: 153-165, 2000.

De Felice, F. G., Vieira, M. N., Bomfim, T. R., Decker, H., Velasco, P. T., Lambert, M. P., Viola, K. L., Zhao, W. Q., Ferreira, S. T., Klein, W. L. Protection of synapses against Alzheimer's-linked toxins: insulin signaling prevents the pathogenic binding of Abeta oligomers. *Proc Natl Acad Sci U S A*. 106: 1971-1976, 2009.

de la Torre, J. C. Vascular basis of Alzheimer's pathogenesis. *Ann N Y Acad Sci.* 977: 196-215, 2002.

de la Torre, J. C. Is Alzheimer's disease a neurodegenerative or a vascular disorder? Data, dogma, and dialectics. *Lancet Neurol*. 3: 184-190, 2004.

de la Torre, J. C. Critically attained threshold of cerebral hypoperfusion: can it cause Alzheimer's disease? *Ann N Y Acad Sci*. 903: 424-436, 2000.

Deane, R., Du, Y. S., Submamaryan, R. K., LaRue, B., Jovanovic, S., Hogg, E., Welch, D., Manness, L., Lin, C., Yu, J., Zhu, H., Ghiso, J., Frangione, B., Stern, A., Schmidt, A. M., Armstrong, D. L., Arnold, B., Liliensiek, B., Nawroth, P., Hofman, F., Kindy, M., Stern,

D., Zlokovic, B. RAGE mediates amyloid-beta peptide transport across the blood-brain barrier and accumulation in brain. *Nat Med.* 9: 907-913, 2003.

Deane, R., Wu, Z., Sagare, A., Davis, J., Du, Y. S., Hamm, K., Xu, F., Parisi, M., LaRue, B., Hu, H. W., Spijkers, P., Guo, H., Song, X., Lenting, P. J., Van Nostrand, W. E., Zlokovic, B. V. LRP/amyloid beta-peptide interaction mediates differential brain efflux of Abeta isoforms. *Neuron.* 43: 333-344, 2004.

DeLegge, M. H., Smoke, A. Neurodegeneration and inflammation. *Nutr Clin Pract.* 23: 35-41, 2008.

DeMattos, R. B., Bales, K. R., Cummins, D. J., Dodart, J. C., Paul, S. M., Holtzman, D. M. Peripheral anti-A beta antibody alters CNS and plasma A beta clearance and decreases brain A beta burden in a mouse model of Alzheimer's disease. *Proc Natl Acad Sci U S A.* 98: 8850-8855, 2001.

DeMattos, R. B., Bales, K. R., Cummins, D. J., Paul, S. M., Holtzman, D. M. Brain to plasma amyloid-beta efflux: a measure of brain amyloid burden in a mouse model of Alzheimer's disease. *Leuk Lymphoma.* 295: 2264-2267, 2002.

Dheen, S. T., Kaur, C., Ling, E. A. Microglial activation and its implications in the brain diseases. *Curr Med Chem.* 14: 1189-1197, 2007.

Di, C. M. Beta amyloid peptide: from different aggregation forms to the activation of different biochemical pathways. *Eur Biophys J.* 2009.

Dickson, D. W., Mattiace, L. A. Astrocytes and microglia in human brain share an epitope recognized by a B-lymphocyte-specific monoclonal antibody (LN-1*). Am J Pathol.* 135: 135-147, 1989.

Donahue, J. E., Flaherty, S. L., Johanson, C. E., Duncan, J. A., III, Silverberg, G. D., Miller, M. C., Tavares, R., Yang, W., Wu, Q., Sabo, E., Hovanesian, V., Stopa, E. G. RAGE, LRP-1, and amyloid-beta protein in Alzheimer's disease. *Acta Neuropathol.* 112: 405-415, 2006.

Douglas, J. L., Gustin, J. K., Dezube, B., Pantanowitz, J. L., Moses, A. V. Kaposi's sarcoma: a model of both malignancy and chronic inflammation. *Panminerva Med.* 49: 119-138, 2007.

Duyckaerts, C., Potier, M. C., Delatour, B. Alzheimer disease models and human neuropathology: similarities and differences. Acta Neuropathol. 115: 5-38, 2008.

Esiri, M. M. The interplay between inflammation and neurodegeneration in CNS disease. *J Neuroimmunol.* 184: 4-16, 2007.

Fiala, M., Liu, Q. N., Sayre, J., Pop, V., Brahmandam, V., Graves, M. C., Vinters, H. V. Cyclooxygenase-2-positive macrophages infiltrate the Alzheimer's disease brain and damage the blood-brain barrier. *Eur J Clin Invest.* 32: 360-371, 2002.

Fonseca, M. I., Zhou, J., Botto, M., Tenner, A. J. Absence of C1q leads to less neuropathology in transgenic mouse models of Alzheimer's disease. *J Neurosci.* 24: 6457-6465, 2004.

Foster, J. K., Verdile, G., Bates, K. A., Martins, R. N. Immunization in Alzheimer's disease: naive hope or realistic clinical potential? *Mol Psychiatry.* 14: 239-251, 2009.

Galimberti, D., Fenoglio, C., Lovati, C., Venturelli, E., Guidi, I., Corra, B., Scalabrini, D., Clerici, F., Mariani, C., Bresolin, N., Scarpini, E. Serum MCP-1 levels are increased in mild cognitive impairment and mild Alzheimer's disease. *Neurobiol Aging*. 27: 1763-1768, 2006a.

Galimberti, D., Schoonenboom, N., Scheltens, P., Fenoglio, C., Bouwman, F., Venturelli, E., Guidi, I., Blankenstein, M. A., Bresolin, N., Scarpini, E. Intrathecal chemokine synthesis in mild cognitive impairment and Alzheimer disease. Arch Neurol. 63: 538-543, 2006b.

Giunta, B., Fernandez, F., Nikolic, W. V., Obregon, D., Rrapo, E., Town, T., Tan, J. Inflammaging as a prodrome to Alzheimer's disease. *J Neuroinflammation*. 5:51.: 51, 2008.

Gomez-Mejiba, S. E., Zhai, Z., Akram, H., Pye, Q. N., Hensley, K., Kurien, B. T., Scofield, R. H., Ramirez, D. C. Inhalation of environmental stressors & chronic inflammation: Autoimmunity and neurodegeneration. *Mutat Res*. 674: 62-72, 2009.

Griffin, R., Nally, R., Nolan, Y., McCartney, Y., Linden, J., Lynch, M. A. The age-related attenuation in long-term potentiation is associated with microglial activation. *J Neurochem*. 99: 1263-1272, 2006.

Heneka, M. T., O'Banion, M. K. Inflammatory processes in Alzheimer's disease. *J Neuroimmunol*. 184: 69-91, 2007.

Hirsch-Reinshagen, V., Wellington, C. L. Cholesterol metabolism, apolipoprotein E, adenosine triphosphate-binding cassette transporters, and Alzheimer's disease. *Curr Opin Lipidol*. 18: 325-332, 2007.

Holtzman, J. L. Amyloid-beta vaccination for Alzheimer's dementia. *Lancet*. 372: 1381-1382, 2008.

Hung, L. W., Ciccotosto, G. D., Giannakis, E., Tew, D. J., Perez, K., Masters, C. L., Cappai, R., Wade, J. D., Barnham, K. J. Amyloid-beta peptide (Abeta) neurotoxicity is modulated by the rate of peptide aggregation: Abeta dimers and trimers correlate with neurotoxicity. *J Neurosci*. 28: 11950-11958, 2008.

Itagaki, S., McGeer, P. L., Akiyama, H. Presence of T-cytotoxic suppressor and leucocyte common antigen positive cells in Alzheimer's disease brain tissue. *Neurosci Lett*. 91: 259-264, 1988.

Itagaki, S., McGeer, P. L., Akiyama, H., Zhu, S., Selkoe, D. Relationship of microglia and astrocytes to amyloid deposits of Alzheimer disease. *J Neuroimmunol*. 24: 173-182, 1989.

Jana, M., Palencia, C. A., Pahan, K. Fibrillar amyloid-beta peptides activate microglia via TLR2: implications for Alzheimer's disease. J Immunol. 181: 7254-7262, 2008.

Jander, S., Schroeter, M., Saleh, A. Imaging inflammation in acute brain ischemia. *Stroke*. 38: 642-645, 2007.

Jensen, M. T., Mottin, M. D., Cracchiolo, J. R., Leighty, R. E., Arendash, G. W. Lifelong immunization with human beta-amyloid (1-42) protects Alzheimer's transgenic mice against cognitive impairment throughout aging. *Neuroscience*. 130: 667-684, 2005.

Johnston, J. A., Liu, W. W., Coulson, D. T., Todd, S., Murphy, S., Brennan, S., Foy, C. J., Craig, D., Irvine, G. B., Passmore, A. P. Platelet beta-secretase activity is increased in Alzheimer's disease. *Neurobiol Aging*. 29: 661-668, 2008.

Kalback, W., Watson, M. D., Kokjohn, T. A., Kuo, Y. M., Weiss, N., Luehrs, D. C., Lopez, J., Brune, D., Sisodia, S. S., Staufenbiel, M., Emmerling, M., Roher, A. E. APP transgenic mice Tg2576 accumulate Abeta peptides that are distinct from the chemically modified and insoluble peptides deposited in Alzheimer's disease senile plaques. *Biochemistry.* 41: 922-928, 2002.

Kong, W., Mou, X., Liu, Q., Chen, Z., Vanderburg, C. R., Rogers, J. T., Huang, X. Independent component analysis of Alzheimer's DNA microarray gene expression data. *Mol Neurodegener.* 4: 5, 2009.

Koutsavlis, A. T., Wolfson, C. Elements of mobility as predictors of survival in elderly patients with dementia: findings from the Canadian Study of Health and Aging. *Chronic Dis Can.* 21: 93-103, 2000.

Kung H-C, Hoyert DL, Xu J, Murphy SL. Deaths: Final Data for 2005. *Centers for Disease Control;* 2008. p. 1-121.

Kuo, Y. M., Beach, T. G., Sue, L. I., Scott, S., Layne, K. J., Kokjohn, T. A., Kalback, W. M., Luehrs, D. C., Vishnivetskaya, T. A., Abramowski, D., Sturchler-Pierrat, C., Staufenbiel, M., Weller, R. O., Roher, A. E. The evolution of A beta peptide burden in the APP23 transgenic mice: implications for A beta deposition in Alzheimer disease. *Mol Med.* 7: 609-618, 2001.

Kuo, Y. M., Crawford, F., Mullan, M., Kokjohn, T. A., Emmerling, M. R., Weller, R. O., Roher, A. E. Elevated A beta and apolipoprotein E in A betaPP transgenic mice and its relationship to amyloid accumulation in Alzheimer's disease. *Mol Med.* 6: 430-439, 2000.

Kuo, Y. M., Emmerling, M. R., Woods, A. S., Cotter, R. J., Roher, A. E. Isolation, chemical characterization, and quantitation of A beta 3- pyroglutamyl peptide from neuritic plaques and vascular amyloid deposits. *Biochem Biophys Res Commun.* 237: 188-191, 1997.

Langheinrich, A. C., Bohle, R. M. Atherosclerosis: humoral and cellular factors of inflammation. *Virchows Arch.* 446: 101-111, 2005.

Lee, S. C., Dickson, D. W., Liu, W., Brosnan, C. F. Induction of nitric oxide synthase activity in human astrocytes by interleukin-1 beta and interferon-gamma. *J Neuroimmunol.* 46: 19-24, 1993.

Lemere, C. A., Maier, M., Jiang, L., Peng, Y., Seabrook, T. J. Amyloid-beta immunotherapy for the prevention and treatment of Alzheimer disease: lessons from mice, monkeys, and humans. *Rejuvenation Res.* 9: 77-84, 2006.

Liang, X., Wang, Q., Hand, T., Wu, L., Breyer, R. M., Montine, T. J., Andreasson, K. Deletion of the prostaglandin E2 EP2 receptor reduces oxidative damage and amyloid burden in a model of Alzheimer's disease. *J Neurosci.* 25: 10180-10187, 2005.

Lombardi, V. R., Garcia, M., Cacabelos, R. Microglial activation induced by factor(s) contained in sera from Alzheimer-related ApoE genotypes. *J Neurosci Res.* 54: 539-553, 1998.

Luber-Narod, J., Rogers, J. Immune system associated antigens expressed by cells of the human central nervous system. *Neurosci Lett.* 94: 17-22, 1988.

Lue, L. F., Rydel, R., Brigham, E. F., Yang, L. B., Hampel, H., Murphy, G. M. J., Brachova, L., Yan, S. D., Walker, D. G., Shen, Y., Rogers, J. Inflammatory repertoire of Alzheimer's disease and nondemented elderly microglia in vitro. *Glia.* 35: 72-79, 2001a.

Lue, L. F., Walker, D. G., Brachova, L., Beach, T. G., Rogers, J., Schmidt, A. M., Stern, D., Yan S.D. Involvement of Microglial Receptor for Advanced Glycation Endproducts

(RAGE) in Alzheimer's Disease: Identification of a Cellular Activation Mechanism. *Exp Neurol.* 171: 29-45, 2001b.

Lyons, A., Downer, E. J., Crotty, S., Nolan, Y. M., Mills, K. H., Lynch, M. A. CD200 ligand receptor interaction modulates microglial activation in vivo and in vitro: a role for IL-4. *J Neurosci.* 27: 8309-8313, 2007a.

Lyons, A., Griffin, R. J., Costelloe, C. E., Clarke, R. M., Lynch, M. A. IL-4 attenuates the neuroinflammation induced by amyloid-beta in vivo and in vitro. *J Neurochem.* 101: 771-781, 2007b.

Maes, O. C., Xu, S., Yu, B., Chertkow, H. M., Wang, E., Schipper, H. M. Transcriptional profiling of Alzheimer blood mononuclear cells by microarray. *Neurobiol Aging.* 28: 1795-1809, 2007.

Maher, F. O., Martin, D. S., Lynch, M. A. Increased IL-1beta in cortex of aged rats is accompanied by downregulation of ERK and PI-3 kinase. *Neurobiol Aging.* 25: 795-806, 2004.

McGeer, P. L. Amyloid-beta vaccination for Alzheimer's dementia. *Lancet.* 372: 1381-1382, 2008.

McGeer, P. L., Akiyama, H., Itagaki, S., McGeer, E. G. Activation of the classical complement pathway in brain tissue of Alzheimer patients. *Neurosci Lett.* 107: 341-346, 1989.

McGeer, P. L., Itagaki, S., Boyes, B. E., McGeer, E. G. Reactive microglia are positive for HLA-DR in the substantia nigra of Parkinson's and Alzheimer's disease brains. *Neurology.* 38: 1285-1291, 1988.

McGeer, P. L., Itagaki, S., Tago, H., McGeer, E. G. Reactive microglia in patients with senile dementia of the Alzheimer type are positive for the histocompatibility glycoprotein HLA-DR. *Neurosci Lett.* 79: 195-200, 1987.

McGeer, P. L., Schulzer, M., McGeer, E. G. Arthritis and anti-inflammatory agents as possible protective factors for Alzheimer's disease: a review of 17 epidemiologic studies. *Neurology.* 47: 425-432, 1996.

Miller, M. C., Tavares, R., Johanson, C. E., Hovanesian, V., Donahue, J. E., Gonzalez, L., Silverberg, G. D., Stopa, E. G. Hippocampal RAGE immunoreactivity in early and advanced Alzheimer's disease. *Brain Res.* 1230:273-280, 2008.

Morgan, D. Immunotherapy for Alzheimer's disease. *J Alzheimers Dis.* 9: 425-432, 2006.

Morgan, D. Mechanisms of A beta plaque clearance following passive A beta immunization. *Neurodegener Dis.* 2: 261-266, 2005.

Morgan, T. E., Wong, A. M., Finch, C. E. Anti-inflammatory mechanisms of dietary restriction in slowing aging processes. *Interdiscip Top Gerontol.* 35:83-97.: 83-97, 2007.

Morgan, T. E., Xie, Z., Goldsmith, S., Yoshida, T., Lanzrein, A. S., Stone, D., Rozovsky, I., Perry, G., Smith, M. A., Finch, C. E. The mosaic of brain glial hyperactivity during normal ageing and its attenuation by food restriction. *Neuroscience.* 89: 687-699, 1999.

Mott, R. T., Hulette, C. M. Neuropathology of Alzheimer's disease. *Neuroimaging Clin N Am.* 15: 755-65, ix, 2005.

Nicoll, J. A., Barton, E., Boche, D., Neal, J. W., Ferrer, I., Thompson, P., Vlachouli, C., Wilkinson, D., Bayer, A., Games, D., Seubert, P., Schenk, D., Holmes, C. Abeta species removal after abeta42 immunization. *J Neuropathol Exp Neurol.* 65: 1040-1048, 2006.

Nilsson, L. N., Bales, K. R., DiCarlo, G., Gordon, M. N., Morgan, D., Paul, S. M., Potter, H. Alpha-1-antichymotrypsin promotes beta-sheet amyloid plaque deposition in a transgenic mouse model of Alzheimer's disease. *J Neurosci.* 21: 1444-1451, 2001.

Nolan, Y., Maher, F. O., Martin, D. S., Clarke, R. M., Brady, M. T., Bolton, A. E., Mills, K. H., Lynch, M. A. Role of interleukin-4 in regulation of age-related inflammatory changes in the hippocampus. *J Biol Chem.* 280: 9354-9362, 2005.

O'Toole, M., Janszen, D. B., Slonim, D. K., Reddy, P. S., Ellis, D. K., Legault, H. M., Hill, A. A., Whitley, M. Z., Mounts, W. M., Zuberek, K., Immermann, F. W., Black, R. S., Dorner, A. J. Risk factors associated with beta-amyloid(1-42) immunotherapy in preimmunization gene expression patterns of blood cells. *Arch Neurol.* 62: 1531-1536, 2005.

Ophir, G., Amariglio, N., Jacob-Hirsch, J., Elkon, R., Rechavi, G., Michaelson, D. M. Apolipoprotein E4 enhances brain inflammation by modulation of the NF-kappaB signaling cascade. *Neurobiol Dis.* 20: 709-718, 2005.

Orr, J. D. Statins in the spectrum of neurologic disease. *Curr Atheroscler Rep.* 10: 11-18, 2008.

Panza, F., D'introno, A., Capurso, C., Colacicco, A. M., Seripa, D., Pilotto, A., Santamato, A., Capurso, A., Solfrizzi, V. Lipoproteins, vascular-related genetic factors, and human longevity. *Rejuvenation Res.* 10: 441-458, 2007.

Parachikova, A., Agadjanyan, M. G., Cribbs, D. H., Blurton-Jones, M., Perreau, V., Rogers, J., Beach, T. G., Cotman, C. W. Inflammatory changes parallel the early stages of Alzheimer disease. *Neurobiol Aging.* 28: 1821-1833, 2007.

Paraskevas, K. I., Tzovaras, A. A., Briana, D. D., Mikhailidis, D. P. Emerging indications for statins: a pluripotent family of agents with several potential applications. *Curr Pharm Des.* 13: 3622-3636, 2007.

Patton, R. L., Kalback, W. M., Esh, C. L., Kokjohn, T. A., Van Vickle, G. D., Luehrs, D. C., Kuo, Y. M., Lopez, J., Brune, D., Ferrer, I., Masliah, E., Newel, A. J., Beach, T. G., Castano, E. M., Roher, A. E. Amyloid-beta peptide remnants in AN-1792-immunized Alzheimer's disease patients: a biochemical analysis. *Am J Pathol.* 169: 1048-1063, 2006.

Qin, L., Liu, Y., Cooper, C., Liu, B., Wilson, B., Hong, J. S. Microglia enhance beta-amyloid peptide-induced toxicity in cortical and mesencephalic neurons by producing reactive oxygen species. *J Neurochem.* 83: 973-983, 2002.

Ray, S., Britschgi, M., Herbert, C., Takeda-Uchimura, Y., Boxer, A., Blennow, K., Friedman, L. F., Galasko, D. R., Jutel, M., Karydas, A., Kaye, J. A., Leszek, J., Miller, B. L., Minthon, L., Quinn, J. F., Rabinovici, G. D., Robinson, W. H., Sabbagh, M. N., So, Y. T., Sparks, D. L., Tabaton, M., Tinklenberg, J., Yesavage, J. A., Tibshirani, R., Wyss-Coray, T. Classification and prediction of clinical Alzheimer's diagnosis based on plasma signaling proteins. *Nat Med.* 13: 1359-1362, 2007.

Reddy, P. H., McWeeney, S., Park, B. S., Manczak, M., Gutala, R. V., Partovi, D., Jung, Y., Yau, V., Searles, R., Mori, M., Quinn, J. Gene expression profiles of transcripts in amyloid precursor protein transgenic mice: up-regulation of mitochondrial metabolism and apoptotic genes is an early cellular change in Alzheimer's disease. *Hum Mol Genet.* 13: 1225-1240, 2004.

Ricciarelli, R., d'Abramo, C., Massone, S., Marinari, U., Pronzato, M., Tabaton, M. Microarray analysis in Alzheimer's disease and normal aging. *IUBMB Life*. 56: 349-354, 2004.

Rogers, J., Cooper, N. R., Webster, S., Schultz, J., McGeer, P. L., Styren, S. D., Civin, W. H., Brachova, L., Bradt, B., Ward, P., Lieberburg, I. Complement activation by beta-amyloid in Alzheimer disease. *Proc Natl Acad Sci U S A*. 89: 10016-20, 1992.

Roher, A. E., Esh, C., Kokjohn, T. A., Kalback, W., Luehrs, D. C., Seward, J. D., Sue, L. I., Beach, T. G. Circle of willis atherosclerosis is a risk factor for sporadic Alzheimer's disease. *Arterioscler Thromb Vasc Biol.* 23: 2055-2062, 2003.

Roy, A., Jana, A., Yatish, K., Freidt, M. B., Fung, Y. K., Martinson, J. A., Pahan, K. Reactive oxygen species up-regulate CD11b in microglia via nitric oxide: Implications for neurodegenerative diseases. *Free Radic Biol Med.* 45: 686-699, 2008.

Rozovsky, I., Finch, C. E., Morgan, T. E. Age-related activation of microglia and astrocytes: in vitro studies show persistent phenotypes of aging, increased proliferation, and resistance to down-regulation. *Neurobiol Aging*. 19: 97-103, 1998.

Salvioli, S., Capri, M., Valensin, S., Tieri, P., Monti, D., Ottaviani, E., Franceschi, C. Inflamm-aging, cytokines and aging: state of the art, new hypotheses on the role of mitochondria and new perspectives from systems biology. *Curr Pharm Des*. 12: 3161-3171, 2006.

Sawada, M., Imamura, K., Nagatsu, T. Role of cytokines in inflammatory process in Parkinson's disease. *J Neural Transm Suppl*. 373-381, 2006.

Schenk, D., Barbour, R., Dunn, W., Gordon, G., Grajeda, H., Guido, T., Hu, K., Huang, J., Johnson-Wood, K., Khan, K., Kholodenko, D., Lee, M., Liao, Z., Lieberburg, I., Motter, R., Mutter, L., Soriano, F., Shopp, G., Vasquez, N., Vandevert, C., Walker, S., Wogulis, M., Yednock, T., Games, D., Seubert, P. Immunization with amyloid-beta attenuates Alzheimer-disease-like pathology in the PDAPP mouse. *Nature*. 400: 173-177, 1999.

Schenk, D., Hagen, M., Seubert, P. Current progress in beta-amyloid immunotherapy. *Curr Opin Immunol.* 16: 599-606, 2004.

Schenk, D. B., Seubert, P., Grundman, M., Black, R. A beta immunotherapy: Lessons learned for potential treatment of Alzheimer's disease. *Neurodegener Dis*. 2: 255-260, 2005.

Schwab, C., Hosokawa, M., McGeer, P. L. Transgenic mice overexpressing amyloid beta protein are an incomplete model of Alzheimer disease. *Exp Neurol.* 188: 52-64, 2004.

Shie, F. S., Breyer, R. M., Montine, T. J. Microglia lacking E Prostanoid Receptor subtype 2 have enhanced Abeta phagocytosis yet lack Abeta-activated neurotoxicity. *Am J Pathol.* 166: 1163-1172, 2005.

Simi, A., Tsakiri, N., Wang, P., Rothwell, N. J. Interleukin-1 and inflammatory neurodegeneration. Biochem Soc Trans. 35: 1122-1126, 2007.

Small, D. H., Cappai, R. Alois Alzheimer and Alzheimer's disease: a centennial perspective. *J Neurochem*. 99: 708-710, 2006.

Sokolova, A., Hill, M. D., Rahimi, F., Warden, L. A., Halliday, G. M., Shepherd, C. E. Monocyte Chemoattractant Protein-1 Plays a Dominant Role in the Chronic Inflammation Observed in Alzheimer's Disease. *Brain Pathol.* 2008.

Steinman, L. Nuanced roles of cytokines in three major human brain disorders. *J Clin Invest.* 118: 3557-3563, 2008.

Tan, J., Town, T., Crawford, F., Mori, T., DelleDonne, A., Crescentini, R., Obregon, D., Flavell, R. A., Mullan, M. J. Role of CD40 ligand in amyloidosis in transgenic Alzheimer's mice. *Nat Neurosci*. 5: 1288-1293, 2002.

Tan, J., Town, T., Mori, T., Wu, Y., Saxe, M., Crawford, F., Mullan, M. CD45 opposes beta-amyloid peptide-induced microglial activation via inhibition of p44/42 mitogen-activated protein kinase. *J Neurosci*. 20: 7587-7594, 2000.

Togo, T., Akiyama, H., Iseki, E., Kondo, H., Ikeda, K., Kato, M., Oda, T., Tsuchiya, K., Kosaka, K. Occurrence of T cells in the brain of Alzheimer's disease and other neurological diseases. *J Neuroimmunol*. 124: 83-92, 2002.

Uchikado, H., Akiyama, H., Kondo, H., Ikeda, K., Tsuchiya, K., Kato, M., Oda, T., Togo, T., Iseki, E., Kosaka, K. Activation of vascular endothelial cells and perivascular cells by systemic inflammation-an immunohistochemical study of postmortem human brain tissues. *Acta Neuropathol* (Berl). 107: 341-351, 2004.

Venneti, S., Wiley, C. A., Kofler, J. Imaging Microglial Activation During Neuroinflammation and Alzheimer's Disease. *J Neuroimmune Pharmacol*. 2008.

Viles-Gonzalez, J. F., Fuster, V., Badimon, J. J. Links between inflammation and thrombogenicity in atherosclerosis. *Curr Mol Med*. 6: 489-499, 2006.

Vitek, M. P., Brown, C. M., Colton, C. A. APOE genotype-specific differences in the innate immune response. *Neurobiol Aging*. 2007.

Vlad, S. C., Miller, D. R., Kowall, N. W., Felson, D. T. Protective effects of NSAIDs on the development of Alzheimer disease. *Neurology*. 70: 1672-1677, 2008.

Walker, D. G., Kim, S. U., McGeer, P. L. Complement and cytokine gene expression in cultured microglial derived from postmortem human brains. *J Neurosci Res*. 40: 478-493, 1995.

Walker, D. G., Link, J., Lue, L. F., Dalsing-Hernandez, J. E., Boyes, B. E. Gene expression changes by amyloid beta peptide-stimulated human postmortem brain microglia identify activation of multiple inflammatory processes. *J Leukoc Biol*. 79: 596-610, 2006.

Walker, D. G., Dalsing-Hernandez, J. E., Campbell, N. A., Lue, L. F. Decreased expression of CD200 and CD200 receptor in Alzheimer's disease: a potential mechanism leading to chronic inflammation. *Exp Neurol*. 215: 5-19, 2009.

Webster, S., Lue, L. F., Brachova, L., Tenner, A. J., McGeer, P. L., Terai, K., Walker, D. G., Bradt, B., Cooper, N. R., Rogers, J. Molecular and cellular characterization of the membrane attack complex, C5b-9, in Alzheimer's disease. *Neurobiol Aging*. 18: 415-421, 1997.

Webster, S. D., Tenner, A. J., Poulos, T. L., Cribbs, D. H. The mouse C1q A-chain sequence alters beta-amyloid-induced complement activation. *Neurobiol Aging*. 20: 297-304, 1999.

Weeraratna, A. T., Kalehua, A., Deleon, I., Bertak, D., Maher, G., Wade, M. S., Lustig, A., Becker, K. G., Wood, W., III, Walker, D. G., Beach, T. G., Taub, D. D. Alterations in immunological and neurological gene expression patterns in Alzheimer's disease tissues. *Exp Cell Res*. 313: 450-461, 2007.

Wilcock, D. M., Jantzen, P. T., Li, Q., Morgan, D., Gordon, M. N. Amyloid-beta vaccination, but not nitro-nonsteroidal anti-inflammatory drug treatment, increases vascular amyloid and microhemorrhage while both reduce parenchymal amyloid. *Neuroscience*. .: 2006.

Wilcock, D. M., Munireddy, S. K., Rosenthal, A., Ugen, K. E., Gordon, M. N., Morgan, D. Microglial activation facilitates Abeta plaque removal following intracranial anti-Abeta antibody administration. *Neurobiol Dis*. 15: 11-20, 2004a.

Wilcock, D. M., Rojiani, A., Rosenthal, A., Subbarao, S., Freeman, M. J., Gordon, M. N., Morgan, D. Passive immunotherapy against Abeta in aged APP-transgenic mice reverses cognitive deficits and depletes parenchymal amyloid deposits in spite of increased vascular amyloid and microhemorrhage. *J Neuroinflammation*. 1: 24, 2004b.

Wyss-Coray, T. Inflammation in Alzheimer disease: driving force, bystander or beneficial response? *Nat Med*. 12: 1005-1015, 2006.

Wyss-Coray, T., Lin, C., Yan, F., Yu, G. Q., Rohde, M., McConlogue, L., Masliah, E., Mucke, L. TGF-beta1 promotes microglial amyloid-beta clearance and reduces plaque burden in transgenic mice. *Nat Med*. 7: 612-618, 2001.

Xiang, Z., Ho, L., Yemul, S., Zhao, Z., Qing, W., Pompl, P., Kelley, K., Dang, A., Qing, W., Teplow, D., Pasinetti, G. M. Cyclooxygenase-2 promotes amyloid plaque deposition in a mouse model of Alzheimer's disease neuropathology. *Gene Expr*. 10: 271-278, 2002.

Yamamoto, M., Horiba, M., Buescher, J. L., Huang, D., Gendelman, H. E., Ransohoff, R. M., Ikezu, T. Overexpression of monocyte chemotactic protein-1/CCL2 in beta-amyloid precursor protein transgenic mice show accelerated diffuse beta-amyloid deposition. *Am J Pathol*. 166: 1475-1485, 2005.

Yan, S. D., Stern, D., Schmidt, A. M. What's the RAGE? The receptor for advanced glycation end products (RAGE) and the dark side of glucose. *Eur J Clin Invest*. 27: 179-181, 1997.

Zlokovic, B. V. Neurovascular mechanisms of Alzheimer's neurodegeneration. Trends *Neurosci*. 28: 202-208, 2005.

In: Alzheimer's Disease and Dementia (Vol. 4) ISBN:978-1-60876-152-4
Editor: Miao-Kun Sun

Chapter VIII

Cathepsins in Alzheimer's Disease and Dementia: Cathepsin Inhibitors as Potential Anti-Dementic Therapeutics

Azizul Haque[1,2,3], *Naren L. Banik*[1,3,4] *and Swapan K. Ray*[*,1,3,5]
Department of Microbiology and Immunology[1]
Children's Research Institute[2]
Hollings Cancer Center[3]
Department of Neurosciences, Medical University of South Carolina, Charleston, SC 29425, USA[4]
Department of Pathology, Microbiology, and Immunology, University of South Carolina School of Medicine, Columbia, SC 29209, USA[5]

Abstract

Acidic cathepsins play multiple roles in the initiation, development, and progression of pathological events in autoimmunity, malignancies, and neurodegeneration. Cysteinyl and aspartyl cathepsins are significantly upregulated in a number of neurodegenerative diseases including Alzheimer's disease (AD), a leading cause of dementia in the elderly. Increases in expression and activity of cathepsins are also found in AD patients where senile plaques and neuronal loss are marked features of the disease. Cysteinyl and aspartyl cathepsins have also been shown to process amyloid precursor protein (APP) generating toxic amyloid-beta (Aβ) peptide, which is predominantly found in senile plaques in AD. In this chapter, we focus on the recent developments regarding the role of acidic cathepsins in the regulation of cellular and molecular events that contribute to the formation of senile plagues and neuronal loss in AD and dementia. This chapter also

[*]Correspondence: Swapan K. Ray, Ph.D., Department of Pathology, Microbiology, and Immunology, University of South Carolina School of Medicine, Building 2, Room C11, 6439 Garners Ferry Road, Columbia, SC 29209, USA. E-mail: swapan.ray@uscmed.sc.edu

includes the role of cathepsin inhibitors as disease-modifying treatment strategies that may have the potential to halt or prevent AD and dementia.

Keywords: Alzheimer's disease (AD), amyloid precursor protein (APP), amyloid-beta (Aβ) peptide, apoptosis, cathepsins, cathepsin inhibitors, neurodegeneration

Introduction

Alzheimer's disease (AD) is a progressive neurodegenerative disorder and the most common cause of dementia in the elderly population (Mueller-Steiner et al., 2006; van Broeck et al., 2007). Studies suggest that the proteolytic processing of the amyloid precursor protein (APP) results in the production of amyloid-beta (Aβ) peptide. This toxic Aβ peptide plays a crucial role in the pathogenesis of AD (Tagawa et al., 1992; Munger et al., 1995; Hook et al., 2007; LaFerla et al., 2007). Although the general assumption is that Aβ peptide is deposited extracellularly, recent evidence from mouse and human studies suggests that Aβ peptide can also be deposited intraneuronally, influencing the progression of disease. The processing of APP is regulated by the action of the enzymes α-secretase, β-secretase, and γ-secretase, with the later two mediating the amyloidogenic production of Aβ peptides (Tagawa et al., 1991; Evin et al., 1995; Mackay et al., 1997; Tsai et al., 2002). While several species of Aβ peptides of 39-43 amino acids are produced in the brain, production of Aβ1-42 is particularly critical for the pathogenesis of AD.

Inflammatory processes in the central nervous system (CNS) may contribute to neuronal death in a number of neurodegenerative diseases including AD (Cataldo et al., 1990; Cataldo et al., 1995; Nixon et al., 2000; Buckwalter et al., 2006; LaFerla et al., 2007; Ding et al., 2008). The inflammatory process is mainly mediated by the CNS immune cells such as microglia in response to neuronal damage, clearing damaged cells by phagocytosis. While activation of microglia plays a crucial role in brain pathology (Amano et al., 1995; Evin et al. 1995; Nakanishi, 2003), it remains unclear whether activation of microglia provides beneficial or detrimental function in the pathogenesis of neurodegeneration. It is believed that the activation of microglia may result in neuronal damage by releasing cytotoxic molecules such as inflammatory cytokines, reactive oxygen species (ROS), complement proteins, and proteases (Tagawa et al., 1992; Amano et al., 1995; Nakanishi, 2003; Clark et al., 2007). Activation of endolysosomal proteases may also lead to the generation of toxic peptides and ROS that induce neuronal death (Tagawa et al., 1992; Yamashima, 2000; Hook, 2006). Accumulation of these toxic peptides induces a cascade of events such as excessive inflammation, production of ROS, and neuronal apoptosis leading to CNS damage and degeneration (Yamashima, 2000; Benchoua et al, 2004; Hook, 2006; Reynolds et al., 2007). Several molecular chaperones and chaperone-related proteases such as proteasome can also hydrolyse ATP to convert stable and unstable harmful protein aggregates into harmless native refoldable or protease-degradable polypeptides (Hinault et al., 2006; Wang et al., 2007). Molecular chaperones and chaperone-related proteases thus control the delicate balance between native folded functional proteins and aggregation-prone misfolded proteins, which may form during the lifetime leading to cell death. Events such as inflammation and oxidative stress can also lead to caspase activation and neuronal apoptosis.

While endolysosomal cathepsins are implicated in the molecular pathogenesis of AD, specific cathepsins that degrade APP remain largely unknown. Studies suggest that cysteinyl and aspartyl cathepsins can be critical regulators of brain Aβ levels as they process APP (Danzin et al., 1997; Nixon et al., 2001; Hook et al., 2005). Because the CNS is a key target for the development of novel therapeutic agents for the treatment of neurodegenerative diseases, neuroproteases may also be involved in the generation of specific peptide neurotransmitters and toxic peptides in major neurodegenerative diseases such as AD, Huntington disease (HD), and Parkinson's disease (PD) (Mantle et al., 1995; Tsai et al., 2002; Hook, 2006; Kim et al., 2006). Various studies have identified secretory vesicles cathepsin B (Cat B) and cathepsin D (Cat D) as novel β-secretases for production of the neurotoxic Aβ peptide. Inhibition of Cat B has been shown to reduce Aβ peptide levels in brain (Hook et al., 2005, Kim et al., 2006; Hook et al., 2007). Likewise, the γ-secretase complex is an intramembrane aspartyl protease that cleaves its substrates along their transmembrane regions. Sequential proteolytic processing of APP by β-secretase and γ-secretase may produce Aβ peptides, which are the major components of amyloid plaques in the brains of AD patients (Tsai et al., 2002; Hook et al., 2005, Hook et al., 2007).

Endolysosomal Systems in Neurological Disorders and Dementia

Endolysosomes are important organelles having an acidic milieu to maintain cellular metabolism by degrading cellular materials that have exceeded their lifetime or are otherwise no longer useful. Late endosomal and lysosomal enzymes, including cathepsins and some lipid hydrolases, which are secreted following rupture of the lysosomal membrane, can be very harmful to their environment, resulting in pathological destruction of cellular structures (Kagedal et al., 2001 et al., 2006; Qin et al., 2008). Since lysosomes contain catalytic enzymes for degrading proteins, carbohydrates, and lipids, it seems natural that they should participate in cellular death and dismantling (Nilsson et al., 2006; Windelborn et al., 2008). Studies have found that neuronal damage may begin after the release of cathepsins and is prevented by inhibitors of either Cat B or Cat D indicating that the release of cathepsins is an important mediator of severe damage. Endolysosomal cathepsins, including cysteinyl and aspartyl cathepsins, are translated as inactive pro-enzymes and mature to active enzymes via proteolytic cleavage exposure within the acidic environments of late endosomal and lysosomal compartments. This process facilitates the separation of proteinases from essential cellular proteins and contributes to a lysosomal environment necessary for the homeostatic turnover of proteins and other cellular materials. Study also suggests that the release of lysosomal cathepsins into the cytosol may cause cellular damage following a wide variety of insults, while these same proteases normally play a vital homeostatic role within the lysosomal system (Kagedal et al., 2001; Nilsson et al., 2006; Qin et al., 2008). The movement of the lysosomal cysteine protease, Cat B, into the cytosol has also been associated with neuronal death following ischemia in animals.

Aβ peptides are produced by proteolytic processing of APP, resulting in production of Aβ40 and Aβ42 (1–40 and 1–42 residues, respectively) peptides. Proteases referred to as β-secretase and γ-secretase cleave at the N-terminal and C terminal of Aβ within APP to generate Aβ peptides. Aβ peptides then undergo secretion to provide extracellular Aβ that produces neurotoxic effects with aggregation and accumulation of amyloid plaques in AD brains. Thus, compounds that inhibit β-secretase activity are attractive as potential therapeutic agents for AD and dementia. Irreversible epoxysuccinyl cysteine protease inhibitors are known to reduce brain Aβ and β-secretase activity in the guinea pig model of human Aβ production. In this study, acetyl-L-leucyl-L-valyl-L-lysinal (Ac-LVK-CHO) is also shown to significantly reduce brain Aβ and β-secretase activity and brain Aβ in the same animal model. Ac-LVK-CHO is structurally distinct from the epoxysuccinyl inhibitors and is a reversible cysteine protease inhibitor. The results suggest that cysteine protease inhibitors generally, and reversible cysteine protease inhibitors specifically, have potential for development of AD therapeutics.

Alterations in the endolysosomal system may represent a central mechanism in neurodegeneration. The identification of cathepsins in Aβ plaques has revealed broad dysfunction of the lysosomal system in AD. While proteolytic processes are important in the generation of Aβ, it remains unclear how proteolytic pathways are adversely influenced by normal brain aging and by genetic and environmental factors, resulting in increased susceptibility of neurons to injury, amyloidogenesis, and neurodegeneration. Collectively, lysosomal disturbances do add to contributing factors to cause neurological problems in AD (Fig. 1). Studies have identified novel compounds to test whether suppression of the lysosomal proteases blocks production of known precursors to neurofibrillary tangles. It has been reported that an induction of lysosomal dysfunction is possible in cultured hippocampal slices with a selective inhibitor of cysteinyl cathepsins Cat B, Cat L, and Cat S (Bi et al., 1999, 2000, Hook et al., 2007, Hook et al., 2008). Potent non-peptidic inhibitors of the aspartyl protease Cat D have also been identified and shown to block production of the fragments, suggesting that cathepsin inhibitors could be used as a new approach to treat AD.

Proteasomal dysfunction may also lead to the activation of autophagy, a lysosomal pathway for degrading organelles and long-lived proteins (Nixon, 2007; Boland et al., 2008). Alterations in the autophagic system may contribute to major neurodegenerative disorders such as AD, PD, and HD (Mizushima, 2005; Komatsu et al., 2006; Boland et al., 2008). Although basal levels of autophagy have been shown to protect against neurodegeneration, the mechanisms remain elusive. Extracellular Aβ that confers neurotoxicity and modulates synaptic plasticity and memory function is thought to be central to the amyloid hypothesis of AD. Intracellular Aβ may affect a variety of cellular physiology from protein degradation, axonal transport, and autophagy to apoptosis. Autophagy is the one and only tier of defence against the accumulation of inclusion bodies and autophagy functionally declines with increasing age. Autophagy also regulates cell survival as well as individual lifespan (de Duve, 2005; Chu, 2006; Komatsu et al., 2006). The generation of Aβ peptide may take place in autophagic vacuoles, which accumulate in AD brains (Komatsu et al., 2006, Nixon, 2007;

Boland et al., 2008). Thus autophagy may play an important role in the alteration of age-associated diseases including AD and dementia (Fig. 1).

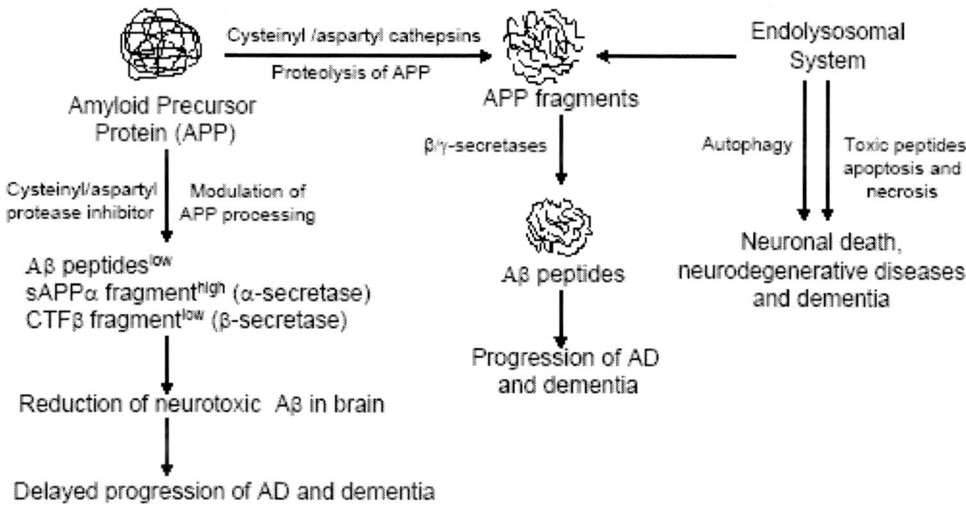

Figure 1. Abnormal regulation of cysteinyl and aspartyl cathepsins in the endolysosomal system may contribute to the pathogenesis of AD and dementia. Endolysosomal functions can be altered by many factors including activation of lysosomal enzymes, oxidative stress, and autophagy. These activities may promote apoptosis or necrosis in neurons and generation of toxic peptides for continuation of neurodegeneration. Cysteinyl and aspartyl cathepsins, mainly Cat B and Cat D, take part in the proteolytic processing of APP and generation of neurotoxic Aβ peptides that can accumulate in the cells initiating a variety of neurologic disorders. These processes can be blocked by cysteinyl and aspartyl cathepsin inhibitors to reduce the harmful effects on neurons.

Cysteinyl and Aspartyl Cathepsins in AD

Cysteinyl and aspartyl cathepsins (A, B, C, D, and L) that degrade axonal and myelin proteins have long been suggested to be involved in degeneration of axons in demyelinating diseases and CNS injuries (Hashim et al., 1969; Benuck et al., 1975; Marks et al., 1977; Banik, 1992). Thus, proper functioning of the cathepsins is critical for normal cellular activity and viability. Studies have reported that cysteinyl and aspartyl cathepsins degrade APP into toxic peptides contributing to the progression of the neurodegenerative process in AD (Fig. 1). Cysteinyl proteases such as Cat B, Cat L, and Cat S are also associated with other neurodegenerative diseases such as epilepsy, PD, and HD (Nixon et al., 2001, Hook et al., 2005; Kim et al., 2006; Nixon et al., 2006; Ma et al., 2007). Secretory vesicle Cat B has been reported as a novel β-secretase for the production of Cat B in neurotoxic Aβ peptide (Mueller-Steiner et al., 2006; Hook et al., 2007). Inhibition of Cat B reduces Aβ peptide levels in brain. Thus, cysteinyl and aspartyl proteases could represent new drug targets for the attenuation of neurodegeneration in AD. Aspartyl Cat D is a ubiquitously expressed lysosomal protease that is involved in proteolytic degradation, cell invasion, and apoptosis

(Deiss et al., 1996; Beneset al., 2008). Cat D has also been implicated in the processing of APP (Ladror et al., 1994) and a Cat D polymorphism may be associated with Aβ deposition in the brain leading to an increased risk of AD (Wisniewski et al., 1998; Nixon et al., 2006). Since Aβ is the main component of the senile plaques that are abundant in AD brain, deposition and clearance of Cat D may be important in AD pathogenesis. Proteolytic processing of APP is also markedly inhibited by aspartyl protease inhibitor (e.g., pepstatin A), suggesting that Cat D is critically involved in the generation of Aβ peptide fragments in AD pathology.

Toxic peptides are also key factors that participate in the development of AD (Bi et al., 1999; Bi et al., 2000; Hook et al., 2007; Hook et al., 2008). Proteolytic cleavage by acidic cathepsins and activation of caspases have also been shown as key players in neurodegeneration that may result in neuronal death in selected brain regions, leading to behavioral deficits, cognitive dysfunction, and other neurologic disorders (Bednarski et al., 1998; Kelly et al., 2005; Dillen et al., 2006; Nixon et al., 2006; Chin et al., 2007). Recent studies in AD have found alterations in systemic immune responses including the presence of activated antigen presenting cells (APC), autoantibodies, abnormal cytokine and chemokine production (Games et al., 2000; Giubilei et al., 2003; Monsonego et al. 2003; Chiappelli et al., 2006; Arbel and Solomon 2007). Activation of APC can also lead to the processing of cathepsins and other proteases that may differentially regulate various neuroinflammatory factors such as AD senile plaques in the brain due to innate immune responses against Aβ peptides (Iribarren et al., 2002; Windisch et al., 2002; Ghochikyan et al., 2006).

Cathepsin Inhibitors as Therapeutic Agents for AD and Dementia

The main clinical features of AD are thought to be neuronal loss and extracellular deposition of amyloid or senile plaques that are composed of toxic Aβ peptide. While age and genetic inheritance are common risk factors for AD, recent evidence suggests that anomalies in the proteolytic processing of APP and the subsequent poor handling of the Aβ peptide may have a central role in the early pathogenesis of the disease (Bi et al., 1999, Bi et al., 2000; Nixon et al., 2000; Hook et al., 2007; Hook et al., 2008). Thus, considerable attention is being focused on the alteration of proteolytic processing of APP for the development of therapies for AD (Fig. 1). For example, molecules that inhibit β-secretase cleavage of APP and thereby reduce extracellular accumulation of brain Aβ, might have potential as AD therapeutics. The regulated secretory pathway of neurons is the major source of extracellular Aβ that accumulates in AD. Extracellular Aβ secreted from that pathway is generated by β-secretase processing of APP (Fig. 1). Previously, cysteinyl protease activity was demonstrated as the major β-secretase activity in regulated secretory vesicles of neuronal chromaffin cells (Nixon et al., 2000; Hook et al., 2005; Nixon et al., 2006; Hook et al., 2007). Immunoelectron microscopic study has shown co-localization of Cat B and Aβ in these secretory vesicles. Studies have demonstrated that in vivo Aβ levels in brain are significantly reduced by the cysteinyl protease inhibitor E64d and the related CA074Me inhibitor, which inhibits Cat B (Hook et al., 2007; Van Broeck et al., 2007). The selective Cat B inhibitor (CA074) may block the conversion of endogenous APP to Aβ in isolated regulated secretory vesicles. In chromaffin cells, CA074Me (a cell permeable form of CA074) is shown to reduce about 50% of the extracellular Aβ released by the regulated secretory pathway, but CA074Me had no effect on Aβ released by the constitutive pathway. Furthermore, CA074Me is shown to inhibit the processing of APP into COOH-terminal β-secretase-like cleavage product (Hook et al., 2005; Mueller-Steiner 2006; Hook et al., 2007). These studies provide evidence for Cat B as a candidate β-secretase in regulated secretory vesicles of neuronal chromaffin cells. These findings also implicate Cat B as a β-secretase in the regulated secretory pathway of brain neurons, suggesting that inhibitors of Cat B may be considered as therapeutic agents to reduce Aβ in AD (Fig. 1). Direct infusion of these cathepsin inhibitors into brains of guinea pigs resulted in reduced levels of Aβ by 50-70% after 30 days of treatment (Zlokovic et al., 1996; Hook et al., 2005). Substantial decreases in Aβ also occurred after only 7 days of inhibitor infusion, with a reduction in both Aβ40 and Aβ42 peptide forms. A prominent decrease in Aβ peptides was also observed in brain synaptosomal nerve terminal preparations after CA074Me treatment. Analyses of APP-derived proteolytic fragments showed that CA074Me reduced brain levels of the CTFβ fragment, and increased amounts of the sAPPα fragment by modulating APP processing. It has been reported that irreversible epoxysuccinyl cysteinyl protease inhibitors can also reduce brain Aβ and β-secretase activity in the guinea pig model of human Aβ production (Zlokovic et al., 1996; Hook et al., 2005). In that study, a reversible cysteinyl protease inhibitor, acetyl-L-Leu-L-Val-L-Lys-aldehyde (Ac-LVK-CHO) was shown to significantly reduce brain Aβ and β-secretase activity. Thus, both reversible and irreversible cysteinyl protease inhibitors possess potentials for the therapeutic efficacy of AD and dementia.

Studies suggest that the amyloid hypothesis is the leading mechanistic theory of AD where an imbalance between production and clearance of Aβ peptides triggers a cascade of events leading to neurodegeneration and dementia. Cat D, which is the lysosomal aspartyl protease, participates in the catabolism, synthesis, and activation of peptides and proteins. Cat D has been implicated in multiple apoptotic events and neurodegenerative diseases including AD (Dreyer et al., 1994; Hoffman et al., 1998) and epilepsy (Hetman at al., 1995). Cat D can initiate and facilitate the caspase cascade of apoptosis. Reports have shown that microinjection of Cat D induces caspase-dependent apoptosis in fibroblasts, while Cat B favors caspase processing activity following exposure to atractyloside (Tagawa et al., 1991; Vancompernolle et al., 1998; Roberg et al., 2002). Interestingly, several reports showed that knockout mice with Cat B, Cat L, and cysteinyl protease suppression affect Cat D levels (Cataldo et al., 1994; Bednarski et al., 1996; 1997; Felbor et al., 2002), suggesting a regulatory role for Cat D. Alterations in the expression levels and activities of Cat B and Cat D have been reported during pathological conditions such as oxidative stress (Cataldo et al., 1995, Cataldo et al., 1997; Nishio et al., 2000; Takuma et al., 2002). Because no endogenous inhibitors have been identified for Cat D, uncontrolled Cat D activity could have detrimental effects on multiple neuronal substrates. Thus, a combination of cysteinyl and aspartyl protease inhibitors may perturb abnormal proteolytic processing and lower the levels of toxic peptides in AD and dementia.

Conclusion

In conclusion, cathepsins play significant roles in the pathogenesis of AD and dementia. Increases in expression and activity of cathepsins cause neuronal death in AD patients. Cathepsins also participate in processing APP to generate toxic Aβ peptides, which are found in senile plaques in AD. Dysregulation of the endolysosomal system seems to be a central mechanism in neurodegeneration in AD and dementia. We have discussed the recent developments regarding the roles of cathepsins in the regulation of cellular and molecular events that contribute to the formation of senile plagues and neuronal death in AD and dementia. Because cathepsin inhibitors appear to be highly promising in preventing abnormal processing of APP and reducing the levels of toxic peptides, they can be used as potential anti-AD and anti-dementic therapeutics.

Acknowledgments

This work was supported in part by the grants from the National Institutes of Health (CA-129560) and Medical University of South Carolina to A.H., R01 grants (NS-41088 and NS-45967) to N.L.B., and also R01 grants (CA-91460 and NS-57811) to S.K.R.

Disclosures

The authors have no financial conflict of interest.

References

Amano, T., Nakanishi, H., Oka, M. and Yamamoto, K. Increased expression of cathepsins E and D in reactive microglial cells associated with spongiform degeneration in the brain stem of senescence-accelerated mouse. *Exp. Neurol.* 136: 171-182, 1995.

Arbel, M., Solomon, B. A novel immunotherapy for Alzheimer's disease: antibodies against the β-secretase cleavage site of APP. *Curr. Alzheimer. Res.* 4: 437-445, 2007.

Banik, N.L. Pathogenesis of myelin breakdown in demyelinating diseases: role of proteolytic enzymes. *Crit. Rev. Neurobiol.* 6: 257-271, 1992.

Bednarski, E. and Lynch, G. Cytosolic proteolysis of tau by cathepsin D in hippocampus following suppression of cathepsins B and L. *J. Neurochem.* 67: 1846-1855, 1996.

Bednarski, E., Lauterborn, J.C., Gall, C.M. and Lynch, G. Lysosomal dysfunction reduces brain-derived neurotrophic factor expression. *Exp. Neurol.* 150: 128-135, 1998.

Benchoua, A., Braudeau, J., Reis, A., Couriaud, C. and Onténiente B. Activation of proinflammatory caspases by cathepsin B in focal cerebral ischemia. *J. Cereb Blood Flow Metab.* 24: 1272-1279, 2004.

Benes, P., Vetvicka, V., and Fusek, M. Cathepsin D - many functions of one aspartic protease. Crit. Rev. Oncol. Hematol. 68:12-28, 2008.

Benuck, M., Marks, N. and Hashim G.A. Metabolic instability of myelin proteins. Breakdown of basic protein induced by brain cathepsin D. *Eur. J. Biochem.* 52: 615-621, 1975.

Bi, X., Haque, T.S., Zhou, J., Skillman, A.G., Lin, B., Lee, C.E., Kuntz, I.D., Ellman, J.A. and Lynch, G. Novel cathepsin D inhibitors block the formation of hyperphosphorylated tau fragments in hippocampus. *J. Neurochem.* 74: 1469-1477, 2000.

Bi, X., Zhou, J. and Lynch, G. Lysosomal protease inhibitors induce meganeurites and tangle-like structures in entorhinohippocampal regions vulnerable to Alzheimer's disease. *Exp. Neurol.* 158: 312-327, 1999.

Boland, B., Kumar, A., Lee, S., Platt, F.M., Wegiel, J., Yu, W.H., and Nixon R.A. Autophagy induction and autophagosome clearance in neurons: relationship to autophagic pathology in Alzheimer's Disease. *J. Neurosci.* 28: 6926-6937, 2008,

Buckwalter, M.S., Coleman, B.S., Buttini, M., Barbour, R., Schenk, D., Games, D., Seubert, P. and Wyss-Coray, T. Increased T cell recruitment to the CNS after amyloid beta 1-42 immunization in Alzheimer's mice overproducing transforming growth factor-beta 1. *J. Neurosci.* 26: 11437-11441, 2006.

Cataldo, A.M. and Nixon, R.A. Enzymatically active lysosomal proteases are associated with amyloid deposits in Alzheimer brain. *Proc. Natl. Acad. Sci. USA.* 87: 3861-3865, 1990.

Chiappelli, M., Tumini, E., Porcellini, E. and Licastro, F. Impaired regulation of immune responses in cognitive decline and Alzheimer's disease: lessons from genetic association studies. *Expert. Rev. Neurother.* 6: 1327-1336, 2006.

Chin, J.H., Ma, L., MacTavish, D. and Jhamandas, J.H. Amyloid beta protein modulates glutamate-mediated neurotransmission in the rat basal forebrain: involvement of presynaptic neuronal nicotinic acetylcholine and metabotropic glutamate receptors. *J. Neurosci.* 27: 9262-9269, 2007.

Chu, C.T. Autophagic stress in neuronal injury and disease. *J. Neuropathol. Exp. Neurol.* 65: 423-432, 2006.

Clark, A.K., Yip, P.K., Grist, J., Gentry, C., Staniland, A.A., Marchand, F., Dehvari, M., Wotherspoon, G., Winter, J., Ullah, J., Bevan, S. and Malcangio, M. Inhibition of spinal microglial cathepsin S for the reversal of neuropathic pain. *Proc. Natl. Acad. Sci. USA.* 104: 10655-10660, 2007.

de Duve, C. The lysosome turns fifty. *Nat. Cell Biol.* 7: 847-849, 2005.

Deiss, L.P., Galinka, H., Berissi, H., Cohen, O. and Kimchi, A. Cathepsin D protease mediates programmed cell death induced by interferon-gamma, Fas/APO-1 and TNF-α, *EMBO J* 15: 3861-3870, 1996.

Dillen, K. and Annaert, W. A two decade contribution of molecular cell biology to the centennial of Alzheimer's disease: are we progressing toward therapy? *Int. Rev. Cytol.* 254: 215-300, 2006.

Ding, J.D., Lin, J., Mace, B.E., Herrmann, R., Sullivan, P. and Bowes Rickman, C. Targeting age-related macular degeneration with Alzheimer's disease based immunotherapies: anti-amyloid-β antibody attenuates pathologies in an age-related macular degeneration mouse model. *Vision. Res.* 48: 339-345, 2008.

Dreyer, R.N., Bausch, K.M., Fracasso, P., Hammond, L.J., Wunderlich, D., Wirak, D.O., Davis, G., Brini, C.M., Buckholz, T.M., Konig, G., Kamarck, M.E. and Tamburini, P.P. Processing of the pre-β-amyloid protein by cathepsin D is enhanced by a familial Alzheimer's disease mutation. *Eur. J. Biochem.* 224: 265-271, 1994.

Evin, G., Cappai, R., Li, Q.X., Culvenor, J.G., Small, D.H., Beyreuther, K. and Masters, C.L. Candidate γ-secretases in the generation of the carboxyl terminus of the Alzheimer's disease βA4 amyloid: possible involvement of cathepsin D. *Biochemistry.* 34: 14185-14192, 1995.

Felbor, U., Kessler, B., Mothes, W., Goebel, H., Ploegh, H.L., Bronson, R.T., Olsen, B.R. Neuronal loss and brain atrophy in mice lacking cathepsins B and L. *Proc. Natl. Acad. Sci. USA.* 99: 7883-7888, 2002.

Games, D., Bard, F., Grajeda, H., Guido, T., Khan, K., Soriano, F., Vasquez, N., Wehner, N., Johnson-Wood, K., Yednock, T., Seubert, P. and Schenk, D. Prevention and reduction of AD-type pathology in PDAPP mice immunized with A beta 1-42. *Ann. NY. Acad. Sci.* 920: 274-284, 2000.

Ghochikyan, A., Petrushina, I., Lees, A., Vasilevko, V., Movsesyan, N., Karapetyan, A., Agadjanyan, M.G., Cribbs, D.H. Aβ-immunotherapy for Alzheimer's disease using mannan-amyloid-β peptide immunoconjugates. *DNA Cell. Biol.* 25: 571-580, 2006.

Giubilei, F., Antonini, G., Montesperelli, C., Sepe-Monti, M., Cannoni, S., Pichi, A., Tisei, P., Casini, A.R., Buttinelli, C., Prencipe, M., Salvetti, M., Ristori and G. Dement. T cell response to amyloid-β and to mitochondrial antigens in Alzheimer's disease. *Geriatr. Cogn. Disord.* 16: 35-38, 2003.

Hashim, G.A. and Eylar E.H. The structure of the terminal regions of the encephalitogenic basic protein from bovine myelin. *Arch. Biochem. Biophys.* 129: 635, 1969.

Hetman, M., Filipkowski, R.K., Domagala, W. and Kaczmarek, L. Elevated cathepsin D expression in kainate-evoked rat brain neurodegeneration. *Exp. Neurol.* 136: 53-63, 1995.

Hinault, M.P., Ben-Zvi, A. and Goloubinoff, P. Chaperones and proteases: cellular fold-controlling factors of proteins in neurodegenerative diseases and aging. *J. Mol. Neurosci.* 30: 249-265, 2006.

Hoffman, K.B., Bi, X., Pam J.T. and Lynch, G. Seizure induced synthesis of fibronectin is rapid and age dependent: implications for long-term potentiation and sprouting. *Neurosci. Lett.* 250: 75–78, 1998.

Hook, V., Kindy, M. and Hook, G. Cysteine protease inhibitors reduce brain beta-amyloid and β-secretase activity in vitro and are potential Alzheimer's disease therapeutics. *Biol. Chem.* 388: 247-252, 2007.

Hook, V., Toneff, T., Bogyo, M., Greenbaum, D., Medzihradszky, K.F., Neveu, J., Lane, W., Hook, G. and Reisine, T. Inhibition of cathepsin B reduces β-amyloid production in regulated secretory vesicles of neuronal chromaffin cells: evidence for cathepsin B as a candidate beta-secretase of Alzheimer's disease. *Biol. Chem.* 386: 931-940, 2005. Erratum in: *Biol. Chem.* 386: 1325, 2005.

Hook, V.Y. Neuroproteases in peptide neurotransmission and neurodegenerative diseases: applications to drug discovery research. *BioDrugs.* 20: 105-119, 2006.

Hook, V.Y., Kindy, M., Hook, G. Inhibitors of cathepsin B improve memory and reduce beta-amyloid in transgenic Alzheimer disease mice expressing the wild-type, but not the Swedish mutant, β-secretase site of the amyloid precursor protein. *J. Biol. Chem.* 283: 7745-7753, 2008.

Iribarren, P., Cui, Y.H., Le, Y. and Wang, J.M. The role of dendritic cells in neurodegenerative diseases. *Arch. Immunol. Ther. Exp. (Warsz).* 50: 187-196, 2002.

Kågedal, K., Johansson, U., Ollinger, K. The lysosomal protease cathepsin D mediates apoptosis induced by oxidative stress. *FASEB J.* 15: 1592-1594, 2001.

Kelly, B.L., Vassar, R. and Ferreira, A. β-Amyloid-induced dynamin 1 depletion in hippocampal neurons. A potential mechanism for early cognitive decline in Alzheimer disease. *J. Biol. Chem.* 280: 31746-31753, 2005.

Kim, Y.J., Sapp, E., Cuiffo, B.G., Sobin, L., Yoder, J., Kegel, K.B., Qin, Z.H., Detloff, P., Aronin, N. and DiFiglia, M. Lysosomal proteases are involved in generation of N-terminal huntingtin fragments. *Neurobiol. Dis.* 22: 346-356, 2006.

Komatsu, M., Kominami, E. and Tanaka, K. Autophagy and neurodegeneration. *Autophagy.* 2: 315-317, 2006.

Ladror, U.S., Snyder, S.W., Wang, G.T., Holzman, T.F., and Krafft, G.A. Cleavage at the amino and carboxyl termini of Alzheimer's amyloid-β by cathepsin D, *J. Biol. Chem.* 269: 18422-18428, 1994.

LaFerla, F.M., Green, K.N. and Oddo, S. Intracellular amyloid-β in Alzheimer's disease. *Nat. Rev. Neurosci.* 8: 499-509, 2007.

Ma, J., Tanaka, K.F., Yamada G. and Ikenaka, K. Induced expression of cathepsins and cystatin C in a murine model of demyelination. *Neurochem. Res.* 32: 311-320, 2007.

Mackay, E.A., Ehrhard, A., Moniatte, M., Guenet, C., Tardif. C., Tarnus, C., Sorokine, O., Heintzelmann, B., Nay, C., Remy, J.M., Higaki, J., Van Dorsselaer, A., Wagner, J., Danzin, C. and Mamont, P. A possible role for cathepsins D, E, and B in the processing of β-amyloid precursor protein in Alzheimer's disease. *Eur. J. Biochem.* 244: 414-425, 1997.

Mantle, D., Falkous, G., Ishiura, S., Perry, R.H. and Perry, E.K. Comparison of cathepsin protease activities in brain tissue from normal cases and cases with Alzheimer's disease, Lewy body dementia, Parkinson's disease and Huntington's disease. *J. Neurol. Sci.* 131: 65-70, 1995.

Marks, N., Grynbaum, A. and Levine, S. Proteolytic enzymes in ordinary, hyperacute, monocytic and passive transfer forms of experimental allergic encephalomyelitis. *Brain Res.* 123: 147-157, 1977.

Mizushima, N. Aβ generation in autophagic vacuoles. *J. Cell. Biol.* 171: 15-17, 2005.

Monsonego, A. and Weiner. H.L. Immunotherapeutic approaches to Alzheimer's disease. *Science* 302: 834-838, 2003.

Mueller-Steiner, S., Zhou, Y., Arai, H., Roberson, E.D., Sun, B., Chen, J., Wang, X., Yu, G., Esposito, L., Mucke, L. and Gan, L. Antiamyloidogenic and neuroprotective functions of cathepsin B: implications for Alzheimer's disease. *Neuron* 51: 703-714, 2006.

Munger, J.S., Haass, C., Lemere, C.A., Shi, G.P., Wong, W.S., Teplow, D.B., Selkoe, D.J. and Chapman, H.A. Lysosomal processing of amyloid precursor protein to Aβ peptides: a distinct role for cathepsin S. *Biochem. J.* 311: 299-305, 1995.

Nakanishi, H. Neuronal and microglial cathepsins in aging and age-related diseases. *Ageing Res. Rev.* 2: 367-381, 2003.

Nilsson, C, Johansson, U, Johansson, A.C., Kågedal, K., Ollinger, K. Cytosolic acidification and lysosomal alkalinization during TNF-α induced apoptosis in U937 cells. *Apoptosis* 11: 1149-1159, 2006.

Nishio, C., Yoshida, K., Nishiyama, K., Hatanaka, H. and Yamada, M. Involvement of cystatin C in oxidative stress-induced apoptosis of cultured rat CNS neurons. *Brain Res.* 873: 252–262, 2000.

Nixon, R.A. and Cataldo, A.M. Lysosomal system pathways: genes to neurodegeneration in Alzheimer's disease. *J. Alzheimers Dis.* 9: 277-289, 2006.

Nixon, R.A., Cataldo, A.M. and Mathews, P.M. The endosomal-lysosomal system of neurons in Alzheimer's disease pathogenesis: a review. *Neurochem. Res.* 25: 1161-1172, 2000.

Nixon, R.A., Mathews, P.M. and Cataldo, A.M. The neuronal endosomal-lysosomal system in Alzheimer's disease. *J. Alzheimers Dis.* 3: 97-107, 2001.

Qin, A.P., Zhang, H.L., Qin, Z.H. Mechanisms of lysosomal proteases participating in cerebral ischemia-induced neuronal death. *Neurosci. Bull.* 24: 117-123, 2008.

Reynolds, A., Laurie, C., Lee., Mosley, R. and Gendelman, H.E. Oxidative stress and the pathogenesis of neurodegenerative disorders. *Int. Rev. Neurobiol.* 82: 297-325, 2007.

Roberg, K., Kagedal K. and Ollinger, K. Microinjection of cathepsin d induces caspase-dependent apoptosis in fibroblasts. *Am. J. Pathol.* 161: 89–96, 2002.

Tagawa, K., Kunishita, T., Maruyama, K., Yoshikawa, K., Kominami, E., Tsuchiya, T., Suzuki, K., Tabira, T., Sugita, H. and Ishiura, S. Alzheimer's disease amyloid beta-clipping enzyme (APP secretase): identification, purification, and characterization of the enzyme. *Biochem. Biophys. Res. Commun.* 177: 377-387, 1991.

Tagawa, K., Maruyama, K. and Ishiura, S. Amyloid β/A4 precursor protein (APP) processing in lysosomes. *Ann. N.Y. Acad. Sci.* 674: 129-137, 1992.

Takuma, K., Kiriu, M., Mori, K., Lee, E., Enomoto, R., Baba, A., Matsuda, T. Roles of cathepsins in reperfusion-induced apoptosis in cultured astrocytes. *Neurochem. Int.* 42: 153-159, 2003.

Tsai, J.Y., Wolfe, M.S. and Xia, W. The search for gamma-secretase and development of inhibitors. *Curr. Med. Chem.* 9: 1087-10106, 2002.

Van Broeck, B., Van Broeckhoven, C. and Kumar-Singh S. Current insights into molecular mechanisms of Alzheimer disease and their implications for therapeutic approaches. *Neurodegener Dis.* 4: 349-365, 2007.

Vancompernolle, K., Herreweghe, F.V., Pynaert, G., Van de Craen, M., De Vos, K., Totty, N., Sterling, A., Fiers, W., Vandenabeele, P. and Grooten, J. Atractyloside-induced release of cathepsin B, a protease with caspase-processing activity. *FEBS Lett.* 438: 150-158, 1998.

Wang, J., Ho, L., Chen, L., Zhao, Z., Zhao, W., Qian, X., Humala, N., Seror, I., Bartholomew, S., Rosendorff, C. and Pasinetti, G.M. Valsartan lowers brain β-amyloid protein levels and improves spatial learning in a mouse model of Alzheimer disease. *J. Clin. Invest.* 117: 3393-3402, 2007.

Windelborn, J.A., Lipton, P. Lysosomal release of cathepsins causes ischemic damage in the rat hippocampal slice and depends on NMDA-mediated calcium influx, arachidonic acid metabolism, and free radical production. *J. Neurochem*. 106: 56-69, 2008.

Windisch, M., Hutter-Paier, B. and Schreiner, E. Current drugs and future hopes in the treatment of Alzheimer's disease. *J. Neural. Transm. Suppl.* 62: 149-164, 2002.

Wisniewski, T., Ghiso, J., Frangione, B. Biology of Aβ amyloid in Alzheimer's disease. *Neurobiol. Dis.* 4: 313-328, 1997. *Erratum in: Neurobiol. Dis.* 5: 65, 1998.

Yamashima, T. Implication of cysteine proteases calpain, cathepsin and caspase in ischemic neuronal death of primates. Prog. *Neurobiol.* 62: 273-295, 2000.

Zlokovic, B.V., Martel, C.L., Matsubara, E., McComb, J.G., Zheng, G., McCluskey, R.T., Frangione, B. and Ghiso, J. Glycoprotein 330/megalin: probable role in receptor-mediated transport of apolipoprotein J alone and in a complex with Alzheimer disease amyloid β at the blood-brain and blood-cerebrospinal fluid barriers. *Proc. Natl. Acad. Sci. USA.* 93: 4229-4234, 1996.

In: Alzheimer's Disease and Dementia (Vol. 4)
Editor: Miao-Kun Sun
ISBN:978-1-60876-152-4

Chapter IX

Role of Gelsolin in Alzheimer's Disease

Lina Ji, Abha Chauhan and Ved Chauhan*
New York State Institute for Basic Research in Developmental Disabilities,
Staten Island, New York, USA

Abstract

Gelsolin, an actin-binding protein, is present both intracellularly (cytoplasmic form) and extracellularly (secretory form in biological fluids). Fibrillar amyloid beta-protein (Aβ) is a major component of amyloid plaques in the brains of individuals with Alzheimer's disease (AD), and adults with Down syndrome. Several reports from our group and other groups have indicated an anti-amyloidogenic role of gelsolin in AD. Our studies showed that both plasma and cytoplasmic gelsolin bind to Aβ, and that plasma gelsolin inhibits the fibrillization of Aβ and solubilizes preformed fibrils of Aβ. In other studies, peripheral administration or transgene expression of plasma gelsolin, or viral-directed overexpression of cytoplamic gelsolin could reduce amyloid load in the transgenic mouse model of AD. Recently, we reported that gelsolin was proteolytically cleaved in the brains of AD patients, and that the levels of a carboxyl-terminus proteolytic fragment of gelsolin were higher in the brains of AD patients as compared to controls, which correlated with the severity of AD. Oxidative damage is considered a major feature in the pathophysiology of AD. Our recent studies showed that the expression of cytoplasmic gelsolin is up-regulated in response to oxidative stress in the cells, suggesting anti-oxidant role of gelsolin. In this article, we review evidence of gelsolin as an anti-amyloidogenic agent that can reduce amyloid load by acting as Aβ-sequestering agent and/or as an inhibitor of Aβ fibrillization.

Keywords: Alzheimer's disease; amyloid beta-protein; anti-amyloidogenic; anti-apoptotic; gelsolin; oxidative stress

---

*Address correspondence to Ved Chauhan, Ph. D., New York State Institute for Basic Research in Developmental Disabilities, 1050 Forest Hill Road, Staten Island, NY 10314, USA, Tel: 718-494-5257; Fax: 718-698-7916; E-mail: ved.chauhan@omr.state.ny.us

Abbreviations

Aβ, amyloid β-protein; AD, Alzheimer's disease; apo, apolipoprotein; APP, β-amyloid precursor protein; CNS, central nervous system; CSF, cerebrospinal fluid; Cys, cysteine; DS, Down syndrome; gelsolin-CTF, carboxyl-terminal fragment of gelsolin; HAT, histone acetyltransferase; HD, Huntington's disease; HDAC, histone deacetylase; PD, Parkinson's disease; PS, presenilin; TSA, trichostatin A

A. Gelsolin

Gelsolin is a multifunctional actin-binding protein. It is present intracellularly as a cytoplasmic protein, and in plasma/cerebrospinal fluid (CSF) as a secreted protein (Kwiatkowski et al., 1988). Both forms of gelsolin originate by the alternative splicing of a single 70 kbp-long gene, and they differ in the length and disulfide structure of the protein. Compared with the cytoplasmic form of gelsolin, its secretory form has a 25 amino acid-signal peptide at its amino-terminus, which facilitates its secretion extracellularly (Yin et al., 1984). There are five cysteine (Cys) residues in gelsolin. All five Cys residues in cytoplasmic gelsolin are free thiols; whereas in plasma gelsolin, three Cys residues at positions 93, 304 and 645 are free thiols and the other two Cys residues at positions 188 and 201 are disulfide-linked (Wen et al., 1996).

The cytoplasmic architecture of cells is maintained by the highly controlled regulation of filament assembly of actin. Gelsolin is expressed in all kinds of cells, and it is involved in cell motility. Gelsolin caps the actin filament's growing end, stimulates its nucleation, and severs the actin filaments (Kwiatkowski, 1999). Two molecules of actin bind to one molecule of gelsolin in a calcium-dependent manner. Gelsolin severs and caps actin in response to calcium, and phosphoinositides bind to gelsolin and block its capping function (Janmey, 1994).

Several reports indicate that cytoplasmic gelsolin acts as an anti-apoptotic protein during apoptosis (Azuma et al., 2000; Koya et al., 2000; Kusano et al., 2000). Compared with wild-type ones, cytoplasmic gelsolin-deficient neurons were more susceptible to apoptosis (Harms et al., 2004). In addition, the knockdown of cytoplasmic gelsolin expression by short interference RNA enhanced cell apoptosis (Qiao et al., 2005; Yermen et al., 2007). Furthermore, an overexpression of cytoplasmic gelsolin in cells inhibited apoptosis induced by Fas antibody (Ohtsu et al., 1997), nutrition deprivation (Yermen et al., 2007) or amyloid β-protein (Aβ) (Qiao et al., 2005). The enhancement of cytoplasmic gelsolin expression has been reported to be protective for neurons under oxygen-glucose deprivation (Meisel et al., 2006). Cytoplasmic gelsolin gets proteolytically cleaved into two fragments by activated caspase or calpain in apoptotic cells (Kamada et al., 1998; Kothakota et al., 1997; Wolf et al., 1999). The molecular mechanism underlying the anti-apoptotic function of cytoplasmic gelsolin is stimulus-specific. Two different pathways, including inhibition of caspase activity (Azuma et al., 2000) and inhibition of the voltage-dependent anion channel activity (Koya et al., 2000), were suggested for different inducers of apoptosis. As reported by Azuma et al., cytoplasmic gelsolin inhibited caspase-3 activity and DNA fragmentation through the formation of a stable phosphatidylinositol 4,5-bisphosphate-gelsolin-caspase complex (Azuma et al., 2000).

A mutation in plasma gelsolin renders it amyloidogenic. Gelsolin-related amyloidosis is a rare hereditary amyloid polyneuropathy, which is a result of Asp187Asn or Asp187Tyr mutation in gelsolin. These mutations cause an aberrant intracellular cleavage of plasma gelsolin that leads to the production of an amyloidogenic 68 kDa- fragment, which deposits as amyloid in the Finish type of amyloidosis (Maury et al., 1997).

Plasma gelsolin is thought to be active in the actin-scavenging system to protect the microcirculation from the effects of long filamentous actin polymers that are released during cell death (Lee and Galbraith, 1992). However, recent evidence indicates that plasma gelsolin may play a variety of other roles such as mediating inflammatory responses by binding to pro-inflammatory compounds (Bucki et al., 2005; Witke et al., 1995), or by altering cell motility and endocytosis (Witke et al., 2001). Plasma gelsolin has been shown to protect against inflammatory reactions associated with injury (Christofidou-Solomidou et al., 2002; Rothenbach et al., 2004).

Gelsolin also plays a protective role in tissue injuries. Compared with wild type mice, gelsolin-knockout mice showed increased brain injury after ischemia (Endres et al., 1999). In addition, an enhancement of gelsolin expression could reduce brain injury in gelsolin-deficient mice (Yildirim et al., 2008). After treatment with Fas antibody Jo2, gelsolin-knockout mice exhibited significantly higher numbers of apoptotic cells in livers and shorter survival time than wild-type mice (Leifeld et al., 2006). The role of gelsolin has also been suggested in tumor suppression (Mullauer et al., 1993). Gelsolin is constitutively expressed throughout the central nervous system (CNS) (Tanaka and Sobue, 1994), and it undergoes cleavage *in vivo* after cerebral ischemia (Endres et al., 1999; Lee et al., 2004). In recent years, accumulating evidence from our and other groups suggests an anti-amyloidogenic role of gelsolin in Alzheimer's disease (AD), which will be reviewed in this chapter.

B. AD and Aβ Fibrillization

AD is by far the most prevalent neurodegenerative disease, affecting an estimated 25 million people worldwide. AD can be classified into an early-onset form (genetic, onset < 60 years) and the more common late-onset form (sporadic, onset > 60 years). AD is characterized by amyloid fibers in senile plaques and in the walls of blood vessels, progressive accumulation of neurofibrillary tangles in neurons, and neuronal cell loss (Wisniewski et al., 1997). Aβ, comprising 39-43 amino acids, is the major component of senile plaques in AD and in adult Down syndrome (DS) (Glenner, 1983). Aβ is produced by the proteolytic cleavage of membrane-associated β-amyloid precursor protein (APP) (Kang et al., 1987). Individuals with DS generally develop AD in their middle age because they have an extra copy of chromosome 21 containing the APP gene (Korenberg et al., 1990). The function of APP is not clear. However, it has been suggested to have role in cell adhesion, intracellular communication, membrane to nucleus communication, and in neurotrophic, and neuroproliferative activity (Turner et al., 2003). The processing of APP can occur by two major pathways. The cleavage of APP at the amino-terminus of the Aβ region by β-secretase

(Vassar et al., 1999), followed by the cleavage at the carboxyl-terminus of Aβ by γ-secretase (Yu et al., 2001), represents the amyloidogenic pathway for processing of APP to produce either Aβ 1-40 or a more hydrophobic Aβ 1-42. Aβ 1-42 is more prone to oligomerization and fibril formation than Aβ 1-40 (Hasegawa et al., 1999; Hilbich et al., 1991). Alternatively, APP can also be processed by α-secretase, which cleaves within the Aβ sequence and does not produce Aβ (Vardy et al., 2005).

Aβ exists in both soluble and fibrillar forms. Soluble Aβ is a normal metabolic product and is present in the CSF and sera of normal individuals and AD patients, and in the conditioned media of many types of cultured cells (Haass et al., 1992; Seubert et al., 1992; Vigo-Pelfrey et al., 1993). A unique feature of Aβ is its ability to aggregate, and to form insoluble fibrils that are deposited extracellularly in the brains of AD patients. Formation of Aβ fibrils is a stepwise process from Aβ monomers to dimers to oligomers, and it involves conformational change of the peptide from α-helical to cross β-sheet structure (Hilbich et al., 1991).

Extensive evidence suggests a causal role of Aβ fibrils in the development of AD (Forloni, 1996). Three genes have been linked to early onset, autosomal dominant forms of AD. A single missense mutation on the APP gene was reported to result in an inheritable form of AD, and the mutations in APP could invariably increase the relative amounts of Aβ 1-42 compared to Aβ 1-40, which suggested that increased concentration and deposition of Aβ can result in AD pathology (Goate et al., 1991; Hardy and Allsop, 1991; Sinha and Lieberburg, 1999; Suzuki et al., 1994). A hereditary form of cerebral hemorrhage with amyloidosis (Dutch type) is associated with a glutamine substitution for glutamic acid, corresponding to residue 22 of Aβ (Levy et al., 1990). Inheritable form of AD also results from mutations in the genes of presenilin (PS). PS is a family of transmembrane proteins that include PS-1 and PS-2, and it functions as a part of the γ-secretase protease complex for the processing of APP. Mutations in PS-1 and PS-2 result in selective processing of APP to produce preferentially Aβ 1-42 rather than Aβ 1-40, and causes early onset AD (Clark and Goate, 1993; Sherrington et al., 1996).

C. Neurotoxicity of Aβ

In vitro studies with synthetic Aβ have shown that Aβ is neurotoxic, and its neurotoxicity is largely dependent on the degree of fibril formation. The intermediates in Aβ fibrillogenesis, namely oligomers and protofilaments of Aβ, are suggested to be more toxic than its fibrillar form (Hartley et al., 1999; Lambert et al., 2001; Serpell et al., 2000; Walsh et al., 1999). Aβ fibrils attached on the culture dish were not toxic to cortical and hippocampal neurons *in vitro*, while Aβ aggregates suspended in culture medium were neurotoxic (Wujek et al., 1996). It was also reported that small diffusible Aβ oligomers kill mature neurons at nanomolar concentrations (Lambert et al., 1998). Furthermore, administration of Aβ oligomers to the animals produced deficits in long-term potentiation, a phenomenon related to memory formation (Walsh et al., 2002). It appears that the toxicity of protofibrils is related to their structure, and not to their sequence (Lansbury, 1999). Protofibrillar material comprising proteins unrelated to Aβ also showed toxicity in cell culture (Bucciantini et al.,

2002), while amyloid fibrils comprising unrelated sequences were nontoxic (Fezoui et al., 2000). Consistent with the observation that cholesterol content of the membrane influences toxicity of Aβ (Arispe and Doh, 2002), amyloid-pore hypothesis suggests that Aβ protofibrils resemble a class of pore-forming bacterial toxins and possibly, result in inappropriate membrane-permeabilization (Kirkitadze and Kowalska, 2005; Lashuel et al., 2002).

D. Aβ-Induced Oxidative Stress

Extensive evidence suggests that oxidative stress plays an important role in neuronal degeneration in AD (reviewd in Chauhan and Chauhan, 2006). On its way to deposition in the brain as plaques, Aβ induces oxidative changes rendering cell insults, as indicated by increased protein oxidation and lipid peroxidation (Chauhan and Chauhan, 2006; Kim et al., 2003; Mohmmad Abdul et al., 2004). Impaired activity of Cu/Zn-superoxide dismutase, an enzyme involved in anti-oxidant defense mechanism, was observed in Thy1-APP751 transgenic mouse model of AD (Schuessel et al., 2005). These animals also showed increased Aβ production and oxidative damage. In addition, the deposition of amyloid plaques was reported to cause the activation of microglia and astrocytes, resulting in the release of pro-inflammatory cytokines and reactive oxygen species (Akama et al., 1998; Hoozemans et al., 2006; Johnstone et al., 1999). Tamagno et al. proposed the existence of a sequence of events in Aβ-induced apoptosis involving simultaneous generation of 4-hydroxynonenal (a lipid peroxidation product) and H_2O_2, and oxidative stress-dependent activation of the mitogen-activated protein kinase, including c-Jun N-terminal kinase and P38 (Tamagno et al., 2003). Other effects of Aβ-mediated oxidative stress are attenuation of functional hyperemia (Park et al., 2004), learning and memory deficits (Jhoo et al., 2004), increased levels of heme oxygenase-1, heat shock protein 72 (Sultana et al., 2005), and high cellular accumulation of apolipoprotein (apo) E (Brendza et al., 2002; Corder et al., 1993; Mazur-Kolecka et al., 2003). Recent evidence suggests that metals concentrated in amyloid deposits may also contribute to the oxidative insults observed in AD brains. Aβ is reported to have copper-reducing ability. The efficacy of Aβ to reduce copper is independent of its aggregation state. In the presence of copper ions, Aβ reduces Cu^{2+} to Cu^{+}, and catalyzes the formation of H_2O_2 that can produce highly toxic hydroxyl radicals (Dikalov et al., 2004). Therefore, Aβ-induced oxidative stress may be increased in the presence of Cu^{2+}.

E. Binding of Gelsolin to Aβ

Our studies showed that conditioned media from several cell lines contain factors that promote the fibrillization of Aβ (Chauhan et al., 1997). However, the fibril formation of Aβ was accelerated only in serum-free cell cultures. The presence of serum in the medium inhibited the formation of Aβ fibrils (Chauhan et al., 1996; Wegiel et al., 1996). In another study, we reported that Aβ fibrillogenesis is also inhibited by CSF (Chauhan et al., 1996). These studies suggested the presence of factors in biological fluids that prevent Aβ fibril formation. Several circulating proteins such as transthyretin, apo E, apo J, and apo A1 have been identified in plasma and CSF, and they were reported to bind to Aβ (Ghiso et al., 1993; Koudinov et al., 1994; Strittmatter et al., 1993).

Accumulating evidence from our laboratory suggests that plasma gelsolin is one of the factors present in biological fluids that can inhibit Aβ fibrillization. When plasma was fortified with different concentrations of Aβ 1-40, and gelsolin immunoprecipitated by monoclonal antibody against gelsolin, Aβ was observed to co-immuniprecipitate along with gelsolin, suggesting the existence of the Aβ-gelsolin complex in plasma. The binding of plasma gelsolin to Aβ was also confirmed by performing the plasma gelsolin overlay assay on Aβ fixed on the nitrocellulose membrane (Chauhan et al., 1999). The binding of Aβ to plasma gelsolin was dependent on the concentrations of both gelsolin and Aβ (Chauhan et al., 1999). Solid phase binding assay using microplates showed that the binding of Aβ with plasma gelsolin is saturable (r = 0.98), and that there are two Aβ-binding sites on gelsolin with the dissociation rate constants (K_d) of 1.38 μM and 2.55 μM. Because the levels of gelsolin in the plasma is in the micromolar range, i.e., 2 μM, the dissociation constant of the Aβ-gelsolin complex falls within the physiological concentration of plasma gelsolin (Paunio et al., 1994).

Recently, we and other group reported that cytoplasmic gelsolin could also bind and form complex with Aβ (Antequera et al., 2009; Ji et al., 2008). The cytoplasmic and plasma forms of gelsolin differ in protein's length and free thiol groups. Since our studies showed that plasma gelsolin could form a complex with synthetic Aβ, it was of interest to study whether cytoplasmic gelsolin could also bind to Aβ. For this purpose, we induced gelsolin expression by H_2O_2 in PC-12 cells. H_2O_2-treatment increased the levels of cytosolic gelsolin. When lysate from the H_2O_2-treated PC-12 cells was fortified with synthetic Aβ 1-40, and Aβ 1-40 was immunoprecipitated with 4G8 monoclonal antibody against Aβ, cytoplasmic gelsolin was observed in the co-immunoprecipitate (Ji et al., 2008). The co-immunoprecipitation of both cytoplasmic/plasma gelsolin and Aβ indicates that structural differences between plasma and cytoplasmic gelsolin do not play a key role in their complex formation with Aβ (Ji et al., 2008).

F. Gelsolin Inhibits the Fibril Formation of Aβ, and Also Defibrillizes the Preformed Aβ Fibrils

Since gelsolin is present in the plasma and CSF, and it binds to Aβ, it was envisioned that gelsolin could affect the fibrillogenesis of Aβ. In fact, plasma gelsolin was found to inhibit the fibrillization of Aβ in an *in vitro* study (Ray et al., 2000). When aged Aβ samples at the fifth and seventh days of incubation were stained with Congo red, they produced a specific green birefringence when observed under polarized light, indicating that Aβ was in the fibrillar form. The green birefringence was not observed in the Aβ sample incubated with plasma gelsolin, indicating that the fibrillization of Aβ was completely inhibited in the presence of plasma gelsolin. The samples containing aged Aβ 1-40 or Aβ 1-42 alone, and corresponding Aβ samples incubated with plasma gelsolin after 7 days of incubation were also examined by *electron microscope* in negative staining (Ray et al., 2000). Aβ 1-40 and Aβ 1-42 formed a dense network of fibrils with morphology similar to that reported previously (Chauhan et al., 1997). Plasma gelsolin inhibited the fibril formation of both Aβ 1-40 and Aβ 1-42 by more than 90% of that observed for Aβs in the absence of plasma gelsolin (Ray et al., 2000). These *in vitro* studies indicated that plasma gelsolin inhibits the formation of β-pleated sheet structure and fibril formation of Aβ. We also observed that gelsolin defibrillizes the preformed fibrils of synthetic Aβ. After mixing plasma gelsolin with the preformed fibrils, the status of the fibrils was analyzed by Congo red staining and *electron microscope* on different days. The results showed that plasma gelsolin can defibrillize the preformed fibrils of Aβ in a time-dependent manner (Ray et al., 2000).

G. Reduction of Amyloid Load by Gelsolin in Transgenic Mouse Model of AD

The accumulation of Aβ is one of the fundamental pathological events in AD, and its elevation and aggregation are associated with several detrimental cellular responses (Small et al., 2001). Brain/periphery Aβ dynamics has been suggested to play a crucial role in the pathogenesis of AD. One therapeutic approach proposed to reduce amyloid load for the treatment of AD has been the immunization with synthetic Aβ peptide or administration of antibodies against Aβ peptides (Das et al., 2003; DeMattos et al., 2001). It was observed that anti-Aβ antibodies could significantly influence Aβ-transfer between the brain and plasma in the transgenic mouse model of AD (DeMattos et al., 2001). The Fab fragment of anti-Aβ antibody, which lacks immunomodulative effects, was found to bind Aβ and reduce brain Aβ levels significantly (Bacskai et al., 2002). It was suggested that the sequestration of Aβ in the periphery by antibodies might shift the equilibrium of Aβ from the CNS to the periphery, thereby reducing Aβ levels in the brain (Bacskai et al., 2001; DeMattos et al., 2001). Aβ immunization could also effectively reduce amyloid deposition in Fc receptor-gamma chain (-/-) knock-out mice (Das et al., 2003). However, subsequent clinical trials of actively administered Aβ peptides had to be suspended because of adverse response in the patients. There were also several problems associated with immunotherapy. Therefore, other compounds such as enoxaparin and ganglioside GM1 with a high binding affinity for Aβ were tried for peripheral sequestration of Aβ. Long-term peripheral treatment with enoxaparin, a low molecular weight heparin analog, significantly lowered the number of cortical Aβ deposits and total Aβ concentration of brain in APP-transgenic mice. Moreover, enoxaparin could reduce the toxicity and pro-inflammatory activity of Aβ (Bergamaschini et al., 2004). This effect may be attributed to the ability of enoxaparin to bind Aβ in the periphery, resulting in alteration of the Aβ periphery/brain dynamics. Ganglioside GM1 also has an affinity for Aβ (Choo-Smith and Surewicz, 1997). APP/PS transgenic mice administered peripherally with GM1 showed a substantial decrease in aggregated Aβ1-40 and Aβ1-42 in the brain (Matsuoka et al., 2003).

Plasma gelsolin is well suited as a peripherally expressed therapeutic agent because it contains an internal signal peptide directing gelsolin to be secreted into the blood system from any peripheral location. Plasma gelsolin is known to bind Aβ via two sites under normal physiological conditions (Chauhan et al., 1999). The anti-amyloidogenic role of plasma gelsolin was confirmed in two independent studies on a transgenic mouse model of AD.

Matsuoka et al. showed that peripheral administration of plasma gelsolin resulted in significant reduction of amyloid load in the brains of APP/PS-transgenic mice (Matsuoka et al., 2003). In another study, peripheral transgene expression of plasma gelsolin in a transgenic mouse model of AD led to reduced accumulation of amyloid plaques (Hirko et al., 2007).

Although it is widely accepted that Aβ fibrillization extracellularly is one of the main events in the pathology of AD, intracellular accumulation of Aβ has also been observed (Glabe, 2001; Knauer et al., 1992). Yuyama et al. suggested that intracellular nuclei of Aβ might be responsible for the extracellular Aβ deposition (Yuyama et al., 2006). Recently, it was reported that viral-directed overexpression of cytoplasmic gelsolin reduced brain Aβ burden in APP/PS transgenic mice (Antequera et al., 2009). Since gelsolin can bind to Aβ, gelsolin may affect the fibrillogenesis both extracellularly and intracellularly.

H. Cleavage of Gelsolin in the Brains of Patients with AD: Role of Apoptosis

We recently studied whether gelsolin levels are affected in the frontal cortex of individuals with AD compared to age-matched controls. Interestingly, we observed a 48 kDa-gelsolin band in addition to a 90 kDa-gelsolin band (full-length) in the brains from individuals with AD (Ji et al., 2009). The densitometric analysis of the protein bands showed that the levels of full-length gelsolin were similar between AD and age-matched control groups. However, the amount of 48 kDa-gelsolin fragment in the brain was 10-fold higher in the AD group as compared to control group.

Several studies indicate that apoptosis may contribute to the neuronal loss in AD. Apoptosis is also reported to be a major form of neuronal cell death in APP/PS-transgenic mice modeling AD-like neurodegeneration (Yang et al., 2008). Apoptotic genes, such as c-Fos, c-Jun and Bak are considered to be critical in the apoptotic cascades of AD (Sajan et al., 2007). Gelsolin is known to be proteolytically cleaved by activated caspase-3 during apoptosis, resulting in the carboxyl-terminal fragment of gelsolin (gelsolin-CTF) (Kothakota et al., 1997). Therefore, it was envisioned that the 48 kDa- gelsolin fragment in AD brain may be a product of apoptosis. As a positive control of gelsolin-CTF, we induced apoptosis in human SH-SY5Y cells by H_2O_2 and A23187 (calcium ionophore) (Ji et al., 2009). Apoptosis was confirmed by the appearance of cleaved poly (ADP-ribose) polymerase and DNA ladder. Using recombinant gelsolin-CTF as a protein marker, human frontal cortex and apoptotic SH-SY5Y cells were simultaneously probed for gelsolin. As expected, the gelsolin's proteolytic fragments in brains and apoptotic cells had the same molecular weight, i.e., 48 kDa as that of the recombinant gelsolin-CTF. These results suggest that 48 kDa fragment of gelsolin observed in the AD brains originates from the proteolysis of gelsolin. It was of particular interest to observe a positive correlation between the appearance of gelsolin-CTF in frontal cortex and severity of AD. In another study, depletion of dietary n-3 polyunsaturated fatty acid has been reported to aggravate Aβ-driven oxidative stress, and result in significant cleavage of gelsolin in the brain of transgenic mouse model of AD

(Tg2576), compared with wild type mice (Calon et al., 2005). Taken together, these studies suggest that there may be a link among neuronal apoptosis, oxidative stress, and gelsolin cleavage in AD.

I. Epigenetic Control of Gelsolin Expression

Acetylation and deacetylation of histones regulate the expression of genes. A schematic diagram for regulation of the expression of genes is shown in Fig. 1. Gelsolin expression is also epigenetically regulated. The inhibition of histone deacetylase (HDAC) increases the expression of gelsolin (Eun et al., 2007). Hoshikawa et al. reported an approximately seven to twelve-fold increase in the levels of gelsolin in Hela cells treated with trichostatin A (TSA), a HDAC-inhibitor, for 24 h (Hoshikawa et al., 1994). Similarly, sodium butyrate inhibited the activity of HDAC and increased the expression of gelsolin (Kamitani et al., 2002). In addition, Mielnicki et al. reported a role for epigenetic changes in chromatin structure leading to down-regulation of gelsolin expression in human breast cancer (Mielnicki et al., 1999). Kamitani et al. (2002) also suggested that the treatment of human glioma cells with TSA suppresses cell growth by decreasing DNA synthesis, and that associated molecular mechanisms responsible for these effects include increased histone acetylation as well as enhanced expression of gelsolin.

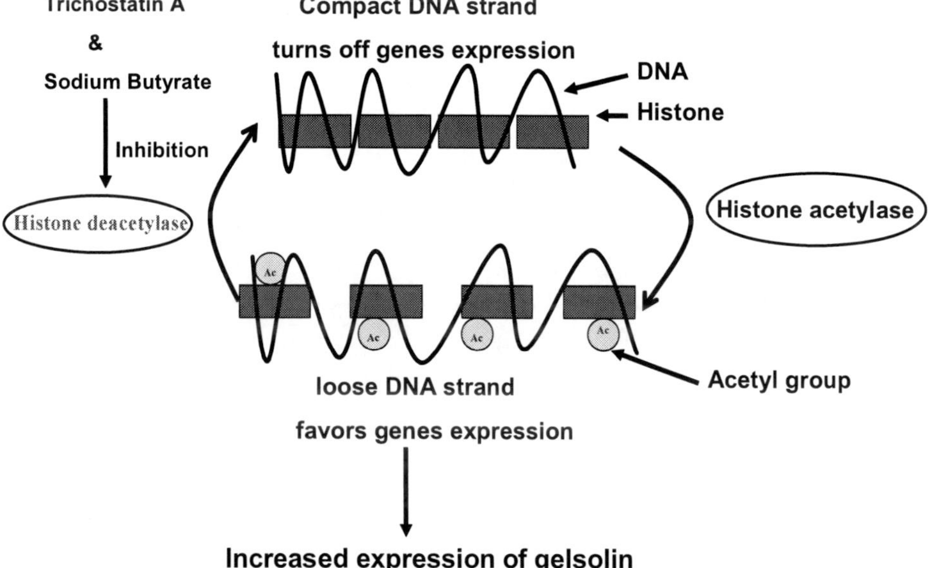

Figure 1. Inhibition of histone deacetylation by TSA and sodium butyrate. A strand of DNA winds around histone proteins. When histones are acetylated by histone acetyltransferase (HAT), the strand begins to loosen, which allows gene expression. After a short period, the histones are deacetylated by HDAC, which causes the gene expression to stop. TSA and sodium butyrate bind to HDAC and inhibit its function. As a result, the histones remain acetylated and gene expression (gelsolin expression) is activated.

J. Potential Role of HDAC Inhibitors as herapeutic Agents for Neurodegenerative Disorders

A role for HDAC in neurodegenerative disorders first became apparent by experiments showing the ability of HDAC inhibitors to rescue lethality and photoreceptor neurodegeneration in a Drosophila model of polyglutamine disease (Steffan et al., 2001). Studies have also demonstrated that HDAC inhibitors could significantly extend survival and improve both the clinical and neuropathological phenotypes in transgenic mouse model of amyotrophic lateral sclerosis (Ryu et al., 2005). These findings were extended to the mouse models of Huntington's disease (HD) by several laboratories, which showed that treatment with HDAC inhibitors could attenuate neuronal loss, increase motor function, and extend survival in a transgenic mouse model of HD (Ferrante et al., 2003; Gardian et al., 2005; Hockly et al., 2003).

Recent studies suggest that HDAC inhibitors may also represent a promising therapeutic strategy to ameliorate the progressive neurodegeneration associated with Parkinson's disease (PD). The initial link between PD and epigenetic dysregulation came from a Drosophila model of PD. Kontopoulos et al. demonstrated that nuclear targeting of α-synuclein promotes its toxicity and that sequestration of α-synuclein to the cytoplasm is protective. It was further shown that α-synuclein binds directly to histones, reduces levels of acetylated histone H3, and inhibits HAT-mediated acetyltransferase activity (Kontopoulos et al., 2006). Administration of HDAC inhibitors *in vivo* or *in vitro* rescued α-synuclein-induced toxicity (Kontopoulos et al., 2006). These reports suggest potential benefit of HDAC inhibitors as therapeutic agents in PD.

Although no direct demonstration of amelioration of synaptic plasticity or cognitive impairments has been documented for AD, recent studies from the laboratory of Fischer et al. showed that HDAC inhibitors restore histone acetylation status, induce sprouting of dendrites, increase number of synapses, and reinstate learning behavior and access to long-term memories in a mouse model of neurodegeneration (Fischer et al., 2007). Increased histone acetylation by HDAC inhibitors were suggested to have broad effects on genes expression involved in inflammation, cognitive functions, and neuronal loss, resulting in amelioration of neuronal degeneration and learning behavior (Alarcon et al., 2004; Korzus et al., 2004; Kumar et al., 2005; Levenson et al., 2004; Ryu et al., 2005). Taken together, above studies suggest that inhibitors of HDAC by increasing expression of gelsolin may also be a suitable therapeutic avenue for neurodegeneration associated with amyloid plaque formation, and learning and memory impairment in AD.

K. Concluding Remarks

Gelsolin can function as an anti-amyloidogenic protein besides controlling actin polymerization and inhibiting apoptosis. By virtue of binding to Aβ and inhibiting Aβ fibrillogenesis, gelsolin can shift the equilibrium of Aβ from CNS to the periphery, and reduce the amyloid load in the brain. Both cytoplasmic and secretory gelsolin can bind to Aβ, and therefore, inhibit Aβ fibrillogenesis extracellularly as well as intracellularly. In AD, gelsolin is cleaved into 48 kDa-fragment (gelsolin-CTF) in the brain, and there is a correlation between levels of gelsolin-CTF and the severity of AD. With its multiple functions as anti-amyloidogenic, anti-apoptotic and anti-oxidant protein, gelsolin can serve to reduce neuronal cell loss and amyloid load, and may help in delaying the progression or preventing the development of AD. A summary of involvement of gelsolin in AD is shown in Table 1. Gelsolin expression can be increased by genetic manipulation or by epigenetic control, i.e., by inhibition of HDAC. Our future studies will be directed towards increasing gelsolin levels by epigenetic control, and studying its beneficial effects towards reducing amyloid load in AD-transgenic animals.

Table 1. Summary of major research highlights regarding involvement of gelsolin in AD

Gelsolin and AD	Research findings	References
Interaction of gelsolin with Aβ	Plasma and cytoplasmic gelsolin bind to Aβ	(Antequera et al., 2009; Chauhan et al., 1999; Hirko et al., 2007; Ji et al., 2008)
	Plasma gelsolin inhibits Aβ fibrillization and defibrillizes its preformed fibrils	(Ray et al., 2000)
	Intraperitoneal administration of plasma gelsolin results in significant reduction of amyloid load in the brains of APP/PS-transgenic mice	(Matsuoka et al., 2003)
	Transgene expression of plasma geslolin reduces the amyloid load in APP/PS-transgenic mouse model of AD	(Hirko et al., 2007)
	Viral-directed overexpression of cytoplasmic gelsolin reduces brain Aβ burden in APP/PS-transgenic mouse model of AD	(Antequera et al., 2009)
Gelsolin and its neuroprotective role	Cytoplasmic gelsolin inhibits the neurotoxicity of Aβ	(Qiao et al., 2005)
	Gelsolin-deficient neurons are susceptible to apoptosis, as compared with wild-type neurons, and the enhancement of gelsolin expression is protective for neurons.	(Harms et al., 2004; Meisel et al., 2006)
	Compared with wild-type mice, gelsolin-knockout mice showed increased brain injury after ischemia, while enhanced gelsolin expression in gelsolin-deficient mice could reduce brain injury.	(Endres et al., 1999; Yildirim et al., 2008)
Gelsolin and oxidative stress	Oxidative stress up-regulates expression of cytoplasmic gelsolin	(Ji et al., 2008)
Cleavage of gelsolin in AD brain	Gelsolin is proteolytically cleaved resulting in its 48 kDa gelsolin-CTF in the brains of individuals with AD.	(Ji et al., 2009)

References

Akama, K. T., Albanese, C., Pestell, R. G., Van Eldik, L. J. Amyloid beta-peptide stimulates nitric oxide production in astrocytes through an NFkappaB-dependent mechanism. *Proc Natl Acad Sci U S A* 95: 5795-5800, 1998.

Alarcon, J. M., Malleret, G., Touzani, K., Vronskaya, S., Ishii, S., Kandel, E. R., Barco, A. Chromatin acetylation, memory, and LTP are impaired in CBP+/- mice: a model for the cognitive deficit in Rubinstein-Taybi syndrome and its amelioration. *Neuron* 42: 947-959, 2004.

Antequera, D., Vargas, T., Ugalde, C., Spuch, C., Molina, J. A., Ferrer, I., Bermejo-Pareja, F., Carro, E. Cytoplasmic gelsolin increases mitochondrial activity and reduces Abeta burden in a mouse model of Alzheimer's disease. *Neurobiol Dis*, 2009 (in press).

Arispe, N., Doh, M. Plasma membrane cholesterol controls the cytotoxicity of Alzheimer's disease Abeta (1-40) and (1-42) peptides. *FASEB J* 16: 1526-1536, 2002.

Azuma, T., Koths, K., Flanagan, L., Kwiatkowski, D. Gelsolin in complex with phosphatidylinositol 4,5-bisphosphate inhibits caspase-3 and -9 to retard apoptotic progression. *J Biol Chem* 275: 3761-3766, 2000.

Bacskai, B. J., Kajdasz, S. T., McLellan, M. E., Games, D., Seubert, P., Schenk, D., Hyman, B. T. Non-Fc-mediated mechanisms are involved in clearance of amyloid-beta in vivo by immunotherapy. *J Neurosci* 22: 7873-7878, 2002.

Bacskai, B. J., Kajdasz, S. T., Christie, R. H., Carter, C., Games, D., Seubert, P., Schenk, D., Hyman, B. T. Imaging of amyloid-beta deposits in brains of living mice permits direct observation of clearance of plaques with immunotherapy. *Nat Med* 7: 369-372, 2001.

Bergamaschini, L., Rossi, E., Storini, C., Pizzimenti, S., Distaso, M., Perego, C., De Luigi, A., Vergani, C., De Simoni, M. G. Peripheral treatment with enoxaparin, a low molecular weight heparin, reduces plaques and beta-amyloid accumulation in a mouse model of Alzheimer's disease. *J Neurosci* 24: 4181-4186, 2004.

Brendza, R. P., Bales, K. R., Paul, S. M., Holtzman, D. M. Role of apoE/Abeta interactions in Alzheimer's disease: insights from transgenic mouse models. *Mol Psychiatry* 7: 132-135, 2002.

Bucciantini, M., Giannoni, E., Chiti, F., Baroni, F., Formigli, L., Zurdo, J., Taddei, N., Ramponi, G., Dobson, C. M., Stefani, M. Inherent toxicity of aggregates implies a common mechanism for protein misfolding diseases. *Nature* 416: 507-511, 2002.

Bucki, R., Georges, P. C., Espinassous, Q., Funaki, M., Pastore, J. J., Chaby, R., Janmey, P. A. Inactivation of endotoxin by human plasma gelsolin. *Biochemistry* 44: 9590-9597, 2005.

Calon, F., Lim, G. P., Morihara, T., Yang, F., Ubeda, O., Salem, N., Jr., Frautschy, S. A., Cole, G. M. Dietary n-3 polyunsaturated fatty acid depletion activates caspases and decreases NMDA receptors in the brain of a transgenic mouse model of Alzheimer's disease. *Eur J Neurosci* 22: 617-626, 2005.

Chauhan, A., Pirttila, T., Mehta, P., Chauhan, V. P., Wisniewski, H. M. Effect of cerebrospinal fluid from normal and Alzheimer's patients with different apolipoprotein E phenotypes on in vitro aggregation of amyloid beta-protein. *J Neurol Sci* 141: 54-58, 1996.

Chauhan, A., Chauhan, V. P., Rubenstein, R., Wegiel, J., Wisniewski, H. M. Media from rhabdomyosarcoma and neuroblastoma cell cultures stimulate in vitro aggregation and fibrillization of amyloid beta-protein. *Neurochem Res* 22: 227-232, 1997.

Chauhan, V., Chauhan, A. Oxidative stress in Alzheimer's disease. *Pathophysiology* 13: 195-208, 2006.

Chauhan, V. P., Ray, I., Chauhan, A., Wisniewski, H. M. Binding of gelsolin, a secretory protein, to amyloid beta-protein. *Biochem Biophys Res Commun* 258: 241-246, 1999.

Chauhan, V. P., Ray, I., Chauhan, A., Wegiel, J., Wisniewski, H. M. Metal cations defibrillize the amyloid beta-protein fibrils. *Neurochem Res* 22: 805-809, 1997.

Choo-Smith, L. P., Surewicz, W. K. The interaction between Alzheimer amyloid beta(1-40) peptide and ganglioside GM1-containing membranes. *FEBS Lett* 402: 95-98, 1997.

Christofidou-Solomidou, M., Scherpereel, A., Solomides, C. C., Christie, J. D., Stossel, T. P., Goelz, S., DiNubile, M. J. Recombinant plasma gelsolin diminishes the acute inflammatory response to hyperoxia in mice. *J Investig Med* 50: 54-60, 2002.

Clark, R. F., Goate, A. M. Molecular genetics of Alzheimer's disease. *Arch Neurol* 50: 1164-1172, 1993.

Corder, E. H., Saunders, A. M., Strittmatter, W. J., Schmechel, D. E., Gaskell, P. C., Small, G. W., Roses, A. D., Haines, J. L., Pericak-Vance, M. A. Gene dose of apolipoprotein E type 4 allele and the risk of Alzheimer's disease in late onset families. *Science* 261: 921-923, 1993.

Das, P., Howard, V., Loosbrock, N., Dickson, D., Murphy, M. P., Golde, T. E. Amyloid-beta immunization effectively reduces amyloid deposition in FcRgamma-/- knock-out mice. *J Neurosci* 23: 8532-8538, 2003.

DeMattos, R. B., Bales, K. R., Cummins, D. J., Dodart, J. C., Paul, S. M., Holtzman, D. M. Peripheral anti-A beta antibody alters CNS and plasma A beta clearance and decreases brain A beta burden in a mouse model of Alzheimer's disease. *Proc Natl Acad Sci U S A* 98: 8850-8855, 2001.

Dikalov, S. I., Vitek, M. P., Mason, R. P. Cupric-amyloid beta peptide complex stimulates oxidation of ascorbate and generation of hydroxyl radical. *Free Radic Biol Med* 36: 340-347, 2004.

Endres, M., Fink, K., Zhu, J., Stagliano, N. E., Bondada, V., Geddes, J. W., Azuma, T., Mattson, M. P., Kwiatkowski, D. J., Moskowitz, M. A. Neuroprotective effects of gelsolin during murine stroke. *J Clin Invest* 103: 347-354, 1999.

Eun, D. W., Ahn, S. H., You, J. S., Park, J. W., Lee, E. K., Lee, H. N., Kang, G. M., Lee, J. C., Choi, W. S., Seo, D. W., Han, J. W. PKCepsilon is essential for gelsolin expression by histone deacetylase inhibitor apicidin in human cervix cancer cells. *Biochem Biophys Res Commun* 354: 769-775, 2007.

Ferrante, R. J., Kubilus, J. K., Lee, J., Ryu, H., Beesen, A., Zucker, B., Smith, K., Kowall, N. W., Ratan, R. R., Luthi-Carter, R., Hersch, S. M. Histone deacetylase inhibition by sodium butyrate chemotherapy ameliorates the neurodegenerative phenotype in Huntington's disease mice. *J Neurosci* 23: 9418-9427, 2003.

Fezoui, Y., Hartley, D. M., Walsh, D. M., Selkoe, D. J., Osterhout, J. J., Teplow, D. B. A de novo designed helix-turn-helix peptide forms nontoxic amyloid fibrils. *Nat Struct Biol* 7: 1095-1099, 2000.

Fischer, A., Sananbenesi, F., Wang, X., Dobbin, M., Tsai, L. H. Recovery of learning and memory is associated with chromatin remodelling. *Nature* 447: 178-182, 2007.

Forloni, G. Neurotoxicity of beta-amyloid and prion peptides. *Curr Opin Neurol* 9: 492-500, 1996.

Gardian, G., Browne, S. E., Choi, D. K., Klivenyi, P., Gregorio, J., Kubilus, J. K., Ryu, H., Langley, B., Ratan, R. R., Ferrante, R. J., Beal, M. F. Neuroprotective effects of phenylbutyrate in the N171-82Q transgenic mouse model of Huntington's disease. *J Biol Chem* 280: 556-563, 2005.

Ghiso, J., Matsubara, E., Koudinov, A., Choi-Miura, N. H., Tomita, M., Wisniewski, T., Frangione, B. The cerebrospinal-fluid soluble form of Alzheimer's amyloid beta is complexed to SP-40,40 (apolipoprotein J), an inhibitor of the complement membrane-attack complex. *Biochem J* 293 (Pt 1): 27-30, 1993.

Glabe, C. Intracellular mechanisms of amyloid accumulation and pathogenesis in Alzheimer's disease. *J Mol Neurosci* 17: 137-145, 2001.

Glenner, G. G. Alzheimer's disease. The commonest form of amyloidosis. *Arch Pathol Lab Med* 107: 281-282, 1983.

Goate, A., Chartier-Harlin, M. C., Mullan, M., Brown, J., Crawford, F., Fidani, L., Giuffra, L., Haynes, A., Irving, N., James, L., et al. Segregation of a missense mutation in the amyloid precursor protein gene with familial Alzheimer's disease. *Nature* 349: 704-706, 1991.

Haass, C., Schlossmacher, M. G., Hung, A. Y., Vigo-Pelfrey, C., Mellon, A., Ostaszewski, B. L., Lieberburg, I., Koo, E. H., Schenk, D., Teplow, D. B., et al. Amyloid beta-peptide is produced by cultured cells during normal metabolism. *Nature* 359: 322-325, 1992.

Hardy, J., Allsop, D. Amyloid deposition as the central event in the aetiology of Alzheimer's disease. *Trends Pharmacol Sci* 12: 383-388, 1991.

Harms, C., Bosel, J., Lautenschlager, M., Harms, U., Braun, J. S., Hortnagl, H., Dirnagl, U., Kwiatkowski, D. J., Fink, K., Endres, M. Neuronal gelsolin prevents apoptosis by enhancing actin depolymerization. *Mol Cell Neurosci* 25: 69-82, 2004.

Hartley, D. M., Walsh, D. M., Ye, C. P., Diehl, T., Vasquez, S., Vassilev, P. M., Teplow, D. B., Selkoe, D. J. Protofibrillar intermediates of amyloid beta-protein induce acute electrophysiological changes and progressive neurotoxicity in cortical neurons. *J Neurosci* 19: 8876-8884, 1999.

Hasegawa, K., Yamaguchi, I., Omata, S., Gejyo, F., Naiki, H. Interaction between A beta(1-42) and A beta(1-40) in Alzheimer's beta-amyloid fibril formation in vitro. *Biochemistry* 38: 15514-15521, 1999.

Hilbich, C., Kisters-Woike, B., Reed, J., Masters, C. L., Beyreuther, K. Aggregation and secondary structure of synthetic amyloid beta A4 peptides of Alzheimer's disease. *J Mol Biol* 218: 149-163, 1991.

Hirko, A. C., Meyer, E. M., King, M. A., Hughes, J. A. Peripheral transgene expression of plasma gelsolin reduces amyloid in transgenic mouse models of Alzheimer's disease. *Mol Ther* 15: 1623-1629, 2007.

Hockly, E., Richon, V. M., Woodman, B., Smith, D. L., Zhou, X., Rosa, E., Sathasivam, K., Ghazi-Noori, S., Mahal, A., Lowden, P. A., Steffan, J. S., Marsh, J. L., Thompson, L. M., Lewis, C. M., Marks, P. A., Bates, G. P. Suberoylanilide hydroxamic acid, a histone deacetylase inhibitor, ameliorates motor deficits in a mouse model of Huntington's disease. *Proc Natl Acad Sci U S A* 100: 2041-2046, 2003.

Hoozemans, J. J., Veerhuis, R., Rozemuller, J. M., Eikelenboom, P. Neuroinflammation and regeneration in the early stages of Alzheimer's disease pathology. *Int J Dev Neurosci* 24: 157-165, 2006.

Hoshikawa, Y., Kwon, H. J., Yoshida, M., Horinouchi, S., Beppu, T. Trichostatin A induces morphological changes and gelsolin expression by inhibiting histone deacetylase in human carcinoma cell lines. *Exp Cell Res* 214: 189-197, 1994.

Janmey, P. A. Phosphoinositides and calcium as regulators of cellular actin assembly and disassembly. *Annu Rev Physiol* 56: 169-191, 1994.

Jhoo, J. H., Kim, H. C., Nabeshima, T., Yamada, K., Shin, E. J., Jhoo, W. K., Kim, W., Kang, K. S., Jo, S. A., Woo, J. I. Beta-amyloid (1-42)-induced learning and memory deficits in mice: involvement of oxidative burdens in the hippocampus and cerebral cortex. *Behav Brain Res* 155: 185-196, 2004.

Ji, L., Chauhan, A., Chauhan, V. Cytoplasmic gelsolin in pheochromocytoma-12 cells forms a complex with amyloid beta-protein. *Neuroreport* 19: 463-466, 2008.

Ji, L., Chauhan, A., Wegiel, J., Essa, M. M., Chauhan, V. Gelsolin is Proteolytically Cleaved in the Brains of Individuals with Alzheimer's Disease. *J Alzheimers Dis*, 2009 (in press).

Johnstone, M., Gearing, A. J., Miller, K. M. A central role for astrocytes in the inflammatory response to beta-amyloid; chemokines, cytokines and reactive oxygen species are produced. *J Neuroimmunol* 93: 182-193, 1999.

Kamada, S., Kusano, H., Fujita, H., Ohtsu, M., Koya, R. C., Kuzumaki, N., Tsujimoto, Y. A cloning method for caspase substrates that uses the yeast two-hybrid system: cloning of the antiapoptotic gene gelsolin. *Proc Natl Acad Sci U S A* 95: 8532-8537, 1998.

Kamitani, H., Taniura, S., Watanabe, K., Sakamoto, M., Watanabe, T., Eling, T. Histone acetylation may suppress human glioma cell proliferation when p21 WAF/Cip1 and gelsolin are induced. *Neuro Oncol* 4: 95-101, 2002.

Kang, J., Lemaire, H. G., Unterbeck, A., Salbaum, J. M., Masters, C. L., Grzeschik, K. H., Multhaup, G., Beyreuther, K., Muller-Hill, B. The precursor of Alzheimer's disease amyloid A4 protein resembles a cell-surface receptor. *Nature* 325: 733-736, 1987.

Kim, H. C., Yamada, K., Nitta, A., Olariu, A., Tran, M. H., Mizuno, M., Nakajima, A., Nagai, T., Kamei, H., Jhoo, W. K., Im, D. H., Shin, E. J., Hjelle, O. P., Ottersen, O. P., Park, S. C., Kato, K., Mirault, M. E., Nabeshima, T. Immunocytochemical evidence that amyloid beta (1-42) impairs endogenous antioxidant systems in vivo. *Neuroscience* 119: 399-419, 2003.

Kirkitadze, M. D., Kowalska, A. Molecular mechanisms initiating amyloid beta-fibril formation in Alzheimer's disease. *Acta Biochim Pol* 52: 417-423, 2005.

Knauer, M. F., Soreghan, B., Burdick, D., Kosmoski, J., Glabe, C. G. Intracellular accumulation and resistance to degradation of the Alzheimer amyloid A4/beta protein. *Proc Natl Acad Sci U S A* 89: 7437-7441, 1992.

Kontopoulos, E., Parvin, J. D., Feany, M. B. Alpha-synuclein acts in the nucleus to inhibit histone acetylation and promote neurotoxicity. *Hum Mol Genet* 15: 3012-3023, 2006.

Korenberg, J. R., Kawashima, H., Pulst, S. M., Allen, L., Magenis, E., Epstein, C. J. Down syndrome: toward a molecular definition of the phenotype. *Am J Med Genet Suppl* 7: 91-97, 1990.

Korzus, E., Rosenfeld, M. G., Mayford, M. CBP histone acetyltransferase activity is a critical component of memory consolidation. *Neuron* 42: 961-972, 2004.

Kothakota, S., Azuma, T., Reinhard, C., Klippel, A., Tang, J., Chu, K., McGarry, T. J., Kirschner, M. W., Koths, K., Kwiatkowski, D. J., Williams, L. T. Caspase-3-generated fragment of gelsolin: effector of morphological change in apoptosis. *Science* 278: 294-298, 1997.

Koudinov, A., Matsubara, E., Frangione, B., Ghiso, J. The soluble form of Alzheimer's amyloid beta protein is complexed to high density lipoprotein 3 and very high density lipoprotein in normal human plasma. *Biochem Biophys Res Commun* 205: 1164-1171, 1994.

Koya, R. C., Fujita, H., Shimizu, S., Ohtsu, M., Takimoto, M., Tsujimoto, Y., Kuzumaki, N. Gelsolin inhibits apoptosis by blocking mitochondrial membrane potential loss and cytochrome c release. *J Biol Chem* 275: 15343-15349, 2000.

Kumar, A., Choi, K. H., Renthal, W., Tsankova, N. M., Theobald, D. E., Truong, H. T., Russo, S. J., Laplant, Q., Sasaki, T. S., Whistler, K. N., Neve, R. L., Self, D. W., Nestler, E. J. Chromatin remodeling is a key mechanism underlying cocaine-induced plasticity in striatum. *Neuron* 48: 303-314, 2005.

Kusano, H., Shimizu, S., Koya, R. C., Fujita, H., Kamada, S., Kuzumaki, N., Tsujimoto, Y. Human gelsolin prevents apoptosis by inhibiting apoptotic mitochondrial changes via closing VDAC. *Oncogene* 19: 4807-4814, 2000.

Kwiatkowski, D. J. Functions of gelsolin: motility, signaling, apoptosis, cancer. *Curr Opin Cell Biol* 11: 103-108, 1999.

Kwiatkowski, D. J., Mehl, R., Yin, H. L. Genomic organization and biosynthesis of secreted and cytoplasmic forms of gelsolin. *J Cell Biol* 106: 375-384, 1988.

Lambert, M. P., Viola, K. L., Chromy, B. A., Chang, L., Morgan, T. E., Yu, J., Venton, D. L., Krafft, G. A., Finch, C. E., Klein, W. L. Vaccination with soluble Abeta oligomers generates toxicity-neutralizing antibodies. *J Neurochem* 79: 595-605, 2001.

Lambert, M. P., Barlow, A. K., Chromy, B. A., Edwards, C., Freed, R., Liosatos, M., Morgan, T. E., Rozovsky, I., Trommer, B., Viola, K. L., Wals, P., Zhang, C., Finch, C. E., Krafft, G. A., Klein, W. L. Diffusible, nonfibrillar ligands derived from Abeta1-42 are potent central nervous system neurotoxins. *Proc Natl Acad Sci U S A* 95: 6448-6453, 1998.

Lansbury, P. T., Jr. Evolution of amyloid: what normal protein folding may tell us about fibrillogenesis and disease. *Proc Natl Acad Sci U S A* 96: 3342-3344, 1999.

Lashuel, H. A., Hartley, D., Petre, B. M., Walz, T., Lansbury, P. T., Jr. Neurodegenerative disease: amyloid pores from pathogenic mutations. *Nature* 418: 291, 2002.

Lee, S. H., Kwon, H. M., Kim, Y. J., Lee, K. M., Kim, M., Yoon, B. W. Effects of hsp70.1 gene knockout on the mitochondrial apoptotic pathway after focal cerebral ischemia. *Stroke* 35: 2195-2199, 2004.

Lee, W. M., Galbraith, R. M. The extracellular actin-scavenger system and actin toxicity. *N Engl J Med* 326: 1335-1341, 1992.

Leifeld, L., Fink, K., Debska, G., Fielenbach, M., Schmitz, V., Sauerbruch, T., Spengler, U. Anti-apoptotic function of gelsolin in fas antibody-induced liver failure in vivo. *Am J Pathol* 168: 778-785, 2006.

Levenson, J. M., O'Riordan, K. J., Brown, K. D., Trinh, M. A., Molfese, D. L., Sweatt, J. D. Regulation of histone acetylation during memory formation in the hippocampus. *J Biol Chem* 279: 40545-40559, 2004.

Levy, E., Carman, M. D., Fernandez-Madrid, I. J., Power, M. D., Lieberburg, I., van Duinen, S. G., Bots, G. T., Luyendijk, W., Frangione, B. Mutation of the Alzheimer's disease amyloid gene in hereditary cerebral hemorrhage, Dutch type. *Science* 248: 1124-1126, 1990.

Matsuoka, Y., Saito, M., LaFrancois, J., Saito, M., Gaynor, K., Olm, V., Wang, L., Casey, E., Lu, Y., Shiratori, C., Lemere, C., Duff, K. Novel therapeutic approach for the treatment of Alzheimer's disease by peripheral administration of agents with an affinity to beta-amyloid. *J Neurosci* 23: 29-33, 2003.

Maury, C. P., Sletten, K., Totty, N., Kangas, H., Liljestrom, M. Identification of the circulating amyloid precursor and other gelsolin metabolites in patients with G654A mutation in the gelsolin gene (Finnish familial amyloidosis): pathogenetic and diagnostic implications. *Lab Invest* 77: 299-304, 1997.

Mazur-Kolecka, B., Kowal, D., Sukontasup, T., Dickson, D., Frackowiak, J. The effect of oxidative stress on accumulation of apolipoprotein E3 and E4 in a cell culture model of beta-amyloid angiopathy (CAA). *Brain Res* 983: 48-57, 2003.

Meisel, A., Harms, C., Yildirim, F., Bosel, J., Kronenberg, G., Harms, U., Fink, K. B., Endres, M. Inhibition of histone deacetylation protects wild-type but not gelsolin-deficient neurons from oxygen/glucose deprivation. *J Neurochem* 98: 1019-1031, 2006.

Mielnicki, L. M., Ying, A. M., Head, K. L., Asch, H. L., Asch, B. B. Epigenetic regulation of gelsolin expression in human breast cancer cells. *Exp Cell Res* 249: 161-176, 1999.

Mohmmad Abdul, H., Wenk, G. L., Gramling, M., Hauss-Wegrzyniak, B., Butterfield, D. A. APP and PS-1 mutations induce brain oxidative stress independent of dietary cholesterol: implications for Alzheimer's disease. *Neurosci Lett* 368: 148-150, 2004.

Mullauer, L., Fujita, H., Ishizaki, A., Kuzumaki, N. Tumor-suppressive function of mutated gelsolin in ras-transformed cells. *Oncogene* 8: 2531-2536, 1993.

Ohtsu, M., Sakai, N., Fujita, H., Kashiwagi, M., Gasa, S., Shimizu, S., Eguchi, Y., Tsujimoto, Y., Sakiyama, Y., Kobayashi, K., Kuzumaki, N. Inhibition of apoptosis by the actin-regulatory protein gelsolin. *Embo J* 16: 4650-4656, 1997.

Park, L., Anrather, J., Forster, C., Kazama, K., Carlson, G. A., Iadecola, C. Abeta-induced vascular oxidative stress and attenuation of functional hyperemia in mouse somatosensory cortex. *J Cereb Blood Flow Metab* 24: 334-342, 2004.

Paunio, T., Kangas, H., Kalkkinen, N., Haltia, M., Palo, J., Peltonen, L. Toward understanding the pathogenic mechanisms in gelsolin-related amyloidosis: in vitro expression reveals an abnormal gelsolin fragment. *Hum Mol Genet* 3: 2223-2229, 1994.

Qiao, H., Koya, R. C., Nakagawa, K., Tanaka, H., Fujita, H., Takimoto, M., Kuzumaki, N. Inhibition of Alzheimer's amyloid-beta peptide-induced reduction of mitochondrial membrane potential and neurotoxicity by gelsolin. *Neurobiol Aging* 26: 849-855, 2005.

Ray, I., Chauhan, A., Wegiel, J., Chauhan, V. P. Gelsolin inhibits the fibrillization of amyloid beta-protein, and also defibrillizes its preformed fibrils. *Brain Res* 853: 344-351, 2000.

Rothenbach, P. A., Dahl, B., Schwartz, J. J., O'Keefe, G. E., Yamamoto, M., Lee, W. M., Horton, J. W., Yin, H. L., Turnage, R. H. Recombinant plasma gelsolin infusion attenuates burn-induced pulmonary microvascular dysfunction. *J Appl Physiol* 96: 25-31, 2004.

Ryu, H., Smith, K., Camelo, S. I., Carreras, I., Lee, J., Iglesias, A. H., Dangond, F., Cormier, K. A., Cudkowicz, M. E., Brown, R. H., Jr., Ferrante, R. J. Sodium phenylbutyrate prolongs survival and regulates expression of anti-apoptotic genes in transgenic amyotrophic lateral sclerosis mice. *J Neurochem* 93: 1087-1098, 2005.

Sajan, F. D., Martiniuk, F., Marcus, D. L., Frey, W. H., 2nd, Hite, R., Bordayo, E. Z., Freedman, M. L. Apoptotic gene expression in Alzheimer's disease hippocampal tissue. *Am J Alzheimers Dis Other Demen* 22: 319-328, 2007.

Schuessel, K., Schafer, S., Bayer, T. A., Czech, C., Pradier, L., Muller-Spahn, F., Muller, W. E., Eckert, A. Impaired Cu/Zn-SOD activity contributes to increased oxidative damage in APP transgenic mice. *Neurobiol Dis* 18: 89-99, 2005.

Serpell, L. C., Sunde, M., Benson, M. D., Tennent, G. A., Pepys, M. B., Fraser, P. E. The protofilament substructure of amyloid fibrils. *J Mol Biol* 300: 1033-1039, 2000.

Seubert, P., Vigo-Pelfrey, C., Esch, F., Lee, M., Dovey, H., Davis, D., Sinha, S., Schlossmacher, M., Whaley, J., Swindlehurst, C., et al. Isolation and quantification of soluble Alzheimer's beta-peptide from biological fluids. *Nature* 359: 325-327, 1992.

Sherrington, R., Froelich, S., Sorbi, S., Campion, D., Chi, H., Rogaeva, E. A., Levesque, G., Rogaev, E. I., Lin, C., Liang, Y., Ikeda, M., Mar, L., Brice, A., Agid, Y., Percy, M. E.,

Clerget-Darpoux, F., Piacentini, S., Marcon, G., Nacmias, B., Amaducci, L., Frebourg, T., Lannfelt, L., Rommens, J. M., St George-Hyslop, P. H. Alzheimer's disease associated with mutations in presenilin 2 is rare and variably penetrant. *Hum Mol Genet* 5: 985-988, 1996.

Sinha, S., Lieberburg, I. Cellular mechanisms of beta-amyloid production and secretion. *Proc Natl Acad Sci U S A* 96: 11049-11053, 1999.

Small, D. H., Mok, S. S., Bornstein, J. C. Alzheimer's disease and Abeta toxicity: from top to bottom. *Nat Rev Neurosci* 2: 595-598, 2001.

Steffan, J. S., Bodai, L., Pallos, J., Poelman, M., McCampbell, A., Apostol, B. L., Kazantsev, A., Schmidt, E., Zhu, Y. Z., Greenwald, M., Kurokawa, R., Housman, D. E., Jackson, G. R., Marsh, J. L., Thompson, L. M. Histone deacetylase inhibitors arrest polyglutamine-dependent neurodegeneration in Drosophila. *Nature* 413: 739-743, 2001.

Strittmatter, W. J., Weisgraber, K. H., Huang, D. Y., Dong, L. M., Salvesen, G. S., Pericak-Vance, M., Schmechel, D., Saunders, A. M., Goldgaber, D., Roses, A. D. Binding of human apolipoprotein E to synthetic amyloid beta peptide: isoform-specific effects and implications for late-onset Alzheimer disease. *Proc Natl Acad Sci U S A* 90: 8098-8102, 1993.

Sultana, R., Ravagna, A., Mohmmad-Abdul, H., Calabrese, V., Butterfield, D. A. Ferulic acid ethyl ester protects neurons against amyloid beta- peptide(1-42)-induced oxidative stress and neurotoxicity: relationship to antioxidant activity. *J Neurochem* 92: 749-758, 2005.

Suzuki, N., Cheung, T. T., Cai, X. D., Odaka, A., Otvos, L., Jr., Eckman, C., Golde, T. E., Younkin, S. G. An increased percentage of long amyloid beta protein secreted by familial amyloid beta protein precursor (beta APP717) mutants. *Science* 264: 1336-1340, 1994.

Tamagno, E., Robino, G., Obbili, A., Bardini, P., Aragno, M., Parola, M., Danni, O. H2O2 and 4-hydroxynonenal mediate amyloid beta-induced neuronal apoptosis by activating JNKs and p38MAPK. *Exp Neurol* 180: 144-155, 2003.

Tanaka, J., Sobue, K. Localization and characterization of gelsolin in nervous tissues: gelsolin is specifically enriched in myelin-forming cells. *J Neurosci* 14: 1038-1052, 1994.

Turner, P. R., O'Connor, K., Tate, W. P., Abraham, W. C. Roles of amyloid precursor protein and its fragments in regulating neural activity, plasticity and memory. *Prog Neurobiol* 70: 1-32, 2003.

Vardy, E. R., Catto, A. J., Hooper, N. M. Proteolytic mechanisms in amyloid-beta metabolism: therapeutic implications for Alzheimer's disease. *Trends Mol Med* 11: 464-472, 2005.

Vassar, R., Bennett, B. D., Babu-Khan, S., Kahn, S., Mendiaz, E. A., Denis, P., Teplow, D. B., Ross, S., Amarante, P., Loeloff, R., Luo, Y., Fisher, S., Fuller, J., Edenson, S., Lile, J., Jarosinski, M. A., Biere, A. L., Curran, E., Burgess, T., Louis, J. C., Collins, F., Treanor, J., Rogers, G., Citron, M. Beta-secretase cleavage of Alzheimer's amyloid precursor protein by the transmembrane aspartic protease BACE. *Science* 286: 735-741, 1999.

Vigo-Pelfrey, C., Lee, D., Keim, P., Lieberburg, I., Schenk, D. B. Characterization of beta-amyloid peptide from human cerebrospinal fluid. *J Neurochem* 61: 1965-1968, 1993.

Walsh, D. M., Klyubin, I., Fadeeva, J. V., Cullen, W. K., Anwyl, R., Wolfe, M. S., Rowan, M. J., Selkoe, D. J. Naturally secreted oligomers of amyloid beta protein potently inhibit hippocampal long-term potentiation in vivo. *Nature* 416: 535-539, 2002.

Walsh, D. M., Hartley, D. M., Kusumoto, Y., Fezoui, Y., Condron, M. M., Lomakin, A., Benedek, G. B., Selkoe, D. J., Teplow, D. B. Amyloid beta-protein fibrillogenesis.

Structure and biological activity of protofibrillar intermediates. *J Biol Chem* 274: 25945-25952, 1999.

Wen, D., Corina, K., Chow, E. P., Miller, S., Janmey, P. A., Pepinsky, R. B. The plasma and cytoplasmic forms of human gelsolin differ in disulfide structure. *Biochemistry* 35: 9700-9709, 1996.

Wisniewski, T., Ghiso, J., Frangione, B. Biology of A beta amyloid in Alzheimer's disease. *Neurobiol Dis* 4: 313-328, 1997.

Witke, W., Li, W., Kwiatkowski, D. J., Southwick, F. S. Comparisons of CapG and gelsolin-null macrophages: demonstration of a unique role for CapG in receptor-mediated ruffling, phagocytosis, and vesicle rocketing. *J Cell Biol* 154: 775-784, 2001.

Witke, W., Sharpe, A. H., Hartwig, J. H., Azuma, T., Stossel, T. P., Kwiatkowski, D. J. Hemostatic, inflammatory, and fibroblast responses are blunted in mice lacking gelsolin. *Cell* 81: 41-51, 1995.

Wolf, B. B., Goldstein, J. C., Stennicke, H. R., Beere, H., Amarante-Mendes, G. P., Salvesen, G. S., Green, D. R. Calpain functions in a caspase-independent manner to promote apoptosis-like events during platelet activation. *Blood* 94: 1683-1692, 1999.

Wujek, J. R., Dority, M. D., Frederickson, R. C., Brunden, K. R. Deposits of A beta fibrils are not toxic to cortical and hippocampal neurons in vitro. *Neurobiol Aging* 17: 107-113, 1996.

Yang, D. S., Kumar, A., Stavrides, P., Peterson, J., Peterhoff, C. M., Pawlik, M., Levy, E., Cataldo, A. M., Nixon, R. A. Neuronal apoptosis and autophagy cross talk in aging PS/APP mice, a model of Alzheimer's disease. *Am J Pathol* 173: 665-681, 2008.

Yermen, B., Tomas, A., Halban, P. A. Pro-survival role of gelsolin in mouse beta-cells. *Diabetes* 56: 80-87, 2007.

Yildirim, F., Gertz, K., Kronenberg, G., Harms, C., Fink, K. B., Meisel, A., Endres, M. Inhibition of histone deacetylation protects wildtype but not gelsolin-deficient mice from ischemic brain injury. *Exp Neurol* 210: 531-542, 2008.

Yin, H. L., Kwiatkowski, D. J., Mole, J. E., Cole, F. S. Structure and biosynthesis of cytoplasmic and secreted variants of gelsolin. *J Biol Chem* 259: 5271-5276, 1984.

Yu, C., Kim, S. H., Ikeuchi, T., Xu, H., Gasparini, L., Wang, R., Sisodia, S. S. Characterization of a presenilin-mediated amyloid precursor protein carboxyl-terminal fragment gamma. Evidence for distinct mechanisms involved in gamma -secretase processing of the APP and Notch1 transmembrane domains. *J Biol Chem* 276: 43756-43760, 2001.

Yuyama, K., Yamamoto, N., Yanagisawa, K. Chloroquine-induced endocytic pathway abnormalities: Cellular model of GM1 ganglioside-induced Abeta fibrillogenesis in Alzheimer's disease. *FEBS Lett* 580: 6972-6976, 2006.

Acknowledgments

This work was supported in part by the funds from the New York State Office of Mental Retardation and Developmental Disabilities, and by NIH Grant No. AG020992.

In: Alzheimer's Disease and Dementia (Vol. 4)
Editor: Miao-Kun Sun
ISBN:978-1-60876-152-4

Chapter X

Declarative Memory Impairment and Hippocampal Atrophy in Parkinson's Disease

Carme Junque*
Department of Psychiatry and Clinical Psychobiology, University of Barcelona, Spain

Abstract

Memory deficits in Parkinson's disease (PD) are seen in the early stages of the disease even in non-medicated patients. The deficits progress over time, are more prevalent in patients with visual hallucinations, and have predictive value for the evolution to dementia. Memory deficits are seen isolated or in combination with deficits in other cognitive domains. Classically the pattern of memory impairment in PD has been described as typical of subcortical dementia, that is, impaired recall with preserved recognition. This pattern has been considered secondary to the executive deficits caused by the neurochemical fronto-striatal dysfunctions. However, recent meta-analyses and empirical data have questioned this classical pattern. The alteration of recognition is similar to that of free recall. Moreover, evidence mainly from neuropathological and structural magnetic resonance imaging studies clearly demonstrates that there are hippocampal gray matter reductions that directly explain the declarative memory deficits. Hippocampal reductions are observed by neuroradiological visual rating scales and are also seen in volumetric and voxel-based morphometry studies. By contrast, both functional magnetic resonance studies and PET studies conclude that working memory deficits seem to depend on the dysfunctions in the fronto-striatal circuitry and are sensitive to dopaminergic and non-dopaminergic pharmacological treatments and also to electrical transcranial stimulation.

*Correspondence: Carme Junque, Department of Psychiatry and Clinical Psychobiology. University of Barcelona, Casanova 143 (08036) Barcelona, Spain, Phone: (+34) 93 402 45 70 // Fax: (+34) 93 403 52 94, E-mail: cjunque@ub.edu

Abbreviations

AD: Alzheimer's disease
AVLT: Auditory verbal learning test
CA: Cornus Ammon
CERAD: Consortium to eEstablish a rRegistry for Alzheimer dDisease
CFQ: Cognitive fFailures qQuestionnaire
CVLT: California vVerbal lLearning tTest
EMQ: Everyday mMemory qQuestionnaire
fMRI: Functional magnetic resonance imaging
MCI: Mild cognitive impairment
MRI: Magnetic resonance imaging
PD: Parkinson's disease
PDD: Parkinson's disease with dementia
PD-VH+. Parkinson's disease with visual hallucinations
PD-VH- Parkinson's disease without visual hallucinations
PET: Positron emission tomography
ROI: Region of interest
SR: Selective rReminding
SRRT: Serial reaction time task
VBM Voxel based morphometry
WMS: Wechsler mMemory sScale

Introduction

Parkinson's disease (PD) is a neurodegenerative illness that is classically characterized by movement disorders. However, in the last decade several studies have concluded that the disease is strongly associated with dementia and several specific cognitive deficits such as memory impairment (Aarsland et al., 2003, 2004, 2005, 2008). Indeed, at twenty years of disease evolution, 83% of patients suffer from dementia (Hely et al., 2008). Cognitive deficits in PD mainly involve memory, visuospatial and frontal lobe dysfunctions (Emre, 2003; Verbaan et al., 2007; Caballoll, Marti and Tolosa, 2007). Recently, the term mild cognitive impairment (MCI) in Parkinson's disease has been proposed for non-demented PD patients with neuropsychological dysfunctions, this being similar to the construct of mild cognitive impairment proposed by Petersen et al. (2001) as a precursor of Alzheimer's disease. The criterion for defining MCI in PD is cognitive performance more than 1.5 standard deviations below either the mean of the control group or the normative data from neuropsychological tests. The MCI profile in PD can involve one or multiple cognitive domains. Caviness et al. (2007) found that 31% of their sample of PD patients met the criteria for MCI, and observed that the most frequently abnormal cognitive domain was frontal/executive dysfunctions, followed by amnesic deficit. Moreover, the diagnosis of MCI in PD seems to predict evolution to dementia (Janvin et al., 2006).

Memory impairment in PD is very relevant because it is seen even in the early stages of the disease (Muslimovic et al., 2005), it progresses over time (Muslimovic et al. 2007), it is more pronounced in patients with visual hallucinations (Grossi et al., 2005; Ramirez-Ruiz et al., 2006; Ozer et al., 2007), and it predicts evolution to dementia (Levy et al., 2002).

Memory is not a unitary function. Indeed, memory disorders can arise from lesions or dysfunctions of cortical and subcortical gray matter structures, as well as from white matter changes. According to Squire and Zola's (1996) model of memory, medial temporal lesions cause deficits of declarative memory, whereas basal ganglia lesions cause deficits of procedural learning. Working memory is a function that maintains information on-line and depends basically on the parieto-frontal networks, as well as on fronto-striatal circuitry (D'Esposito, 2007; Hillary, 2008). Since PD patients have gray matter loss in the medial temporal lobe and fronto-temporo-parietal regions (Burton et al., 2004; Nagano-Saito et al., 2005; Ramirez-Ruiz et al., 2005; Feldmann et al., 2008) it is reasonable to expect deficits in declarative, procedural and working memory.

The classical memory profile reported in PD follows that described for all the so-called "subcortical dementias", namely that memory deficits are due not to encoding problems but, rather, to impaired recall of information. In turn, this impaired information recall results from a primary deficit in executive functions. According to this model, patients perform worse than controls on recall tasks that require active retrieval of information due to their impairment in the manipulation of stored data. The difference in patients' scores on spontaneous recall versus stimuli recognition has been used to support this hypothesis (Brown and Marsden, 1988; Taylor et al., 1986). However, the validity of this model has recently been undermined by results from both meta-analyses and new empirical data (Whittington, Podd and Kan, 2000; Beatty et al., 2003; Higginson, 2005; Whittington et al., 2006).

In order to determine the origin of memory and other cognitive dysfunctions in PD, neuropsychological research over the last two decades has focused on the neurochemical model of cognitive dysfunctions in PD, which is mainly based on information about cortico-striatal loops (Alexander, DeLong and Strick, 1986). According to this model, memory dysfunctions arise from frontal dysfunctions caused by neurochemical disturbance in these loops. Basically, the direct and indirect loss of dopamine in the prefrontal cortex is thought to be responsible for executive dysfunctions, i.e. impairment in accessing, planning and organizing information. In turn, these dysexecutive symptoms impede the normal functioning of memory (Owen, 2004). More recently, it has been proposed that cognitive dysfunction in PD arises from a disruption of the dopamine-acetylcholine synaptic balance. In support of a role for cholinergic systems, research in PD patients has found neural cell loss in the nucleus basalis of Meynert and reductions in cortical cholinergic markers. These cholinergic deficits may cause memory disturbances. In turn, dopamine deficits could explain the impairment in the reinforcement mechanisms of learning processes (Schott et al., 2007). Because dopamine and acetylcholine interact at the anatomical, biochemical and physiological level to induce long-lasting changes in synaptic strength, some authors have proposed a convergent biochemical model for cognitive dysfunctions associated with PD (Calabresi et al., 2006). However, as an alternative or a complement to the neurochemical origin of memory dysfunctions in PD, recent magnetic resonance imaging (MRI) studies have demonstrated several cerebral gray matter reductions in PD involving the hippocampal and parahippocampal regions, and these could directly explain the memory loss associated with the disease progression.

Declarative Memory Deficits in PDd

Declarative memory refers to remembering personal events, cultural history, semantic information and other facts that we can be explicitly aware of and thus report, or "declare", either verbally or nonverbally (as when pressing a button in a test paradigm). Declarative memory has been classified into semantic and episodic memories and facts and events. It is a function that depends on the integrity of temporal medial structures, basically the hippocampus (Squire and Zola, 1996).

Clinically, declarative memory deficits can be assessed by asking subjects to learn lists of words (Dubois et al., 2007). The variables that are usually recorded are learning (sum of words recalled in five trials), long-term retention (recall of information after a period of time), forgetting (percentage of words lost between learning and long-term retention) and recognition (words correctly identified in a passive auditory task). In recognition tasks a distinction can be made between two types of error: false positives (confabulation) and false negatives (omission). The most widely-used tests involving word lists are Rey's Auditory Verbal Learning Test (RAVLT), the California Verbal Learning Test (CVLT), the Selective Reminding (SR) test, and the list of the Consortium to Establish a Registry for Alzheimer Disease (CERAD). Other tests of declarative memory taken from the Wechsler Memory Scale (WMS) are paired associative learning and story recall (see Lezak et al., 2004 for a description of the tests and references).

Visual memory tests are less widely used because most of them involve motor functions during the copy phase (i.e. Rey's complex figures, visual memory from the WMS) and are thus not appropriate for PD patients. To assess visual declarative memory in PD the recommended tests are those such as Warrington's facial recognition test or the face recognition subtest from the WMS IVII, as these do not require motor functions.

There is extensive evidence of declarative memory deficits in PD (for reviews, see Dubois and Pillon, 1997; Troster, 2008). As mentioned above, the subcortical dementia model (Cummings and Benson, 1984) considers that these deficits are severe on free recall testing but mild for recognition. Thus, declarative memory deficits in PD have been suggested to be secondary to retrieval rather than encoding impairments per se. However, recent evidence has cast serious doubt on the validity of this model. For example, Troster (2008) analyzed the statistical power of the retrieval deficit hypothesis and concluded that evidence was lacking. Similarly, Whittington, Podd and Kan (2000) performed a meta-analysis of recognition memory in PD and concluded that deficits in recognition memory are seen not only in demented PD patients but also in non-demented patients. Likewise, a study by Beaty et al. (2003) using z scores found no differences between free recall and recognition in demented and non-demented PD patients. In a large sample of patients (n=99) Higginson et al. (2005) showed that the performance of demented and non-demented PD patients on measures of cued recall and delayed recognition were not significantly better than those obtained for free recall. These results suggest that memory deficits in PD are not solely due to retrieval problems, and they fail to support the classical concept of subcortical dementia in PD patients. Similar findings were reported by Whittington et al. (2006). These investigators developed two tasks of recognition memory (abstract stimuli and nouns) with two levels of complexity (easy and difficult). They found that PD patients were impaired in both verbal and non-verbal recognition, although patients in the early stages of the disease performed similarly to controls on the easy task. Ceiling effects could explain these results, as might the preservation of recognition in PD that has been previously reported in the literature.

Remote memory (recall of information from the remote past) is typically preserved in PD, although it is impaired in PD patients with dementia (Troster, 2008). In summary, the concept of a subcortical memory profile is not supported by recent neuropsychological studies, or by data from structural MRI studies. In this regard, several recent MRI studies report decreased gray matter in neocortical structures (Burton et al., 2004; Summerfield et al., 2005; Nagano-Saito et al., 2005; Beyer et al., 2007; Feldmann et al., 2008).

Although memory deficits in PD are accompanied by other neuropsychological deficits, they are in themselves of special relevance. A recent study of cognitive deficits performed with a large sample of 196 untreated PD patients showed that those with the largest effect size were verbal memory deficits. Moreover, one third of patients with mild cognitive impairment are of the amnestic type (Aarsland et al., 2008). In a longitudinal study including 180 patients with a re-assessment period of between 3 and 5 years, Williams-Gray et al. (2007) showed that spatial recognition memory was the function with the highest percentage of patients impaired (37%) at follow-up. However, memory was not the best predictor of evolution to dementia; the best predictors were pentagon copying and verbal semantic fluency, both of which are tests that assess the posterior region of the cortex (temporo-parietal). Similar results were found in a meta-analysis of 25 longitudinal studies involving 901 initially non-demented PD patients. During a mean follow-up interval of 29 months, significant declines were detected in visuoconstructive skills (d=.32) and memory (d=.29) (Muslimovic et al., 2007).

The presence of visual hallucinations (VH) is very frequent in PD and is a marker for evolution to dementia (Aarsland et al., 2003). Patients with VH have more marked memory deficits compared with patients without hallucinations on measures of recognition of faces previously seen and percentage of forgetting (Ramirez-Ruiz et al., 2006; Ozer et al., 2006). Interestingly, patients with visual hallucinations, but not those without VH, differed from controls on tests of face memory recognition (Warrington's recognition test), as well as on a test of facial identification (Benton's Facial Recognition Test) (Ramirez Ruiz et al., 2006). These findings are consistent with the increased degeneration of gray matter in the temporal and parietal associative visual areas in patients with VH (Ramirez-Ruiz et al., 2007a). Moreover, in patients with VH, visual memory for faces shows a significant decline at one-year follow up, whereas patients without hallucinations and age-matched controls showed no significant decline over the same time period. This involution was not selective for visual memory, as similar results were observed for verbal learning, delayed recall and recognition (Ramirez-Ruiz et al., 2007b).

Neuropsychological tests have provided clear evidence of memory impairment in PD. However, such tests may lack ecological validity, in other words, there is no correspondence between test performance and the problems faced in daily living activities. The question remains, therefore, as to how memory deficits affect everyday life. In this regard, self-report questionnaires such as the Cognitive Failures Questionnaire (CFQ) and the Everyday Memory Questionnaire (EMQ) indicate that PD is associated with impaired retrieval processes; for example, patients have difficulty in recalling important details from the previous day and they also forget where they have put certain objects (newspapers, glasses, etc.) (Poliakoff and Smith-Spark, 2008). At all events, it is clear that memory deficits do affect the quality of life of patients.

Another important question is the possible reversibility of memory deficits in PD after treatment. Treatment effects not only have clinical relevance but also implications as regards the physiopathological mechanism of cognitive deficits. If dopaminergic deficits are responsible for the memory deficits in PD, these might remit after L-dopa administration, similar to what occurs with motor deficits. The effects of L-dopa on cognitive function in Parkinson's disease are very complex, and both positive and negative effects have been observed for cognitive flexibility and working memory (for a review, see Cools, 2006). As regards declarative memory, Cooper et al. (1992) found no changes in declarative memory after dopamine therapy in de novo patients, although Kulisevsky et al. (2000) did observe significant improvements at 6- and 12-month follow up in a study that assessed patients six times over a period of two years. Although this study used alternative forms of the RALVLT list, the design did not control for difficulties of the list or practice effects.

As regards neurosurgical and neurophysiological treatments, a decline in verbal memory has been reported in the immediate post-surgery assessment (1 week), although this had returned to normal levels at 3-month follow up (Junque et al., 1999). Similarly, bilateral subthalamic stimulation has also been reported to produce a memory decline that remained stable at 3-month follow up (Alegret et al., 2001), although it was absent at 1-year follow up (Pillon et al., 2000; Alegret et al., 2004) and 4-year follow up (Alegret et al., 2003). Overall, the percentage of patients with a clinically significant decline is around 16% (Higginson et al., 2009). Memory impairment after these treatments may be due to surgical procedures that can cause damage to corticothalamic or mamillothalamic circuits (Frank et al., 2007).

Neuropathological Studies on Hippocampal Degenerative Changes in PD

Parkinson's disease is a widespread degenerative illness affecting the central nervous system. The underlying pathological process progresses slowly but relentlessly and involves multiple neural systems. Components of the limbic and motor systems have been shown to be particularly vulnerable to severe destruction. For example, the entorhinal region and the second sector of Ammon's horn are favored regions for neurodegeneration (Braak and Braak, 2000) and they are involved in the memory system. According to the staging model of Braak et al. (2002, 2003, 2004), neural destruction in stage 3 reaches the magnocellular cholinergic nuclei of the basal forebrain, while in stage 4 it reaches the anteromedial temporal mesocortex, involving several centers of the limbic loop that are essential for memory processing (amygdala, hippocampal formation and entorhinal region). Since motor signs appear and diagnosis is made in Braak stages 3-4 it is reasonable to assume that memory deficits will be observed due to cholinergic dysfunctions in memory systems, as well as to degeneration of the hippocampus. The Braak stages also correlate with the degree of global cognitive decline as assessed by the MMSE. However, specific memory assessment was not examined in these samples (Braak et al., 2005, 2006).

There is consistent neuropathological evidence that the hippocampus is compromised in PD patients. Pathological findings reported in PD patients include the presence of Lewy bodies and Lewy neuritis in CA2 and CA3 hippocampal subfields, and Lewy neurites in the CA2 subfield correlated with dementia (Churchyard and Lees, 1997). Halliday et al. (2008) described the pathological progression of longitudinally followed cases with levodopa-responsive Parkinson's disease who came to autopsy during the Sydney Multicenter Study of Parkinson's disease. In a group of younger onset patients with a typically long clinical course of Parkinson's disease, 50% of cases at 13 years have a limbic distribution of Lewy bodies, while by 18 years all will have at least this pathological phenotype.

There is one negative report of neuronal reductions in PD (Joelving et al., 2006). These authors found no significant differences in cell number or volumes in PD patients when compared with age-matched controls. This negative finding could be due to the small sample size analyzed (8 PD patients) and the heterogeneous characteristics of the sample.

Structural Magnetic Resonance Studies: Visual Inspection and Volumetry

Magnetic resonance (MR) analysis enables in vivo detection and quantification of regional cerebral atrophy of the hippocampus. In PD, hippocampal atrophy has been reported by using several methods for evaluating hippocampal reduction. These methods are visual inspection by expert neuroradiologists, quantification of volume from the sum of the surfaces of the slices covering the entire hippocampus, and automatic methods such as voxel-based morphometry (VBM) analyses.

Using a five-point rating scale of atrophy by visual inspection, Brück et al. (2004) reported that the mean right-sided atrophy in the hippocampus was 1.15 for PD patients and 0.45 for controls. Corresponding figures for the left hippocampus were 1.05 for patients and 0.64 for controls. This study concluded that non-medicated, non-demented patients with early stage PD show hippocampal and prefrontal atrophy with specific patterns of correlations.

The volumetric analysis of regions of interest (ROI) can be performed by means of drawing the selected structure (see fig. 1). The volume of the structure (i.e. hippocampus) must be corrected by the whole brain volume because of inter-individual variability, sex effects and the degree of general atrophy related to age and the degenerative illness. The whole brain volume is obtained by the sum of partial volumes of gray matter, white matter and cerebrospinal fluid obtained from the segmentation of the native MR scans (before spatial normalization). These methods are labor intensive and time-consuming, and are also subject to wide inter-rater and intra-rater variability. Methodologically they require two different operators in order to obtain the inter-rater correlation, or taking two measures of the same structure by the same operator so as to obtain the intra-rater reliability coefficient.

Another method for obtaining volumetric measures of the hippocampus is the stereological analyses provided by the ANALYZE program (see fig. 2). In general, and starting from images with a voxel size of 0.5 mm^3, a rigid grid of 2.5 x 2.5 mm^2 is superimposed onto every coronal slice. Each grid point is then viewed in the orthogonal planes simultaneously. This procedure helps to decide whether a point is contained within the measured structure or not.

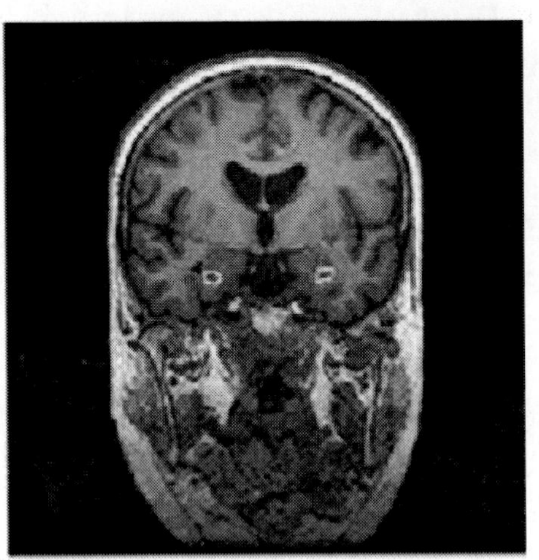

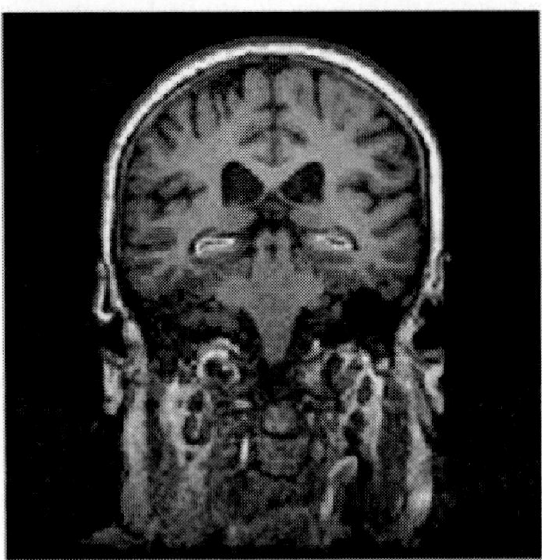

Figure 1. Example of region of interest (ROI) procedure. Manual delineation of the hippocampus performed in the coronal plane.

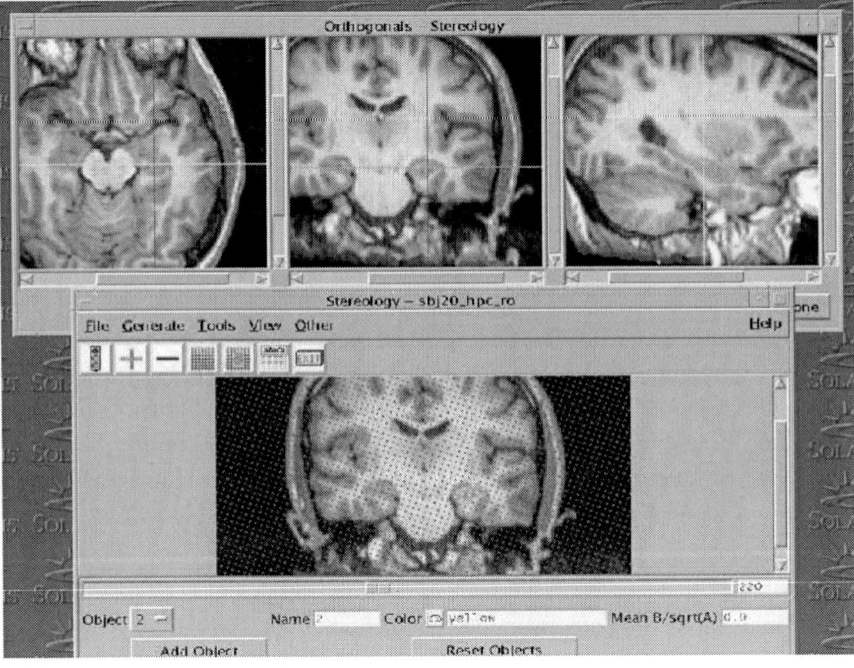

Figure 2. Quantification of the hippocampal volume by stereological procedures.

Reductions in hippocampal volume have also been observed in demented PD patients using the manual ROI approach (Laakso et al., 1996; Junque et al., 2005), as well as in PD patients without dementia (Laakso et al., 1996; Camicioli et al., 2003). Compared to controls of similar age, PD patients show 10% volume reductions in the hippocampus, while the reduction in demented PD patients is 20%. (Junque et al., 2005). These figures are similar to those observed in post-mortem studies (Junque et al., 2005). The atrophy seen in demented PD was less marked than that observed in Alzheimer's disease. According to the effect size analysis for hippocampal atrophy the order would be AD>PDD>PD compared with controls (Laakso et al., 1996).

It is well known that ageing per se produces hippocampal atrophy, and that this is more prominent in subjects with memory deficits and amnesic mild cognitive impairment (Apostolova et al., 2006a, 2006b, 2007). In Parkinson's disease the age effect seems to have an exponential effect. Bouchard et al. (2007) showed that hippocampal volumes in older PD patients (>70), but not in younger non-demented PD patients, differed from normal controls; furthermore, in patients (but not in controls) age was correlated with hippocampal volume. In this study it was reported that hippocampal volume reductions were significant for the hippocampal head but not the body or tail.

Voxel-Based Morphometry Studies

In contrast to the classical, manual ROI approach, voxel-based morphometry (VBM) is an automated image analysis that allows regional patterns of brain volume from T1-weighted magnetic resonance imaging (MRI) scans to be compared between two or more groups of subjects. The standard procedure is relatively unbiased because it examines the differences throughout the whole brain and does not require any a priori assumption concerning which structures to assess. Thus, regional gray matter reductions of the whole brain can be obtained. VBM analyses involve a complex semiautomatic process of segmentation, normalization and smoothing. The group comparison can be selected for what is termed density or concentration (unmodulated images) or volume (modulated images) (Mechelli et al., 2005).

Although VBM processes seem to be automatic there are several steps that involve decisions on the part of investigators and which may affect the final results. Errors in segmentation due to the threshold selected in this step are very frequent in the case of degenerative illness, as white matter loss can be classified as gray matter.

Another issue is that the kernel selected in the smoothing procedure is relevant as regards the potential to detect changes in relatively small structures such as the hippocampus. For example, in whole brain analysis a 12 mm kernel is commonly used, whereas for detection of hippocampal changes the optimal kernel size is between 4 and 8 mm (Honea et al., 2005). The cut-off criteria for statistical significance are also relevant. In VBM studies performed with PD samples the criteria range from uncorrected $p<0.01$ to FWE corrected. Other methodological differences that may explain discrepancies between VBM studies are the program and tests used (parametric or non-parametric), the version used for the analysis and the covariables entered in the analyses (i.e. whole intracranial brain volume, whole gray matter volume, age, gender, illness severity, motor impairment). Finally, discrepancies between studies can also be due to the selection of a standard template or a specific template created with the subjects and controls of the study itself. VBM analysis provides images that represent the clusters of statistical significance in group comparison (see fig 3). Usually the t values are represented in a colored bar in which yellow represent higher statistical differences than red.

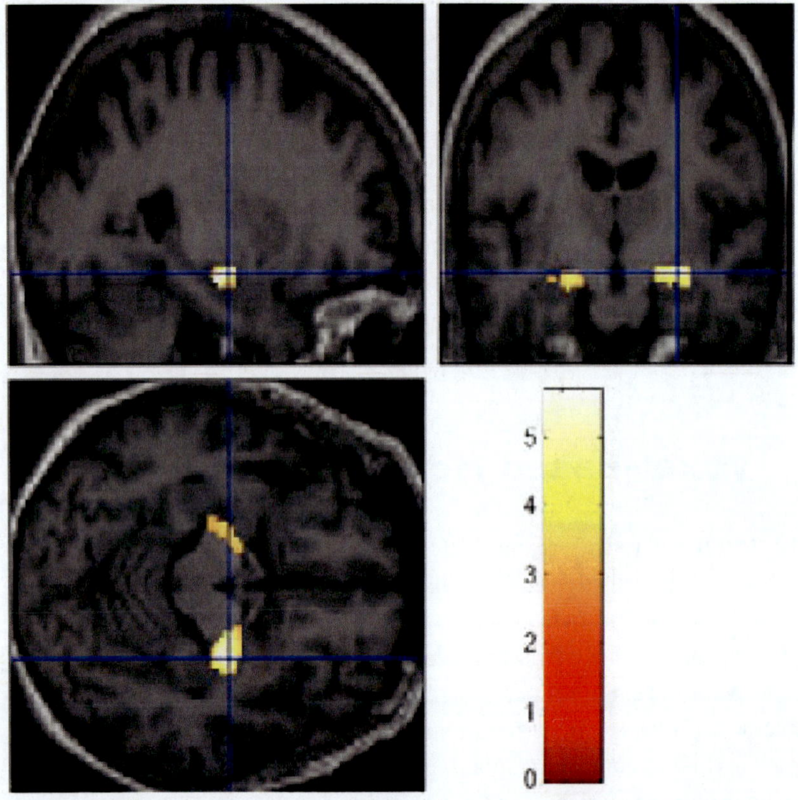

Figure 3. Images illustrating the results of the vVoxel based-morphometry analysis. In yellow the gray matter region of the hippocampus showing decreased concentration in PD patients compared with controls.

Over the last five years voxel-based morphometry has been used in several movement disorders to identify patterns of gray matter atrophy, as well as in an attempt to provide differential diagnosis between similar pathologies such as PD multisystem atrophy and supranuclear palsy (Price et al., 2004; Whitwell and Josephs, 2007). VBM studies have proved to be a useful tool for explaining the origin of cognitive dysfunctions in what are known as subcortical dementias, above and beyond the models based on neurochemical changes proposed in the 1980s and 1990s (Brown and Marsden, 1990).

VBM studies with demented PD patients have shown hippocampal reductions (Burton et al., 2004; Summerfield et al., 2005; Beyer et al., 2007a). Furthermore, demented PD patients have more right hippocampal reductions than do non-demented patients (Nagano-Saito et al., 2005). Hippocampal reductions were also observed in non-demented patients when comparing PD patients with controls and PDD with PD (Summerfield et al., 2005).

In contrast, Nagano-Saito et al. (2005) found no hippocampal differences between non-demented patients and controls, but they did report that advanced non-demented PD patients have gray matter loss in the left parahippocampal region. If we consider that the cerebral locations of VBM procedures are determined by the Talairach coordinates of the maxima, according to the cluster size, then other regions surrounding the reported one may also show a decrease. Moreover, VBM procedures can involve a localization error of up to 5 mm (Mechelli et al., 2005), and such errors increase in atrophic brains. In summary, the involvement of the hippocampus in studies that report reductions in the amygdala or parahippocampal gray matter cannot be ruled out.

As regards the evolution of hippocampal atrophy only two published studies have investigated gray matter changes over time in PD. In a sample of 14 PD patients followed up over 1.4 years Brenneis et al. (2007) failed to observe gray matter changes in any corresponding region. In contrast, patients with multiple system atrophy did show gray matter volume loss over the same time interval in multiple bilateral cortical regions, including the hippocampus. The lack of gray matter degeneration could be due to the relatively young age of patients (mean 59) or other clinical variables not reported in the paper (Hoenh and Yahr stage, years of evolution, presence of hallucinations). In a similar follow-up study, we found that PD patients with and without dementia showed a significant gray matter loss in the hippocampus. This gray matter decrement was accompanied by decreased scores on verbal learning that were statistically significant in demented patients and which showed a trend toward significance in non-demented subjects ($p<0.052$) (Ramirez-Ruiz et al., 2005).

In addition to whole brain analyses VBM also enables researchers to focus automatically on regions of interest by means of the FW Pickatlas tool (Maldjian et al., 2003). This procedure can detect more accurately the gray matter regions that show volume loss within the hippocampus. Using the ROI approach we found that non-demented PD patients with and without visual hallucinations have hippocampal reductions involving the hippocampal head, while demented patients showed reductions in both anterior and posterior hippocampal regions with a relatively spared body (Ibarretxe et al., 2008).

Another interesting application of VBM is individual analysis (see fig 4). Analyzing the MRI significance of single patients with suspected degenerative illness is of enormous clinical interest and is usually done by visual inspection. However, subtle reductions in regions such as the basal ganglia or hippocampus are very difficult to detect by neuroradiological visual inspection. A study by Shiino et al. (2006) showed that by clustering the profiles from individual analysis, several profiles of gray matter loss in AD can be observed. For example, one of the subgroups of subjects showed neocortical reductions without hippocampal changes. As regards subcortical dementias, Muhlau et al. (2009) suggested that statistical parametric maps of GM decreases at the single-subject level in early HD have clinical utility for diagnosis. For example, when comparing the GM density of the caudate nucleus of 19 subjects in the initial stages of HD, 18 of them showed statistically significant changes. Using this method we compared each patient with a control group of 56 subjects and observed significant individual hippocampal reductions in 7 out of 9 (78%) PDD patients, 5 of 16 (31%) PD+VH patients and 5 of 19 (26%) PD-VH patients. All these rates of hippocampal atrophy were statistically significant (Ibarretxe-Bilbao et al., 2008). Although all three groups of PD showed reduction in the hippocampal head the size of the clusters followed the pattern PDD>PD+VH>PD-VH.

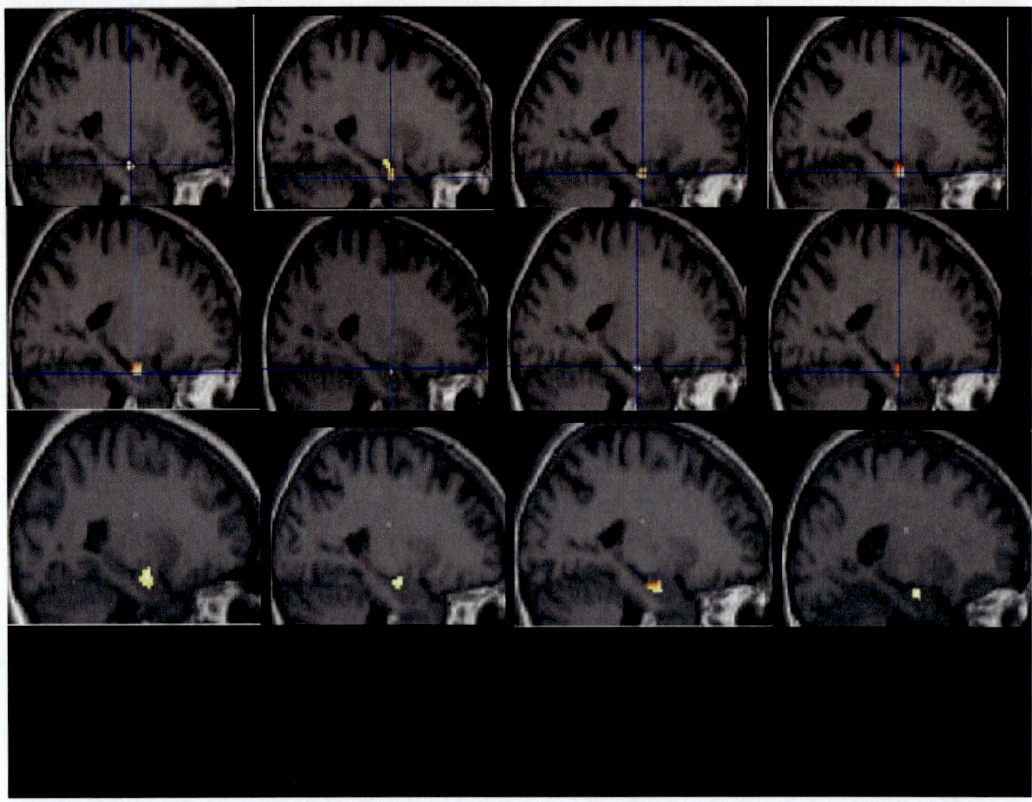

Figure 4. Individual analyses of hippocampal gray matter reduction. Each saggital cut corresponds to a patient compared with the mean of the control group. All the subjects have the gray matter concentration decrease in the anterior region (hippocampal head).

Correlations Between Memory Deficits and Hippocampal Reductions

Riekkinen et al. (1998) selected two tests of hippocampal dysfunction that have been shown to be sensitive to medial temporal lobe structures (delayed matching to sample test and a verbal learning test) and classified the subjects as impaired (one standard deviation below the mean) and non-impaired. They showed that impaired patients had greater hippocampal volume reductions than did patients with normal memory performance. Moreover, there was a trend toward a correlation between hippocampal atrophy and impaired memory performance, but not with frontal lobe performance. In contrast, frontal lobe functions correlated with motor functions but memory did not. Similarly, and using a visual rating scale of MRI atrophy on coronal slices, Brück et al. (2004) found bilateral atrophy of the hippocampus that correlated with verbal memory functions. In this study the correlation seems to be selective since sustained attention was found to be related to prefrontal but not to hippocampal atrophy. A similar procedure was recently used by Jokinen et al. (2009), who also found a correlation between the degree of hippocampal atrophy and declarative memory.

However, not all the published studies have shown selectivity in the correlation analysis. For example, it has been suggested that hippocampal atrophy reflects a general cognitive decline. In this regard, some authors have reported that hippocampal volume correlates with the global score of the Mini Mental State Examination (MMSE) (Camicioli et al., 2003), although others have not found such correlations (Bouchard et al., 2007). As regards particular cognitive domains the correlations between memory loss and hippocampal atrophy are not always specific. For example, some authors have reported similar correlations with memory for both the hippocampus and the amygdala (Junque et al., 2005; Bouchard et al., 2008). This makes sense because both cerebral structures form part of the limbic system and degenerate at a similar stage of the disease. It should also be noted that the results from correlation analyses do not refer to causal relationships. Moreover, in addition to medial temporal lobe reductions, neocortical atrophy can also contribute to a decrease in declarative memory. For example, Camicioli et al. (2009) found that poor memory was associated with GM atrophy in both the left (uncus, middle temporal and fusiform gyri) and right temporal lobes. These structural findings agree with PET studies. Huang et al. (2007) described a cognitive profile in PD that consisted of marked metabolic reductions in bilateral parietal areas, as well as in bilateral premotor areas and a small cluster in the left lateral prefrontal region. This hypometabolism appears to coexist with increased cerebellar metabolism. Furthermore, the pattern of hypo- and hyper-metabolism correlated with declarative memory dysfunctions as assessed by the CAVLT.

Recognition memory is a function that clearly depends on medial temporal lobe integrity (Squire Wixted and Clark, 2007) and it is known to be impaired in Alzheimer's disease. Camicioli et al. (2003) reported that recognition memory correlated with left but not right hippocampal atrophy, whereas recall did not correlate with any hippocampal measure. In this study, recognition memory was evaluated by CERAD word list recall. In contrast, Bouchard et al. (2008), using the California Verbal Learning Test, did observe a correlation between the hippocampus and recall, although recognition scores did not reach statistical significance. Moreover, left hippocampus also correlated with visual memory as assessed by the brief visuospatial memory test. The discrepancies between these studies may be due to task difficulty (ceiling effect on recognition tasks) and clinical characteristics of the samples (years at testing, years of illness evolution, and illness severity).

Hippocampal subdivisions have been related to encoding and retrieval processes (Schacter and Wagner, 1999). Using an ROI analysis of the hippocampus we found (Ibarretxe-Bilbao et al., 2008) that verbal learning correlated with the hippocampal head. This correlation was seen for the whole sample of PD patients, and also for a sub-sample of patients with visual hallucinations. The same relationship was observed in group comparison analyses. Patients with hippocampal reduction observed in the individual analyses performed significantly worse on verbal learning tasks than did patients without hippocampal gray matter reductions. The correlations between hippocampal head and memory were also observed by another research group who looked at delayed recall (Bouchard et al., 2008), and this phenomenon has also been described as a pattern for normal ageing (Hackert et al.,

2002). Thus, there are convergent results as regards the relevance of the hippocampus to gray matter loss when explaining memory impairment.

Working Memory Deficits in PD

Working memory has been described as a brain system that provides temporary storage and manipulation of the information necessary for complex tasks such as language comprehension, learning and reasoning (Baddeley, 1992). Owen et al. (1997) observed that working memory deficits in PD depend on medication, progression and severity of the illness. They designed a task in which patients were required to remember sequences of color-changing boxes on a computer screen. The impaired subjects were those taking medication and who had severe clinical symptoms. A recent review and meta-analysis (Siegert et al., 2008) concluded that there was a clear impairment in working memory in PD, this being small for verbal span but moderate on simple and complex visuospatial tasks, as well as on complex verbal tasks. Future research would need to rule out the role of a primary impairment in visuospatial processing, which could preclude normal functioning on working memory tasks.

Working memory deficits seem to have a clear dopaminergic basis (Nieoullon 2002; Cools, 2006). For example, a recent PET study demonstrated that when training working memory in normal subjects the improvement in memory capacity is associated with changes in the density of cortical dopamine D1 receptors. Fourteen hours of training over 5 weeks was associated with changes in both prefrontal and parietal D1 binding potential (McNab et al., 2009). Although L-dopa does ameliorate the working memory deficit shown by PD patients in terms of manipulating information (shown by both accuracy and reaction time measures) it has no effect on the attentional set-shifting impairment (Lewis et al., 2005). However, it is worth considering whether DA medications might lead to enhancements or impairments of working memory tasks depending on the phase of the tests and the cognitive demands of the task (distracters, shifting or learning) (Moustafa, Sherman and Frank, 2008).

Another stimulant treatment, anodal transcranial direct current stimulation, also improves working memory, although this depends on the intensity and site of stimulation. Specifically, a 2 mA of stimulation in the left dorsolateral prefrontal cortex leads to improvement on a 3-back task (Boggio et al., 2006).

Functional neuroimaging of PD is potentially a very powerful tool to understand the neural substrates of WM deficits in PD. Early fMRI studies showed that WM deficits in PD are accompanied by reduced activity in frontostriatal neural circuitry (Lewis et al., 2003). However, more recent evidence from fMRI studies indicates that WM deficits in PD seem to the related to metabolic changes in basal ganglia, but not to changes in prefrontal cortex (Marklund et al., 2008). Similarly, PET studies have shown an attenuated dopamine release in the dorsal caudate in PD, but preserved levels of medial prefrontal release. Thus, working memory deficits in early PD patients are associated with impaired nigrostriatal dopaminergic function resulting in abnormal processing in the cortico-basal ganglia circuit. In contrast, mesocortical dopaminergic transmission appears to be well preserved in early PD patients (Sawanoto et al., 2008).

Procedural Learning in PD

Procedural learning is a form of non-declarative or implicit memory that refers to the ability to acquire motor or cognitive skills gradually through practice (Cohen and Squire, 1980). Acquisition of such skills is manifested by increased accuracy or speed of performance as a result of repeated exposure to a specific procedure. A characteristic of this learning is the lack of conscious recollection of the rules underlying the tasks. The neuroanatomical substrates underlying procedural learning are not fully understood, although it has been hypothesized that it depends on the striatum (Squire and Zola, 1996). Clinically, procedural learning is assessed by successive repetitions of the Tower of Hanoi, the mirror maze, or the pursuit rotor task (Lezak et al., 2004). In research on motor skill learning the most frequently employed experimental paradigm has been the serial reaction time task (SRTT). The SRTT is a choice reaction-time task in which subjects are required to respond as quickly as possible to the presentation of a visual stimulus appearing at one of several different spatial locations. The location of the stimulus follows a repeating sequence. Although patients do not know that the sequence is repeated they improve their performance for the repeated sequences compared to new ones. Neuroimaging studies have shown that these tasks activate fronto-striatal circuitry (Rauch and Savage, 1997). In PD some studies have found important deficits in procedural learning, while others report no significant differences (Osman et al., 2008). A review and meta-analysis of six studies carried out by Siegert et al. (2006) concluded that PD patients show a clear impairment in implicit memory as assessed by the SRTT. However, research to date has used very small samples and there is a substantial lack of clinical information.

Recently, Muslimovic et al. (2007) carried out an SRTT study with a sample of 95 non-demented PD patients and 44 matched controls. The groups did not differ in their learning rate across blocks of repeating sequence trials. However, PD patients were less efficient than controls in acquiring sequence-specific knowledge, although this impairment had a relatively small effect size (d=0.38). Separating the groups according to severity, the authors found that early non-medicated patients did not differ from controls. These findings indicate that although procedural learning impairment is not an early feature of PD it is likely to emerge with progression of the disease. In treated patients, performance did not correlate with levodopa dosage. Interestingly, in this study SRTT performance did not correlate with measures of declarative memory. These data confirm the dissociation between the two memory systems, although they do not provide conclusive evidence of the relationship between procedural impairment and dopaminergic deficits.

In a PET study designed to determine the neural substrates of procedural learning in PD, Beauchamp et al. (2008) showed that while cognitive skill learning is normally acquired thought frontostriatal circuitry in healthy individuals, patients with PD have increased activity in the hippocampus and dorsolateral prefrontal cortex. This indicates that PD patients are using the circuitry of declarative memory to acquire procedural learning. Thus, there is a compensatory mechanism.

Conclusions

Declarative memory deficits in PD do not follow the pattern described in subcortical dementia. Patients have impaired recall and recognition, and the use of cues raises performance to levels similar to those of controls. Neuropathological and structural magnetic resonance imaging studies reveal degeneration in the hippocampus even in the early stages of the disease; this is seen in demented as well as non-demented and non-treated patients. The hippocampal atrophy is seen mainly in the anterior part and progresses to the whole hippocampus in demented patients. Declarative memory deficits correlate with hippocampal reduction. In contrast, working memory deficits seem to depend on the fronto-striatal dysfunctions and are more sensitive to the effects of levodopa. Finally, procedural memory impairment is not seen in the early stages of the disease and the neural substrate of its impairment is unknown.

References

Aarsland, D, Andersen, K,, Larsen, J,P,, Lolk, A,, Kragh-Sørensen, P. Prevalence and characteristics of dementia in Parkinson disease: an 8-year prospective study. *Arch Neurol.* 60: 387-392, 2003.

Aarsland, D., Andersen. K., Larsen. J.P., Perry, R., Wentzel-Larsen, T., Lolk, A., Kragh-Sørensen, P. The rate of cognitive decline in Parkinson disease. *Arch Neurol.* 61:1906-1911, 2004.

Aarsland, D., Zaccai, J., Brayne, C. A systematic review of prevalence studies of dementia in Parkinon's disease. *Mov Disord.* 20:1255-1263, 2005.

Aarsland, D., Brønnick, K., Larsen, J.P., Tysnes, O.B., Alves, G., For the NorwegianParkWest Study Group. Cognitive impairment in incident, untreated Parkinson disease: The Norwegian Park West Study. *Neurology.* 72:1121-1126, 20092008. (On line)

Alegret, M., Junque, C., Valldeoriola, F., Vendrell, P., Pilleri, M., Ruma, J., Tolosa, E. Effects of bilateral subthalamic stimulation on cognitive function in Parkinson's disease. *Arch Neurol.* 58:1223-1227, 2001.

Alegret, M., Valldeoriola, F., Tolosa, E., Vendrell, P., Junque, C., Martínez, J., Rumia, J. Cognitive effects of unilateral posteroventral pallidotomy: a 4-year follow-up study. *Mov Disord.*18:323-328, 2003.

Alegret, M., Valldeoriola, F., Martí, M., Pilleri, M., Junque, C., Rumia, J., Tolosa, E. Comparative cognitive effects of bilateral subthalamic stimulation and subcutaneous continuous infusion of apomorphine in Parkinson's disease. *Mov Disord.*19:1463-1469, 2004.

Alexander, G.E., DeLong, M.R., Strick ,P.L. Parallel organization of functionally segregated circuits linking basal ganglia and cortex. *Annu Rev Neurosci.*9:357-368,1986.

Apostolova ,L.G., Dinov,I.D., Dutton ,R.A., Hayashi, K.M., Toga, A.W., Cummings, J.L., Thompson PM. 3D comparison of hippocampal atrophy in amnestic mild cognitive impairment and Alzheimer's disease. *Brain.*129:2867-2873, 2006a.

Apostolova, L.G., Dutt, R.A., Dinov, I.D., Hayashi, K.M, Toga, A,W,, Cummings, J.L., Thompson, P.M. Conversion of mild cognitive impairment to Alzheimer disease predicted by hippocampal atrophy maps. *Arch Neurol* .3:693-694, 2006b.

Apostolova ,L.G., Stein,er C.A., Akopya, G.G., Dutton,R.A., Hayashi. K.M., Toga. A.W, Cummings, J.L, Thompson, P.M. Three-dimensional gray matter atrophy mapping in mild cognitive impairment and mild Alzheimer disease. *Arch Neurol*.64:1489-1495, 2007.

Baddeley, A.D. Working memory. *Science*, 255: 556-559, 1992.

Beauchamp, M.H., Dagher, A., Panisset, M., Doyon, J. Neural substrates of cognitive skill learning in Parkinson's disease; *Brain Cog*. 68:134-143, 2008.

Beatty, W.W., Ryder, K.A., Gontkovsky, S.T., Scott, J.G., McSwan, K.L, Bharucha, K.J.

Analyzing the subcortical dementia syndrome of Parkinson's disease using the RBANS. *Arch Clin Neuropsychol*.18:509-250, 2003.

Beyer, M,K, Larsen, J.P., Aarsland, D.. Gray matter atrophy in Parkinson disease with dementia and dementia with Lewy bodies. *Neurology*.9:747-754. 2007a.

Beyer, M.K., Janvin, C.C., Larsen, J.P., Aarsland, D. A magnetic resonance imaging study of patients with Parkinson's disease with mild cognitive impairment and dementia using voxel-based morphometry. *J Neurol Neurosurg Psychiatry*.78:254-259,2007b.

Beyer, M,K,, Aarsland. Grey matter atrophy in early versus late dementia in Parkinson's disease. *Parkinsonism Relat Disord*.14:620-625, 2008.

Bonelli, R.M., Cummings, J.L. Frontal-subcortical dementias. *Neurologist*.14:100-107, 2008.

Boggio, P.S., Ferrucci, R., Rigonatt, S.P., Covre, P., Nitsche, M., Pascual-Leone, A., Fregni, F. Effects of transcranial direct current stimulation on working memory in patients with Parkinson's disease. *J Neurol Sciences*. 249:31-38, 2006.

Bouchard, T.P., Malykhin, N., Martin, W.R., Hanstock CC, Emery DJ, Fisher NJ,

Camicioli RM. Age and dementia-associated atrophy predominates in the hippocampal head and amygdala in Parkinson's disease. *Neurobiol Agin*.29:1027-1039, 2008.

Braak, H., Braak ,E. Pathoanatomy of Parkinson's disease. *J Neurol*.247 Suppl 2:II3-10, 2000.

Braak. H,, Del Tredic, K., Bratzke., Hamm-Clemen, J., Sandmann-Keil, D., Rüb, U. Staging of the intracerebral inclusion body pathology associated with idiopathic Parkinson's disease (preclinical and clinical stages). *J Neurol*. 249 Suppl 3:III/1-5, 2002.

Braak, H., Del Tredici, K,, Rüb, U,, de V, R.A., Jansen Steur, E.N., Braak, E. Staging of brain pathology related to sporadic Parkinson's disease. *Neurobiol Aging*.24:197-211, 2003.

Braak, H, Ghebremedhin. E., Rüb, U., Bratzke, H., Del Tredici, K.. Stages in the development of Parkinson's disease-related pathology. *Cell Tissue Res*.318:121-134, 2004.

Braak, H., Rüb, U., Jansen Steur, E.N., Del Tredici, K., de Vos, R.A. Cognitive status correlates with neuropathologic stage in Parkinson disease. *Neurology*. 64:1404-1410, 2005.

Braak, H., Rüb, U., Del Tredici, K. Cognitive decline correlates with neuropathological stage in Parkinson's disease. *J Neurol Sci*. 248:255-258, 2006.

Brenneis, C., Egger, K., Scherfler, C., Seppi, K., Schocke, M., Poewe, W., Wenning, G.K. Progression of brain atrophy in multiple system atrophy. A longitudinal VBM study. *J Neurol.* 254:191-196, 2007.

Brown,, Marsden, C,D. 'Subcortical dementia': the neuropsychological evidence. *Neuroscience.*25:363-387, 1988.

Brown, R.G., Marsden, C.D. Cognitive function in Parkinson's disease: from description to theory. *TINS.* 13: 21-29,1990.

Brück, A., Kurki, T., Kaasinen, V., Vahlberg, T., Rinne, J.O. Hippocampal and prefrontal atrophy in patients with early non-dementedParkinson's disease is related to cognitive impairment. *J Neurol Neurosurg Psychiatry.* 75:1467-1469, 2004.

Burton, E.J, McKeith, I.G., Burn, D.J., Williams, E.D., O'Brien, J.T. Cerebral atrophy in Parkinson's disease with and without dementia: a comparison with Alzheimer's disease, dementia with Lewy bodies and controls. *Brain.*127:791-800,2004.

Caballol, N., Martí, M.J., Tolosa, E. Cognitive dysfunction and dementia in Parkinson disease. *Mov Disord.* 22 17:358-66, 2007.

Calabresi, C., Picconi, B., Parnetti, .L, Di Filippo, M. A convergent model for cognitive dysfunctions in Parkinson's disease: the critical dopamine-acetylcholine synaptic balance. *Lancet Neurol.* 5:974-983, 2006.

Camicioli, R,, Moore, M.M., Kinney, A., Corbridge, E., Glassberg, K., Kaye. J.A. Parkinson's disease is associated with hippocampal athophy. *Mov Disord.* 18:784-790, 2003.

Camicioli, R., Gee, M., Bouchard, T.P., Fisher, N.J., Hanstock, C.C., Emery, D.J., Martin, W.R. Voxel-based morphometry reveals extra-nigral atrophy patterns associated withdopamine refractory cognitive and motor impairment in parkinsonism. *Parkinsonism Relat Disord.* 15:187-195,2009 Jun 21. [Epub ahead of print]

Caviness, J.N., Driver-Dunckley, E., Connor, D.J., Sabbagh, M.N., Hentz, J.G., Noble, B., Evidente, V.G., Shill, H.A., Adler, C.H. Defining mild cognitive impairment in Parkinson's disease. *Mov Disord.*22:1272-1277, 2007.

Churchyard, A., Lees, A.J. The relationship between dementia and direct involvement of the hippocampus and amygdala in Parkinson's disease. *Neurology.* 49:1570-576, 1997.

Cohen NJ, Squire LR. Preserved learning and retention of pattern-analyzing skill in amnesia: dissociation of knowing how and knowing that. *Science.* 10:207-210, 1980

Cools, R. Dopaminergic modulation of cognitive function-implications for l-DOPA treatment in Parkinson's disease. *Neuroscience and Biobehavioral Reviews.* 30:1-23, 2006.

Cooper, H., Sagar, H.J., Doherty, S.M., Jordan, N., Tidswell, P., Sullivan, E.V. Different effects of dopaminergic and anticholinergic therapies on cognitive and motor function in Parkinson's disease. *Brain.* 115:1701-1725, 1992.

Cummings, J.L., Benson, D.F. Subcortical dementia. Review of an emerging concept. *Arch Neurol.*41:874-879, 1984.

Churchyard, A., Lees, A.J. The relationship between dementia and direct involvement of the hippocampus and amygdala in Parkinson's disease. *Neurology.*49:1570-1576, 1997.

D'Esposito,M. From cognitive to neural models of working memory. *Philos Trans R Soc Lond B Biol Sci.* 362:761-772, 2007.

Dubois, B., Pillon, B. Cognitive deficits in Parkinson's disease. *J Neurol.* 244:2-8, 1997.

Dubois, B., Burn, D., Goetz, C., Aarsland, D., Brown, R.G., Broe, G.A., Dickson, D., Duyckaerts, C., Cummings, J., Gauthier, S., Korczyn, A., Lees, A., Levy, R., Litvan, I., Mizuno,Y., McKeith, I.G., Olanow, C.W., Poewe, W., Sampaio, C., Tolosa E., Emre, M. Diagnostic procedures for Parkinson's disease dementia: recommendations from the movement disorder society task force. *Mov Disord.* 22:2314-2324, 2007.

Emre, M.What causes mental dysfunction in Parkinson's disease? *Mov Disord* .18 Suppl 6:S63-71, 2003.

Feldmann, A., Illes, Z., Kosztolanyi, P., Illes, E., Mike, A., Kover, F., Balas, I., Kovacs, N., Nagy, F. Morphometric changes of gray matter in Parkinson's disease with depression: a voxel-based morphometry study. *Mov Disord.* 23:42-46, 2008.

Frank, M.J., Samanta, J., Moustafa , A.A., Sherman, S.J. Hold your horses: impulsivity, deep brain stimulation, and medication in parkinsonism. *Science.* 318:1309-1312, 2007.

Grossi, D., Trojano, L., Pellecchia, M.T., Amboni, M., Fragassi, N.A., Barone, P. Frontal dysfunction contributes to the genesis of hallucinations in non-demented Parkinsonian patients. *Int J Geriatr Psychiatry.* 20:668–673, 2005.

Ibarretxe-Bilbao, N,, Ramirez-Ruiz, B., Tolosa, E., Marti, M.J., Valldeoriola, F., Bargallo, N., Junque, C. Hippocampal head atrophy predominance in Parkinson's disease with hallucinations and with dementia. *J Neurol.* 255:1324-1331, 2008.

Hackert, V.H., den Heijer, T., Oudkerk, M., Koudstaal, P.J,, Hofman, A., Breteler, M.M.

Hippocampal head size associated with verbal memory performance in nondemented elderly. *Neuroimage.*17:1365-1372, 2002.

Halliday, G., Hely, M., Reid, W., Morris, J.. The progression of pathology in longitudinally followed patients with Parkinson's disease. *Acta Neuropathologica* . 115. 409-420, 2008.

Hely, M.A., Reid, W.G.J., Adena, M.A, Halliday, G.M., Morris, J.G.L. The Sydney multicenter study of Parkinson's disease: The inevitability of dementia at 20 years. *Mov Disord.* 6:837-844, 2008.

Higginson, C.I., Wheelock, V.L., Carroll, K.E., Sigvardt, K.A. Recognition memory in Parkinson's disease with and without dementia: evidence inconsistent with the retrieval deficit hypothesis. *J Clin Exp Neuropsychol.* 27:516-528, 2005.

Higginson, C.I,. Wheelock, V,L,, Levine, D., King, D.S., Pappas, C.T., Sigvardt, K.A. The clinical significance of neuropsychological changes following bilateral subthalamic nucleus deep brain stimulation for Parkinson's disease. *J Clin Exp Neuropsychol* . 31:65-72, 2009.

Hillary, F.G.. Neuroimaging of working memory dysfunction and the dilemma with brain reorganization hypotheses. *J Int Neuropsychol Soc.*14:526-534, 2008.

Honea, R., Crow, T.J., Passingham, D., Mackay, C.E. Regional deficits in brain volume in schizophrenia: a meta-analysis of voxel-based morphometry studies. *Am J Psychiatry.*162:2233-2245, 2005.

Huang C, Tang C, Feigin A, Lesser M, Ma Y, Pourfar M, Dhawan V, Eidelberg D. Changes in network activity with the progression of Parkinson's disease. *Brain.* 130:1834-1846, 2007

Janvin, C.C., Larsen, J.P., Aarsland, D., Hugdahl, K.. Subtypes of mild cognitive impairment in Parkinson's disease: progression to dementia. *Mov Disord.* 21:1343-1349, 2006.

Joelving, F,C, Billeskov, R., Christensen, J.R., West, M., Pakkenberg, B. Hippocampal neuron and glial cell numbers in Parkinson's disease. A stereological study. *Hippocampus*. 16:826-833, 2006.

Jokinen P, Brück A, Aalto S, Forsback S, Parkkola R, Rinne JO. Impaired cognitive performance in Parkinson's disease is related to caudate dopaminergic hypofunction and hippocampal atrophy. *Parkinsonism Relat Disord*. 15:88-93, 2009

Junque, C., Alegret. M., Nobbe, F.A., Valldeoriola, F., Pueyo, R., Vendrell, P., Tolosa, E., Rumia, J., Mercader, J.M. Cognitive and behavioral changes after unilateral, posteroventral pallidotomy: relationship with lesional data from MRI. *Mov Disord*. 14:780-789, 1999.

Junque, C., Ramirez-Ruiz, B., Tolosa, E., Summerfield, C., Marti, M.J, Pastor, P., Gomez-Anson, B., Mercader, J.M. Amygdalar and hippocampal MRI volumetric reductions in Parkinson's disease wit dementia. *Mov Disord*. 20:540-544, 2005.

Kulisevsky, J., Garcia-Sánchez, C., Berthier, M.L., Barbanoj, M., Pascual-Sedano, B., Gironell, A., Estévez-González, A. Chronic effects of dopaminergic replacement on cognitive function in Parkinson's disease: a two-year follow-up study of previously untreated patients. *Mov Disord*. 15:613-626, 2000.

Laakso, M.P., Partanen, K., Riekkinen, P., Lehtovirta, M., Helkala, E.L., Hallikainen, M., Hanninen, T., Vainio, P., Soininen, H. Hippocampal volumes in Alzheimer's disease, Parkinson's disease with and without dementia, and in vascular dementia: An MRI study. *Neurology*. 46:678-68, 1996.

Levy, G., Jacobs. D.M., Tang, M.X., Côté, .LJ., Louis, E.D., Alfaro, B., Mejia, H., Stern, Y., Marder, K. Memory and executive function impairment predict dementia in Parkinson's disease. *Mov Disord*. 17:1221-1226, 2002.

Lewis, S,J,, Dove, A,, Robbins, T,W., Barker, R.A., Owen, A.M. Cognitive impairments in early Parkinson's disease are accompanied by reductions in activity in frontostriatal neural circuitry. *J Neurosc*. 23: 6351-635, 2003.

Lewis, S.J.G., Slabosz, A., Robbins,T.W., Barker, R.A., Owen, A,M. Dopaminergic basis for deficits in working memory but not attentional set-shifting in Parkinson's disease. *Neuropsychologia*. 43: 823-832, 2005.

Lezak, M.D., Howieson, D.B., Loring, D.W. *Neuropsychological Assessment*. 4th Edition. Oxford: Oxford University Press, 2004.

Maldjian, J.A, Laurienti, P.J, Kraft, R.A, Burdette, J.H. An automated method for neuroanatomic and cytoarchitectonic atlas-based interrogation of fMRI data sets. *Neuroimage*. 19:1233-1239, 2003.

Marklund, P., Laarson, A., Elh, E., Linder, J., Riklund, K.A., Forsgren. L., Nyberg. L. Temporal dynamics of basal ganglia under-recruitment in Parkinson's disease: transient caudate abnormalities during updating of working memory. *Brain*. 132:236-246,2009. 2008; (on line)

Mechelli, A., Price, C.J., Friston, K.J., Ashburner, J.. T1 Voxel-based morphometry of the human brain: methods and applications. *Curr Med Imagin Rev*. 1:105-113, 2005.

McNab, F., Varrone, A., Farde, L., Jucaite, A., Bystritsky, P., Forssberg, H., Klingberg, T. Changes in cortical dopamine D1 receptor binding associated with cognitive training *Science*. 323:800-802, 2009.

Mühlau, M., Wohlschläger, A.M., Gaser, C., Valet, M., Weindl, A., Nunnemann, S., Peinemann, A., Etgen, T., Ilg ,R. Voxel-Based Morphometry in individual patients: A pilot study in early Huntington Disease. *AJNR Am J Neuroradiol.* 2008. Dec 12. [Epub ahead of print) 30:539-543,2009

Muslimovic, D., Post, B., Speelman, J.D., Schmand, B. Cognitive profile of patients with newly diagnosed Parkinson disease. *Neurology*. 65:1239-1245, 2005.

Muslimovic, D., Schmand. B., Speelman. J.D., de Haan , R.J. Course of cognitive decline in Parkinson's disease: a meta-analysis. *J Int Neuropsychol So*c. 13:920-932, 2007a.

Muslimovic, D., Post, B., Speelman, J.D., Schmand, B. Motor procedural learning in Parkinson's disease. *Brain.*130:2887-2897, 2007b.

Mustafa, A,A, Sherman, S.J., Frank, M.J. A dopaminergic basis of working memory, learning and attentional shifting in parkinsonism. *Neuropsychologia*. 46; 3144-3156, 2008.

Nagano-Saito, A., Washimi, Y., Arahata ,Y., Kachi, T., Lerch, J.P., Evans, A.C., Dagher, A., Ito, K. Cerebral atrophy and its relation to cognitive impairment in Parkinson disease. *Neurology*. 64:224-229, 2005.

Nieoullon, A. Dopamine and the regulation of cognition and attention. *Prog Neurobiol.*67:53-83, 2002.

Osman, M., Wilkinson, L., Beigi, M., Castaneda, C.S., Jahanshahi, M. Patients with Parkinson's disease learn to control complex systems via procedural as well as non-procedural learning. *Neuropsychologia*. 46:2355-2363, 2008.

Owen, A.M. Cognitive dysfunction in Parkinson's disease: the role of frontostriatal circuitry. *Neuroscientist*. 10:525-537, 2004.

Owen, A.M., Iddon, J.L., Hodges, J.R., Summers, B.A., Robbins, T.W. Spatial and non-spatial working memory at different states of Parkinson's disease. *Neuropsychologia.* 35: 519-532, 1997.

Ozer, F., Meral, H., Hanoglu, L., Ozturk, O., Aydemir, T., Cetin, S., Atmaca, B., Tiras, R. Cognitive impairment patterns in Parkinson's disease with visual hallucinations. *J Clin Neurosci*. 14:742-746, 2007.

Petersen, R.C., Doody, R., Kurz, A., Mohs, R.C., Morris, J.C., Rabins, P.V., Ritchie, K., Rossor, M., Thal, L., Winblad, B. Current concepts in mild cognitive impairment. *Arch Neurol* . 58:1985-1992, 2001.

Pillon, B., Ardouin, C., Damier. P., Krack, P., Houeto, J.L., Klinger ,H., Bonnet, A.M., Pollak, P,. Benabid, A.L., Agid, Y. Neuropsychological changes between "off" and "on" STN or GPi stimulation in Parkinson's disease. *Neurology.* 55:411-418, 2000.

Poliakoff, E., Smith-Spark, J.H. Everyday cognitive failures and memory problems in Parkinson's patients without dementia. *Brain Cogn.* 67:340-35, 2008.

Price, S., Paviour, D., Scahill, R., Stevens, J., Rossor, M., Lees, A., Fox, N. Voxel-based morphometry detects patterns of atrophy that help differentiate progressive supranuclear palsy and Parkinson's disease. *Neuroimage*. 23: 63-669, 2004.

Ramirez-Ruiz, B., Marti, M.J., Tolosa, E., Bartres-Faz, D., Summerfield, C., Salgado-Pineda, P., Gomez-Anson, B., Junque, C. Longitudinal evaluation of cerebral morphological changes in Parkinson's disease with and without dementia. *J Neurol.* 252:1345-1352, 2005.

Ramirez-Ruiz, B, Junque, C., Marti, M.J., Vallderiola. F., Tolosa, E. Neuropsychological deficits in Parkinson's disease patients with visual hallucinations. *Mov Disord*. 21:1483-1487, 2006.

Ramirez-Ruiz, B., Martí, M.J., Tolosa, E., Gimenez, M., Bargallo, N., Valldeoriola, F., Junque, C. Cerebral atrophy in Parkinson's disease patients with visual hallucinations *Eur J Neurol.* 14: 750-756, 2007a.

Ramirez-Ruiz, B., Junque, C., Marti, M.J, Valldeoriola, F., Tolosa, E. Cognitive changes in Parkinson's disease patients with visual hallucinations. *Dement Geriatr Cogn Disord.* 23:281-288, 2007b.

Rauch SL, Savage CR. Neuroimaging and neuropsychology of the striatum. Bridging basic science and clinical practice. *Psychiatr Clin North Am*;20:741-768. 1997

Riekkinen, P., Kejonen, K., Laakso, M.P., Soininen, K., Partanen, K., Riekkinen, M. Hippocampal atrophy is related to impaired memory, but not frontal functions in non-demented Parkinson's disease patients. *Neuroreport*. 9:1507-1511,1998.

Sawamoto, N., Piccini, P., Hotton, G., Pavese, N., Thielemans, K., Brooks, D.J. Cognitive deficits and striato-frontal dopamine release in Parkinson's disease. *Brain*. 131:1294-302, 2008.

Schacter, D.L., Wagner,.A.D. Medial temporal lobe activations in fMRI and PET studies of episodic encoding and retrieval. *Hippocampus*.9:7-24, 1999.

Schott, B.H., Niehaus,L, Wittmann, B., Schütze, H., Seidenbecher, C.I, Heinze, H.J., Düze,l E. sAgeing and early-stage Parkinson's disease affect separable neural mechanism of mesolimbic reward processing. *Brain*. 130: 2412-2424, 2007.

Shiino, A., Watanabe, T., Maeda, K., Kotani, E., Akiguchi, I., Matsuda, M.. Four subgroups of Alzheimer's disease based on patterns of atrophy using VBM and a unique pattern for early onset disease. *Neuroimage*. 33:17-26, 2006.

Siegert R.J., Weatherall, M., Taylor. K.D., Abernethy, D.A. A meta-analysis of performance on simple span and more complex working memory tasks in Parkinson's disease. *Neuropsychology*. 22:450-461, 2008.

Siegert, R.J,. Taylor, K.D., Weatherall, M., Abernethy, D.A. Is implicit sequence learning impaired in Parkinson's disease? A meta-analysis. *Neuropsychology*. 20:490-495, 2006.

Squire, L.R., Zola, S.M.. Structure and function of declarative and nondeclarative memory systems. *Proc Natl Acad Sci U S A*. 93:13515-13522, 1996.

Squire, L.R., Wixted, J..T, Clark, R.E. Recognition memory and the medial temporal lobe: a new perspective. *Nat Rev Neurosci*. 8:872-883, 2007.

Summerfield, C., Junque, C., Tolosa, E., Salgado-Pineda, P., Gomez-Anson, B., Marti M.J., Pastor, P., Ramirez-Ruíz, B., Mercader. J. Structural brain changes in Parkinson disease with dementia: a voxel-based morphometry study. *Arch Neurol*. 62:281-285, 2005.

Taylor A.E., Saint-Cyr, J.A., Lang, A.E. Frontal lobe dysfunction in Parkinson's disease. The cortical focus of neostriatal outflow. *Brain*. 109:845-883, 1986.

Troster, A.L. Neuropsychological characteristics of dementia with Lewy bodies and Parkinson'sdisease with dementia: differentiation, early detection, and implications for"mild cognitive impairment" and biomarkers. *Neuropsychol Rev*.18:103-119, 2008.

Verbaan, D., Marinus, J., Visser ,M., van Rooden, S.M., Stiggelbout ,A.M., Middelkoop, H.A., van Hilten, J.J. Cognitive impairment in Parkinson's disease. *J Neurol Neurosurg Psychiatry*. 78:1182-1187, 2007.

Williams-Gray, C.H, Foltynie, T., Brayne, C.E.G., Robbins, T.W., Barker, R.A. Evolution of cognitive dysfunction in an incident Parkinson’s disease cohort. *Brain*. 130:1787-1798, 2007.

Whittington, C.J., Podd, J., Kan, M.M. Recognition memory impairment in Parkinson's disease: power and meta-analyses. *Neuropsychology*. 14:233-246, 2000.

Whittington, C.J., Podd, J., Stewart-Williams, S. Memory deficits in Parkinson's disease. *J Clin Exp Neuropsychol*. 28:738-754, 2006.

Whitwell, J,L,, Josephs, K.A. Voxel-based morphometry and its application to movement disorders. *Parkinsonism Relat Disord*.13 Suppl 3:S406-416, 2007.

In: Alzheimer's Disease and Dementia (Vol. 4)
Editor: Miao-Kun Sun
ISBN:978-1-60876-152-4

Chapter XI

Fronto-Temporal Dementia

Alfredo Postiglione,* ***Graziella Milan and Sabina Pappatà***

Dementia Study Center, Department of Clinical and Experimental Medicine, University of Naples "Federico II" and ASL Napoli 1, Naples, Italy

Abstract

Frontotemporal dementia includes several neurodegenerative diseases with predominant frontal and temporal lobes degeneration (FTLD), and, most commonly, presents with two classical forms. The first with changes in personal and social conduct, often associated with disinhibition, is the behavioural or frontal variant FTD (bv-FTLD), while the forms with predominant language impairment recognize two syndromes: primary progressive non-fluent aphasia (PNFA) and semantic dementia (SD). New pathological and genetic studies have given more insights on the great variability observed in FTLD patients . There are two major immunocytochemical subdivisions of FTLD: tauopathies with an accumulation of intraneuronal hyperphosphorylated Tau and pathologies with intraneuronal inclusions immunoreactive to ubiquitin (FTLD-U); the latter have been associated with the identification of TDP-43 as the major ubiquinated protein component of the inclusions. Two major genetic mutations are involved in the FTLD: tau mutations (MAPT) and, more recently, mutations in the progranulin gene (PGRN) on chromosome 17. Many studies found the presence of identifiable relationship between genetic mutations and clinical expression. There is evidence that MAPT and PGRN mutations could be present in various forms of bv-FTLD with characteristic clinical features, while the clinical expression of PNFA seems more linked to PRGN mutation carriers and that of SD to MAPT mutation carriers. Future research has to answer to many unresolved questions.

** Address for correspondence: Alfredo Postiglione, MD, Department of Clinical and Experimental Medicine, University of Naples "Federico II", Via S. Pansini 5, 80131 Naples, Italy, Tel.: +39 081 7463689, Fax: +39 081 5466152, e-mail: alfposti@unina.it

* Institute of Biostructures & Bioimaging, CNR, Naples, Italy

Keywords: Frontotemporal dementia – behaviour – genetic diseases - neuroimaging

Abbreviation List

AAA-ATPase ATPases associate with a variety of activities;
AD Alzheimer's disease;
aFTLD-U FTLD atypical FTLD with ubiquitinated inclusions,
AGD argyrophilic grain disease,
APO-E4 apolipoprotein E4;
APP amyloid precursor protein;
BIBD basophilic inclusions body disease;
bv-FTLD behavioural- fronto-temporal lobe degeneration;
CBD corticobasal degeneration,
CHMP2B charged multivescicular body protein 2B;
DLDH dementia lacking distinctive histopathology,
FBI frontal behavioral inventory;
^{18}*FDG-PET* Fluorodeoxyglucose- Positron emission tomography;
FTD-3 frontotemporal dementia linked to chromosome 3,
FTLD frontotemporal lobar degeneration,
FTLD-IF FTLD intermediate filament,
FTLD-MND Frontotemporal lobar degeneration with motor neuron disease;
FTLD-ni FTLD no inclusions,
FTLDP frontotemporal lobar degeneration with parkinsonism;
FTLDP-17 frontotemporal lobe dementia with Parkinson linked to chromosome 17,
FTLD-TDP FTLD nuclear TAR DNA binding protein,
FTLD-U FTLD with ubiquitinated inclusions,
FTLD-UPS FTLD ubiquitin proteosome system,
IBMPFD Inclusion body myopathy with Paget's disease of bone and frontotemporal dementia
IFT74 Intraflagellar transport protein;
LBD Lewy body dementia;
MAPT microtubule-associated protein tau;
MRI magnetic resonance imaging;
MSTD multiple system taupathy with dementia,
NIFID neuronal intermediate filament inclusions,
PET Positron emission tomography;
PGRN progranulin;
PiD Pick disease,
PNFA Primary progressive non fluent aphasia;
PS1 Presenilin 1;
PS2 Presenilin 2;
PSP progressive supranuclear palsy;
3R, 4R 3-4 repeats;

SD Semantic Dementia; *MND* Motor neuron disease;
SPECT Single-photon emission computerized tomography;
TDP-43 TDP-43 Transactivation response DNA binding protein of 43 kDa;
UPS Ubiquitin-proteasome system;
VCP valosin-containing protein;

Introduction

In the last ten years there has been an increased scientific interest on frontotemporal dementia due to its complexity and variability in the clinical presentation and to recent progress in molecular and genetic biology. It is evident that the term is not consistent, but includes several neurodegenerative diseases with predominant frontal and temporal lobes degeneration (FTLD), and, most commonly, presents with two classical forms. The first is characterized by changes in personal and social conduct, often associated with disinhibition, i.e., the behavioural or frontal variant FTD (bv-FTLD), while the forms with predominant language impairment recognizes two syndromes: primary progressive non-fluent aphasia (PNFA) and semantic dementia (SD). A proportion of patients will develop parkinsonism as part of their disease or will exhibit wide large clinical phenotypes, in some cases rare and difficult to diagnose, that could be also considered as variants of FTLD (Kipps et al., 2007).

Contributions from molecular genetic basis about hereditary FTLD (about 20%-50% of FTLD patients are associated with autosomal dominant inheritance) have enormously enlarged the complexity of the disease that is linked to several chromosomal loci including those in chromosome 17, chromosome 9 and chromosome 3. New insights in the neuropathology of FTLD have also stimulated new nosologic criteria based on tauopathies and on recent immunohistochemical, biochemical and genetic advances.

Epidemiology of FTLD was previously based on pathological studies, but, after the publication of the consensus diagnostic criteria from the Lund and Manchester group (Brun et al., 1994), many clinical studies have been published aiming to know the incidence, prevalence, age at onset, gender influence and risk factors. Currently, most clinicians and research investigations rely on Consensus Criteria by Neary et al., published in 1998 (table 1) (Neary et al., 1998). Clinical-based studies have the bias of exploring the disease in psychiatric hospitals or in Memory Clinics or in particular settings, where the memory disturbance is not predominant in the FTLD patient, at least at the beginning of the disease. One retrospective community-based study found an annual incidence rate of zero in the age group 40-64 years and 11/100.000 for the whole population (Andreasen et al., 1999). The Rochester Epidemiology Project calculated an annual incidence rates for FTLD of 2.2/100.000 in the age group 40-49, 3.3/100.000 for ages 50-59, and 8.9/100.000 for age 60-69 years (Knopman et al., 2004). Three prospective community-based studies in UK and Netherlands calculated a prevalence of 15.1, 15.4 and 6.7/100.000, respectively (Ratnavalli et al, 2002; Harvey et al., 2003; Rosso et al., 2003). Regarding age of onset, FTLD is commonly a pre-senile disorder (45-65 years) , although it appears that late-onset FTLD is commoner than expected (about 25% of cases or more). New molecular insights have provided new evidence on the age of onset of FTLD, as later reported. Also for gender, there is no evidence for a definite difference incidence between sexes. The prognosis of FTLD has a median survival of 6.0 years, but there is a great variability according to the clinical phenotype: patients with motor neuron disease (MND) have a median life expectancy of 2 years from symptoms onset, patients with tau-positive pathology of 9.0 years and tau-negative of 5.0 years (Graham et al., 2007).

Table 1. Clinical diagnostic features of FTD, PNFA and SD (Neary et al., 1998, modified)

FTD	PNFA	SD
CORE DIAGNOSTIC FEATURES		
Insidious onset an gradual progression Early decline in social interpersonal conduct Early impairment in regulation of personal conduct Early emotional blunting Early loss of insight	Insidious onset an gradual progression Non fluent spontaneous speech with at least one of the following: agrammatism, phonemic paraphasias, anomia	Insidious onset an gradual progression Progressive, fluent, empty spontaneous speech Loss of word meaning, manifest by impairment naming *and* comprehension Semantic paraphasias *and/or* Prosopoagnosia *and/or* associative agnosia Preserved perceptual matching and drawing reproduction Preserved single-word repetition Preserved ability to read aloud and write to dictation orthographically regular words
	SUPPORTIVE DIAGNOSTIC FEATURES	
Behavioral disorder Decline in personal hygiene and grooming Mental rigidity and inflexibility Distractibility and impersistence Hyperorality and dietary changes Perseverative and stereotyped behavior Utilization behavior	Early preservation of social skills Late behavioral changes similar to FTD	Loss of sympathy and empathy Narrowed preoccupations Parsimony
Speech and language Altered speech output (aspontaneity, economy and press of speech) Stereotypy of speech Echolalia Perseveration Mutism	Stuttering or oral apraxia Impaired repetition Alexia, agraphia Early preservation of word meaning Late mutism	Press of speech Idiosyncratic word usage Absence of phonemic paraphasias Surface dyslexia and dysgraphia Preserved calculation
Physical signs Primitive reflexes Incontinence Akinesia, rigidity and tremor Low and labile blood pressure	Late controlateral primitive reflexes, akinesia, rigidity and tremor	Absent or late primitive reflexes Akinesia, rigidity and tremor

FTD frontotemporal dementia, *PNFA* progressive nonfluent aphasia, *SD* semantic dementia.

However, it should be taken into account that it is almost impossible to accurately date the onset of symptoms, which may represent an exaggeration of pre-existent personality traits. Major risk factors are head trauma (3.3 fold increased risk) and thyroid disease (2.5 fold increase). It is evident that new epidemiological studies are needed, since it seems evident that the diagnosis of FTLD is generally underestimated. Moreover, new longitudinal studies must be conducted correlating genotypes and clinical variability. This necessity is due to the difficulty of diagnosis in large prospective studies, where behavioural changes could not be identified as pathological at their early onset, also for the influence of social and cultural environment. Another bias may be given by the large number of FTLD variants that frequently are reported in the literature making a correct diagnosis even more difficult.

Neuropathology and Genetics

New pathological and genetic studies have given even more insights on the great variability observed in FTLD patients, as on the age at onset, duration of disease and clinical features. Examination of the brain of a patient with FTLD reveals symmetrical atrophy of the frontal or temporal lobes, or both. In some cases, there is an asymmetry of atrophy and an atrophy of the basal ganglia and loss of pigmentation from the substantia nigra. There are two immunocytochemical subdivisions of FTLD: tauopathies with an accumulation of intraneuronal hyperphosphorylated Tau and pathologies with intraneuronal inclusions immunoreactive to ubiquitin (FTLD-U) (Cairns et al., 2007): the conditions associated with FTLD-U have been linked by the identification of TAR DNA binding protein (TDP-43) as the major ubiquinated protein component of the inclusions ((Neumann et al.,2006) and four TDP-43 subtypes are now described (Cairns et al., 2007).

Tau, also known as microtubule-associated protein tau (MAPT) is involved in the regulation of microtubule assembly and disassembly. Six isoforms are present: three have three microtubule-binding regions (3R) and three have four repeats (4R) (Goedert et al., 1992). Many tau mutations on chromosome 17 exist and affect all tau isoforms, causing mutated proteins that fail to promote microtubule assembly and disassembly or facilitate axonal transport. Some of the mutations increase the propensity of the mutated tau to self-aggregate into neurofibrillary inclusions or Pick's bodies, biochemically composed by predominantly 3R tau. Other tau mutations cause an aggregation of excess tau formed into neurofibrils composed of 4R tau. All tau mutations alter the ability of neurons to assembly and disassembly microtubules and, therefore, disrupt axonal transport (Neary et al., 2005). Mutations in the microtubule-associated protein tau gene (MAPT) account for 5-10% of FTLD. More recently mutations in the progranulin gene on chromosome 17 (PGRN, OMIN *138945, 1.7 Mb centromeric to MAPT) were found in approximately 10-20% of FTLD with all the PGRN mutation families sharing the ubiquitin-positive tau-negative inclusion bodies in both nucleus and cytoplasm (Baker et al., 2006; Cruts et al., 2006). PGRN codes for progranulin, the precursor of granulin proteins, a 593 amino acid glycoprotein containing 7.5 cysteine-rich tandem repeats. Progranulin is a secreted growth factor expressed in many tissues and is implicated in development, wound repair, inflammation and tumourgenesis (Ahmed et al., 2007). It is highly expressed in the central nervous system (Daniel et al.,

2000), but its function is still unknown. The ubiquitin-positive inclusions in FTLD-U patients with PGRN mutations do not contain progranulin, since neurodegeneration is caused from partial loss of progranulin function rather than the aggregation of the mutant protein, with TAR DNA binding protein (TDP-43) as the major ubiquinated protein component of the inclusions in patients with or without PGRN mutations (Neumann eta al., 2006). The PGRN Leu271LeufsX10 mutations seems to be one of the most common mutation worldwide and found in the Brescia cohort in the 15% of patients with bv-FTLD and in 27% of those with the familial form and in 29% of patients with FTLD-MND and in the 50% of those with the familial form (Benussi et al., 2009).

Mutations in valosin-containing protein (VCP) gene are present in rare forms of FTLD associated with myopathy and Paget's disease of bone (IBMPFD, inclusion body myopathy with Paget disease of bone and frontotemporal dementia). The VCP gene is located on the short (p) arm of chromosome 9 at position 13.3. The product of VCP gene (p97, cdc48) is a hexameric protein, member of the AAA-ATPase superfamily and is involved in numerous essential cellular pathways, including membrane fusions, nuclear traffic, cell proliferation, protein folding, degradation of proteins by the ubiquitin-proteaseome system (UPS) and activation of membrane-bond transcription factors. VCP plays a pivotal role in the degradation of proteins by the ubiquitin proteasome system and interacts with many different cellular proteins involved in this function. Patients with VCP gene mutations have an unique neuropathological form of FTLD, where the ubiquinated inclusions are not composed of the mutated VCP, but rather TDP-43. About 90% of affected patients have myopathy or muscle weakness particularly of the shoulder and hip girdles, which can lead to loss of walking ability and even death for complications of respiratory and cardiac failure. About 50% of the patients have also Paget disease of the bone and bone pain, enlargement and high risk of fractures (Watts et al., 2004; Kimonis et al., 2008).

A charged multivescicular body protein 2B (CHMP2B) gene mutation causes FTLD linked to chromosome 3 in a large Danish family by dysregulating the endosomal secretory complex. These patients are ubiquitin-positive, but TDP-43 negative (Skibinski et al., 2005). In one family, a genetic locus for FTLD has been described in the intraflagellar transport protein 74 (IFT74) gene of chromosome 9p. IFT74 is a protein localised to the intracellular vesicle compartment and is responsible of the transport of materials into and along dendrites and axons. The neuropathology is similar (ubiquitin-positive and TDP-43-positive) to other families with and without motor neuron disease (MND) linked to chromosome 9p (Momeni et al., 2006; Morita et al., 2006).

The apolipoprotein E-4 (APOE-E4) genotype is a major risk factor for Alzheimer's disease (AD), but this is not the case in most association studies with FTLD (Srinivasan et al., 2006). A recent report found evidence that APOE-E4 genotype delays age of clinical onset by around 6 years (Beck et al., 2008). Genetic mutations of amyloid precursor protein (APP) and presenilin 2 (PS2) are not risk factors for FTLD. Cases have been associated with mutations in the gene encoding presenilin 1 (PS1): usually they are patients overlapping AD and FTLD diagnosis (Tang-Wai et al., 2002; Mendez et al., 2006; Zekanovski et al., 2006).

Since the most recent genetic and neuropathological studies can predict clinical categories, the Consortium for Frontotemporal Lobar Degeneration has suggested new nosological criteria for the diagnosis of FTLD (Cairns et al., 2007): 1. Tauopathy (with associated neuron loss and gliosis) and insoluble tau with a predominance of 3R tau, the most likely diagnoses are: FTLD with Pick bodies and FTLD with MAPT mutation; 2. Tauopathy (with associated neuron loss and gliosis) and insoluble tau with a predominance of 4R tau, the most likely diagnoses are: corticobasal degeneration (CDB), progressive supranuclear palsy (PSP), argyrophilic grain disease (i.e., FTLD with parkinsonism linked to chromosome 17), sporadic multiple system tauopathy with dementia, FTLD with MAPT mutations; 3. Tauopathy (with associated neuron loss and gliosis) and insoluble tau with a predominance of 3R and 4R tau, the most likely diagnoses are: neurofibrillary tangle dementia, FTLD with MAPT mutation; 4. Frontotemporal neuronal loss and gliosis without tau- or ubiquitin/P62-positive inclusions, the most likely diagnosis is: FTLD; 5. TDP-43 proteinopathy with ubiquitin/P62-positive inclusions, tau-negative inclusions, the most likely diagnoses are: FTLD-U with and without MND, FTLD-U with PGRN mutations, FTLD-U with VCP mutation, FTLD-U linked to chromosome 9p and other and not yet identified TDP-43 proteinopathies; 6. Frontotemporal neuronal loss and gliosis with ubiquitin/P62-positive inclusions, TDP-43- and tau-negative inclusions, the most likely diagnoses are: FTLD-U with CHMP2B mutation, basophilic inclusion body disease (BIBD), other yet unidentified FTLD-U forms;

Table 2. Recommended nomenclature for frontotemporal lobar degenerations (Mackenzie et al., 2009)

Current Terminology	New Terminology	Major pathological Subtypes
Tau-positive FTLD	FTLD-tau	PiD
		CBD
		PSP
		AGD
		MSTD
		Unclassifiable
Tau-negative FTLD		
FTLD-U		
TDP-43 positive	FTLD-TDP	Type 1-4
		Unclassifiable
TDP-43-negative	FTLD-UPS	aFTLD-U
		FTD-3
NIFID	FTLD-IF	
DLDH	FTLD-ni	
Other		
BIBD	BIBD	

FTLD frontotemporal lobar degeneration, *PiD* Pick disease, *CBD* Corticobasal degeneration, *PSP* progressive supranuclear palsy, *AGD* argyrophilic grain disease, *MSTD* multiple system tauopathy with dementia. *FTLD-U* FTLD with ubiquitinated inclusions, *FTLD-TDP* FTLD nuclear TAR DNA binding protein, *FTLD-UPS* FTLD ubiquitin proteasome system, *aFTLD-U* FTLD atypical FTLD with ubiquitinated inclusions, *FTD-3* frontotemporal dementia linked to chromosome 3, *NIFID* neuronal intermediate filament inclusions, *FTLD-IF* FTLD intermediate filament, *DLDH* dementia lacking distinctive histopathology, *FTLD-ni* FTLD no inclusions, BIBD basophilic inclusions body disease. Pathological subtypes indicate characteristics pattern of pathology, not the clinical syndrome. FLDTP-17 is not listed as a pathological subtype because cases with different MAPT mutations do not have a consistent pattern of pathology. These cases would all be FTLD-tau, but further subtyping would vary.

7. Frontotemporal neuronal loss and gliosis with ubiquitin/P62 and alfa-internexin-positive inclusions, the most likely diagnosis is the neuronal intermediate filament inclusion disease (NIFID). Due to the most recent scientific data, which have shown that a significant proportion of sporadic FTLD are TDP-43 negative and that TDP-43 positive inclusions are present also in other neurodegenerative conditions, such AD, LBD and some primary tauopathies, a new and more simple protein-based nomenclature has been proposed (table 2) (Mackenzie et al., 2009).

The present evidence of genetic defects involving genes encoding proteins with different functions as the causes for the various types of hereditary FTLD suggests that there is no single pathway leading to the cellular and anatomic damage seen in FTLD and each genetic mutation may contribute to the variability in the clinical presentation of FTLD patients. Genetic involvement could be better elucidated by genealogical studies, which could find the ancestor founder of the genetic mutation. One example of a large genealogical investigation is shown in figure 1 (Novelli et al., 2008).

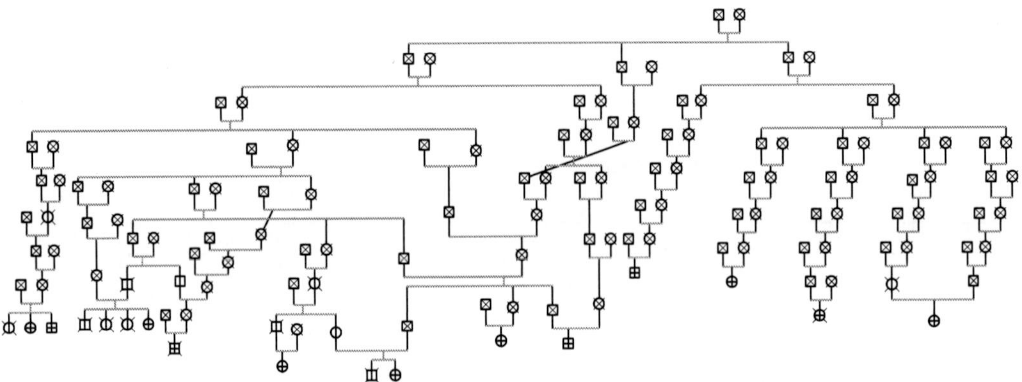

□ Male ○ Female, ⊞ ⊕ Affected; ◫ ⦶ Affected by hearsay, ⊠ ⊗ Dead.

Figure 1. This is a large genealogical pedigree starting from twelve FTLD patients and going back to the seventeen century up to a common ancestor in a Calabrian genetic isolated population. Eleven affected patients were also identified by familial and anamnestic hearsay. For genealogical reconstruction the following sources were used: 1) birth, marriage and death data from Municipal Archives (from 1809 on), 2) the baptism, marriage, burial records and the Status Animarum records of Parish Registers of Local Church (before 1809 until 1700 because some registers were destroyed during the French invasion of the Kingdom of Naples in 1799), 3) the data of Catasto Onciario for 1753 located in the State Archive of Naples; 4) Notarial Archives for 1680 and 1700 located in State Archive of Cosenza (Novelli et al., 2008).

Clinical Presentation

The predominant feature in bv-FTLD is alteration in the patient's social conduct and personality which becomes gradually evident to family, friends and colleagues and induces a medical visit to a neurologist, geriatrician or even more frequently to a psychiatrics. Each of these medical contexts may have a different clinical approach to the disease and, therefore, consensus criteria need to be continuously verified and refreshed. Patients with bv-FTLD frequently have a variable degree of language impairment, as well as those with language deficits have behavioural changes. Symptoms onset is gradual and insidious and insight is generally impaired, while patients with language impairment commonly recognize their deficits. Apathy is characterized by passivity, inertia or inactivity together with social withdrawal. Disinhibition is an early symptom, and seems to be more prevalent in those with right predominant frontal and temporal lobe dysfunction. Distractibility, abnormal eating behaviour, stereotypic and ritualistic behaviours are also frequent, as well as neglect of self-care and loss of empathy for the emotional concerns of others. Mental rigidity is also frequent with lack of creativity and inability to take the viewpoints of others. Dysexecutive symptoms, such as impaired organization, planning and goal setting are frequent at first presentation in bv-FTLD patients who progress over time (Hornberger et al., 2008). Language disturbances such as reduced verbal output, echolalia and verbal stereotypies are frequent. Memory complaints are present in bv-FTLD, but are usually overshadowed by behavioural aspects. Currently, clinical criteria most widely adopted are those by Neary et al., published in 1998 (table 1). However, strict application of these criteria misses a significant proportion of patients, since many core features are not present at the beginning and other supportive features have low prevalence and are not clinically relevant (Mendez et al, 2002; Pijnenburg et al., 2008; Piguet et al., 2009). Moreover, some patients show a rapid disease progression over a few years, while others have little or no progression over a decade. Despite the difficulties on the basis of current clinical diagnosis in identifying at first presentation those progressive versus those non- progressive, it seems that executive dysfunction together with general cognitive and activities of daily living impairment measures appears to be best discriminator factors (Hornberger et al., 2008; Hornberger et al., 2009). Discriminatory examination of those who have progressive FTLD could be MRI: normal or borderline findings at the diagnosis showed longer survival to institutionalization or death than those with definite frontotemporal atrophy (Davies et al., 2006).

Many studies found the presence of identifiable relationship between genetic mutations and clinical expression. Patients with tau-positive FTLD presented more often than other patients visual perceptual-spatial impairment and extra-pyramidal signs together with poor planning and judgement. Those with tau-negative FTLD had greater difficulties with social language, and verbally mediated executive functions (Grossman et al., 2007; Hu et al., 2007). In French patients with bv-FTLD the frequency of PGRN mutations was 5.7%, but increased to 17.9% in familial forms (Le Ber et al., 2008). Families from North America and Belgium had a higher frequency of PGRN mutations of 25% (Baker et al., 2006; Cruts et al., 2006), but patients from Holland and Italy had a lower frequency (4% and 1%, respectively) (Bronner et al., 2007; Bruni et al., 2007). Many neurological signs are associated with PGRN mutations and partially could explain the observed variability in presentation. Visual hallucinations were present in bv-FTLD patients with PGRN mutations at a rate of 25%, while they were present in 2% only of those without PGRN mutations. The presence of hallucinations has been also suggested as discriminatory tool of PGRN mutations in bv-FTLD patients, but a great care should devoted to the differential diagnosis versus Lewy body dementia (LBD), in particular when parkinsonism is associated. However, cognitive symptoms fluctuate in LBD, but not in bv-FTLD with PGRN mutations. Patients with bv-FTLD and PGRN mutations have apraxia at an earlier stage of the disease as compared to those without PGRN mutations, and have an unexpected high frequency (89%) of episodic memory disorders and frontal executive dysfunction (Le Ber et al., 2008). In 223 patients of the Manchester FTLD cohort prevalence rate of PGRN mutations was 5.8% in all cases of FTLD and 17% in familial FTLD, while that of MAPT mutations was 8% and 21% respectively (Pickering-Brown et al., 2008). Most of these patients presented bv-FTLD, but also PNFA. Patients of this cohort with SD and FTLD-MND, despite having ubiquitin/TDP-43 histopathology similar to that of PGRN mutations, did not bear PGRN mutations suggesting different pathogenic mechanisms. In cases with PGRN mutations, patients presented pure bv-FTLD with predominant symptom of apathy and with a language disorder that took form of PNFA. In MAPT cases, patients presented bv-FTLD with predominant social disinhibition and language disorder characterized by semantic loss (Pickering-Brown et al., 2008). In an another cohort of 247 English patients with FTLD (Beck et al., 2008) mean age of onset was 57 years for those with PGRN mutations, 49 years for those with MAPT mutations and 56 years for those FTLD-U, but PGRN-negative. Patients with PGRN mutations had a shorter duration of the disease than other subtypes of FTLD: mean 5±1.0 years versus 12±2.0 years in those with MAPT mutations and mean 9±1.7 years for those FTLD-U PGRN negative. Even in this cohort, patients with PGRN mutations presented bv-FTLD with predominant symptom of apathy and episodic memory impairment. Language disorder was mainly due to decreased spontaneous speech with dynamic aphasia until mutism as the disease progressed. The presence of APOE-E4 genotype delayed the age of onset of clinical symptoms of about 6 years. In a large Calabrian kindred a novel PGRN mutation was found in one family only: it presented a very variable age of onset not explained by APOE-E4 or MAPT haplotypes (Bruni et al., 2007). In these patients language disorders evolved at high rate with final mutism, as well as episodic memory. Extra-pyramidal and pyramidal signs and primitive reflexes were observed at disease onset in PGRN mutation carriers, who became somnolent in the late course of the disease, while phenocopies (phenocopies are environmentally induced phenotype that mimics one caused by genetic factor) (Lein et al.,2007) became severely agitated. Most recently, a PGRN ELISA test was implemented for plasma analysis, and all patients with FTLD PGRN mutations showed significantly reduced levels of PGRN in plasma to about one third of the levels observed in non-PGRN carriers and control individuals. The authors suggest to use plasma PGRN determination as a reliable tool to identify all PGRN mutation carriers in FTLD patients and in asymptomatic individuals at risk (Finch et al., 2009). CHMP2B is a rare cause of familial FTLD and may specific to a Danish pedigree (Cannon et al., 2006). Patients with CHMP2B mutations have a clinical syndrome dominated by personality change and behavioural symptoms, but language, memory, calculation and praxis impairments are also seen in the early course of the disease (Rohrer et al., 2009).

Progressive non-fluent aphasia (PNFA) is a disorder of expressive language with reduced conversation ability and a tendency to speak in shorter sentences. While word comprehension is preserved, patients with PNFA have difficulties in initiating speech, have frequent pauses and prefer to listen rather than start conversation. Word-finding difficulty is present in all cases of PNFA, as well as phonemic errors that produce non-existent words, known as phonemic or verbal paraphasias. Errors are present in spontaneous speech, but also on naming or on repetition of multisyllabic words. In reading aloud patients with PNFA make fewer errors than in spontaneous speech. Onset of the disease is gradual, usually in their 60ies and patients came to clinical observation 2-3 years after beginning of the symptoms. Patients share symptoms with bv-FTLD, in particular personality changes and apathy and have a progressive slowing in the rate and phrase length until complete mutism. A significant group of patients have ubiquitin-positive inclusion and PGRN mutations (4.4% in the French cohort) (Le Ber et al., 2008). In the Manchester cohort, PNFA is more common in PGRN mutations than in cases without, although different language phenotypes could be seen, including dynamic aphasia (Pickering-Brown et al., 2008).

Semantic dementia (SD) is a disorder with loss of ability to name and understand words and to recognise the significance of faces, objects and other sensor stimuli. Patients with SD present anomia with a frequent use of circumlocutions, loss of memory of words with difficulties in remembering the names of persons and objects and a deficit in single-word comprehension both written and spoken. At the beginning the deficit affects less common words, but gradually the patient starts to have problems in various activities, such as using the telephone, following the TV or reading. Memory loss is limited to words, since autobiographical memory is well preserved at least at the beginning, as well as topographical memory and recall of abstract geometrical figures. SD also affects the knowledge of object use: in the early phase of the disease the patient is able to use an object when they have forgotten its name, but he functions better at home than in the clinic. Behavioural and personality changes are prominent and express with emotional withdrawal, depression, disinhibition, apathy, irritability and changing in eating behaviour. Compulsion is a delayed feature and often associated with disinhibition and altered food preference. It has been reported that in the left-predominant SD, visual objects are the target of the compulsive stimulus, while in the right-sided variant, the focus is on letters, words and symbols. In the Manchester cohort of FTLD patients, no subject with PGRN mutations presented SD, which occurred with significantly higher frequency in MAPT mutation cases than in cases with unknown mutation (Pickering-Brown et al., 2008). In the French cohort, no patient with the classic SD syndrome was found to have PGRN mutations (Le Ber et al., 2008). There is evidence that the clinical expression of PNFA is linked to PRGN mutation carriers, but that of SD to MAPT mutation carriers.

FTLD with parkinsonism (FTLDP) is a major syndrome, particularly in those who have symptoms before 65 years. Typical age at onset varies from 25 to 65 years with duration of symptoms from onset to death between 3 and 10 years. Main symptoms are executive dysfunction, altered personality and behaviour with aphasia and parkinsonism. Memory impairment occurs with less frequency as the primary feature. Many patients have mutations in the MAPT gene with tau-positive inclusions in neurons and/or glia. A significant minority of cases with FTLDP-17 do not have any tau-positive inclusions at autopsy, but have mutations in PGRN gene, with a frequency similar to that of MAPT. The PGRN mutations inheritance is autosomal dominant but with reduced penetrance: there are many mutation carriers who are asymptomatic in their 70s and 1 patient has been reported to develop symptom after age 80 years. Patients carrying PGRN mutations have clinical features more variable than those with MAPT mutations: behavioural and cognitive symptoms are commonly present together with memory impairment, limb apraxia, parkinsonism and visuospatial dysfunction. On histological examination, the consistent findings are ubiquitin-positive inclusions with neuronal intranuclear inclusions. FTLDP-17 patients with PGRN mutations have greater parietal involvement than those with MAPT mutations. Furthermore, it has been reported a tendency in some kindreds to a maximal involvement of the same cerebral hemisphere in most or all members of a family, such as progressive aphasia for those with left hemisphere involvement and corticobasal syndrome for those with right hemisphere. In refining the nosological diagnosis of FTLDP-17 it has been suggested to subdivide the disease in FTLDP-17 (MAPT) and FTLDP-17 (PGRN) (Boeve et al., 2008).

FTLD with motor neuron disease (FTLD-MND) begins insidiously in the presenile period, usually in the 60ies. Patients present with personality changes, irritability, obsessions, poor insight and pervasive deficits on executive functions. This psychotic phase lasts for few months and is followed by a tendency to be friendly and calm. Decline in spoken language is affected before the written language and comprehension is also affected. At the clinical observation depending on the predominant symptoms a first diagnosis could be bv-FTD or SD, but the rate of progression of the disease is faster than the two syndromes. After several months or years, the patients present wasting, fasciculations and weakness as well as increased muscle tone and brisk reflexes. Bulbar symptoms are predominant. In either the French and the English cohorts none of the patients with PGRN mutations developed MND during the course of the disease and none of the patients with FTLD-MND had PGRN mutations. Therefore, FTLD-MND syndrome, despite having a basic ubiquitin/TDP-43 histopathology immunohistochemistry, has underlying pathogenic mechanisms different from FTLD-17 (PGRN) (Le Ber et al., 2008; Pickering-Brown et al., 2008).

Beyond the association of FTLD with corticobasal degeneration (CBD) and progressive supranuclear palsy (PSP), other rare syndromes could present symptoms of FTLD. The Fahr's syndrome is a rare syndrome characterised by symmetrical and bilateral intracranial calcification and most cases present with extra-pyramidal symptoms. Two men with Fahr's syndrome have been described with predominant frontal symptoms (Lam et al., 2007). Geschwind's syndrome is present in patients with temporal lobe epilepsy and is characterized by sexual behavioural disorders, hyper-religiosity, hypergraphia and viscosity. A patient affected by FTLD was described with all the personality changes of the syndrome without having epilepsy (Postiglione et al., 2008). The Kluver-Bucy syndrome is characterised by hypersexuality, hyperorality, placidity, visual agnosia, amnesia, hypermetamorphosis, and emotional and nutritional behavioural changes with herpes encephalitis as the most common cause. This form could be also considered a variant of FTLD genetically associated with a mutation of the gene encoding presenilin 1 (PS1) (Tuleja et al., 2008). De Clerambault's syndrome, characterised by erotomania and early and persistent delusion, has been recently considered as a variant of FTLD (Vrieze et al., 2007). The Nasu-Hakola syndrome is characterised by polycystic lipomembranous osteodysplasia with sclerosing leukoencephalopathy and presenile dementia with FTLD features (Madry et al., 2007).

Neuroimaging

Magnetic resonance imaging (MRI), single-photon emission computerised tomography (SPECT) and positron emission tomography (PET) studies have offered new insights in clinical diagnosis, and in understanding the neural basis for cognitive and behavioural impairments and the pathological subtypes. The study of brain metabolism by ^{18}FDG-PET and of brain perfusion by SPECT are valid and reliable tests that increase diagnostic accuracy and can help physicians in making the sometimes difficult clinical distinction between AD and FTLD (Foster et al., 2007), in particular when clinical findings are not definitive and symptoms of different dementias are overlapping. The application to SPECT images of automated voxel-by-voxel statistical analysis of perfusion brain maps has also improved diagnostic accuracy and highlighted the networks that are more specifically involved in FTLD and AD (Varrone et al., 2002). Figure 2 shows ^{18}FDG-PET brain images in two cases of FTLD with typical hypometabolism in the frontal cortex and anterior cingulate.

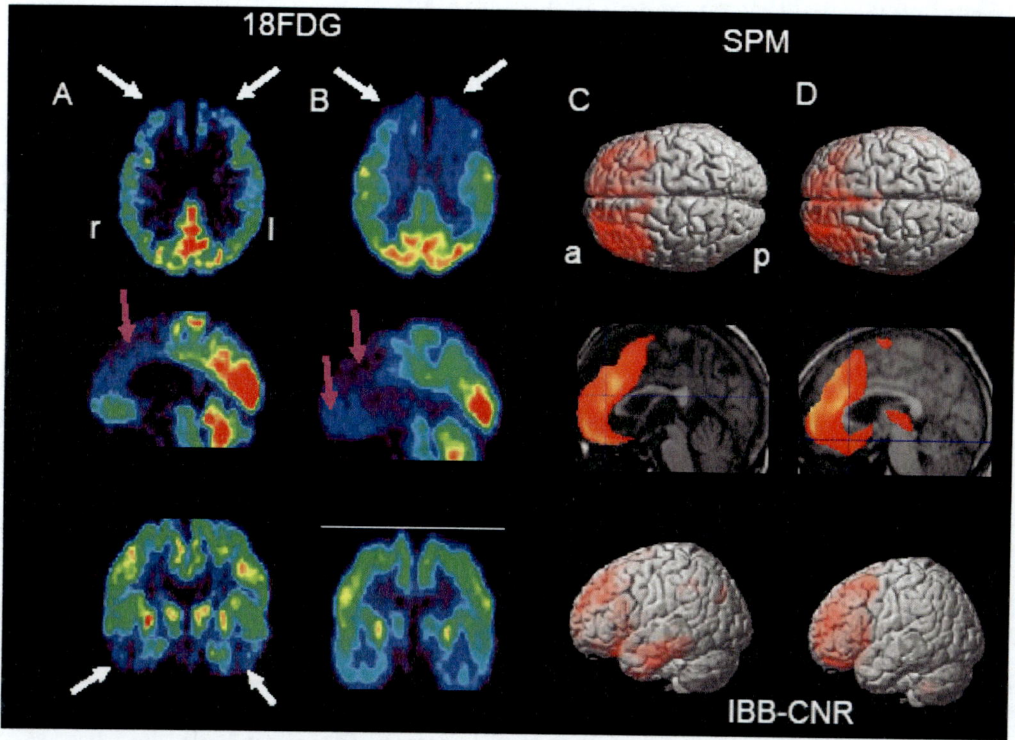

Figure 2. ^{18}FDG-PET images (A,B) and statistical parametric maps of significant metabolic reduction (C,D) obtained in two patients with FTLD. In both patients the typical pattern of hypometabolism involving the prefrontal (lateral and medial) cortex and the anterior cingulate is clearly evident. In patient A there was also a reduced hypometabolism in the lateral temporal cortex. In patient B the metabolic reduction was limited to the frontal cortex but spreads to the fronto-orbital regions. The SPM analysis compared the single subject to a group of normal subjects (n=14, age range: 27-70 years, age was considered in the statistical model of SPM as nuisance covariate) and highlights the location and the extent of metabolic alterations. r=right; l=left; a=anterior; p=posterior

FTLD patients with either PGRN and MAPT mutations showed at MRI grey matter loss in frontal, temporal, and parietal lobes as compared to controls. The loss was predominant in posterior temporal and parietal lobes in PGRN and in anteromedial temporal lobes in MAPT. In the latter the loss was greater when compared to healthy subjects in particular in the median temporal lobes, insula, and in putamen (Whitwell et al., 2009). In the French cohort of FTLD patients with PGRN mutations, cortical atrophy was markedly asymmetric in 76% of mutation carriers, being 48% left and 29% right predominant. SPECT showed significant hypoperfusion bilaterally in the fronto-cingular, the right posterior cortex, including hippocampus, and the inferior parietal cortex, compared to healthy subjects. When compared to patients without PGRN mutations, the hypoperfusion was more significant in the dorsolateral right frontal cortex, the right posterior temporal and inferior parietal cortices, the right hippocampus and the posterior cingulated cortex bilaterally. The author stressed the unexpected hypoperfusion in the hippocampus, probably related to the amnestic syndrome, and the hippocampal degeneration found in PGRN mutation carriers, and in posterior cingulate hypothesizing a deafferentation of the medial temporal cortex, as it probably occurs in AD (Le Ber et al., 2008). In the English cohort MRI showed fronto-temporal-parietal atrophy and those with PGRN mutations showed an asymmetrical atrophy even greater than that observed in the classical asymmetrical SD (Beck et al., 2008). Using the combination of diffusion tensor imaging and fractional anisotrophy Borroni et al. found in patients with bv-FTLD a significant white matter reduction in the superior longitudinal fasciculus, which connects dorsolateral frontal lobe and posterior associative areas, and could explain the observed behavioural impairment. Patients with temporal variant of FTLD showed different white matter reductions bilaterally in the inferior longitudinal fasciculus, in the inferior fronto-occipital fasciculus and in the left superior longitudinal fasciculus. The involvement of the white matter bundles correlates with the atrophy of grey matter and support the role of white matter lesions in the pathological characteristics of FTLD (Borroni et al., 2007).

In patients with FTLDP-17 MRI studies showed frontal and/or temporal atrophy either symmetric or asymmetric, with parenchymal signal changes absent or mild (Boeve et al., 2008). In patients with CHMP2B mutations a generalized atrophy was observed in all cases, included in those who are mutation carriers, but still asymptomatic (Rohrer et al., 2009). SPECT perfusion imaging showed two different patterns of cerebral dysfunction in H1 and H2 tau haplotypes: hypoperfusion in frontal medial and cingulated cortex was predominantly observed in H2-carriers, while a prevalent involvement of posterior parietal regions was seen in H1-carriers (Borroni et al., 2007).

Conclusions and Future Research

FTLD is a common and severe neurodegenerative disorder. The recent progress has revealed increased complexity even higher than that expected, since FTLD is associated with different histological features, different immunochemical characteristics and different genetic basis. However, recent studies have also evidenced clear relationships among genetic mutations, in particular MAPT and PGRN mutations, underlying histopathology and clinical expression.

Beyond the presence of PGRN and MAPT gene mutations in the pathogenesis of FTLD, most cases of familial FTLD still lack any causative genetic mutation. In the Dutch cohort of FTLD patients, 27% had a positive family history, including 11% MAPT and 6% PGRN mutations; in 10% of patients with autosomal dominant inheritance, genetic defect has yet to be identified. The authors suggest future genetic studies in order to identify genetic defects in at least two neuropathological groups, distinguished in familial FTLD-MND and familial FTLD-U with hippocampal sclerosis (Kamphorst et al., 2008). Future research must be dedicated also to the identification of other possible genetic causes of bv-FTLD (Novelli et al., 2008).

Diagnostic criteria should be verified and implemented. It has been suggested to revise the current criteria by Neary et al. (Neary et al., 1998), taking into consideration that the strict application of these criteria misses a significant proportion of patients. Diagnostic accuracy is complicated by patients with features of FTLD, who do not progress in the disease or have a little progression over many years and by the inclusion of "phenocopies", who could dramatically interfere with the sensitivity of the criteria. New and very different variants of FTLD with peculiar features could not be correctly identified and diagnosed. New neuropsychological tests should be able to give an accurate differential diagnosis of FTLD as compared to other dementias. For example, new cut-off values for the frontal behavioral inventory (FBI) (Kertesz et al., 1997) have recently shown a 97% sensitivity and 95% specificity in distinguishing bv-FTLD from non-bv-FTLD patients (Milan et al., 2008). Environmental conditions must be taken into account in new studies, since cultural and socioeconomic conditions could delay the diagnosis of the disease at its early onset, as it occurs for AD.

Neuroimaging investigations must be implemented: ^{18}FDG-PET and SPECT studies have shown to improve the diagnostic accuracy of FTLD, as also recommended by scientific guidelines. New studies will also help understanding the pathological mechanisms underlying different variants of FTLD. New biomarkers for a correct diagnosis should be investigated and checked in clinical practice, as shown by the usefulness of the plasma assessment of PGRN.

Effective treatment of FTLD is still lacking, since currently it is symptomatic only. Selective serotonin reuptake inhibitors (SSRIs) have shown an effect on behaviour symptoms, but not on cognitive decline, and studies have been conducted with trazodone and antipsychotics (Weder et al., 2007). Novel therapeutic compounds will likely study targets linked to disease pathogenesis, such as preventing expression and accumulation of tau protein, with the goal to improve the prognosis of FTLD patients and quality of life.

References

Ahmed Z., Mackenzie I.R., Hutton M.L., Dickson D.W. Progranulin in frontotemporal lobar degeneration and neuroinflammation. *J. Neuroinflammation* 4:7, 2007.

Andreasen N., Blennow K., Sjodin C., Winblad B., Svardsudd K. Prevalence and incidence of clinically diagnosed memory impairments in a geographically defined general population in Sweden. The Pitea Dementia Project. *Neuroepidemiology* 18:144-155, 1999.

Baker M., Mackenzie I.R., Pickering-Brown S.M., Gass J., Rademakers R., Lindholm C., Snowden J., Adamson J., Sadovnick A.D., Rollinson S., Cannon A., Dwosh E., Neary D., Melquist S., Richardson A., Dickson D., Berger Z., Eriksen J., Robinson T., Zehr C., Dickey C.A., Crook R., McGowan E., Mann D., Boeve B., Feldman H., Hutton M.

Mutation in the progranulin cause tau-negative frontotemporal dementia linked to chromosome 17. *Nature* 442:916-919, 2006.

Beck J., Roher J.D., Campbell T., Isaacs A., Morrison K.E., Goodall E.F., Warrington E.K., Stevens J., Revesz T., Holton J., Al-Sarraj S., King A., Scahill R., Warren J.D., Fox N.C., Rossor M.N., Collinge J., Mead S. A distinct clinical, neuropsychological and radiological phenotype is associated with progranulin gene mutations in a large UK series. *Brain* 131:706-720, 2008.

Benussi L., Ghidoni R., Pegoiani E., Moretti D.V., Zanetti O., Binetti G. Progranulin Leu271LeufsX10 is one of the most common FTLD and CBS associated mutations worldwide. *Neurobiol. Dis*. 33:379-385, 2009.

Boeve B.F., Hutton M. Refining frontotemporal dementia with parkinsonism linked to chromosome 17. *Arch. Neurol.* 65:460-464, 2008.

Borroni B., Bramati S.M., Agosti C., Gipponi S., Bellelli G.,Gasparotti R., Garibotto V., Di Luca M., Scifo P., Perani D., Padovani A. Evidence of white matter changes on diffusion tensor imaging in frontotemporal dementia. *Arch. Neurol.* 64:246-251, 2007.

Borroni B., Perani D., Agosti C., Anchisi D., Paghera B., Archetti S., Alberici A., Di Luca M., Padovani A. Tau haplotype influences cerebral perfusion pattern in frontotemporal lobar degeneration and related disorders. *Acta Neurol. Scand.* 117:269-366, 2008.

Bronner J.F., Rizzu P., Seelaar H., van Mil S.E., Anar B., Azmani A., Kaat L.D., Rosso S., Heutink P., van Swieten J.C. Progranulin mutations in Dutch familial frontotemporal lobar degeneration. *Eur. J. Hum. Genet.* 15:369-374, 2007.

Brun A. Consensus statement. Clinical and neuropathological criteria for frontotemporal dementia: Lund and Manchester groups. *J. Neurol. Neurosurg. Psychiatry*. 57:416-418, 1994.

Bruni A.C., Momeni P., Bernardi L., Tomaino C.,Frangipane F.,Elder J., Kawarai T., Sato C., Pradella S., Wakutani Y., Anfossi M., Gallo M., Geracitano S., Costanzo A., Smirne N., Curcio S.A.M., Mirabelli M., Puccio G., Colao R., Maletta R.G., Kertesz A., St. George-Hyslop P., Hardy J., Rogava E. Heterogeneity within a large kindred with frontotemporal dementia. *Neurology* 69:140-147, 2007.

Cairns N.J., Bigio E.H., Mackenzie I.R., Neumann M., Lee V.M., Hatanpaa K.J., White III C.L., Schneider J.A., Grinberg L.T., Halliday G., Duyckaerts C., Lowe J.S., Holm I.E., Tolnay M., Okamoto K., Yokoo H., Murayama S., Woulfe J., Munoz D.G., Dickson D.W., Ince P.G., Trojanowski J.Q., Mann D.M.A. Neuropathological diagnostic and nosologic criteria for frontotemporal lobar degeneration: consensus of the Consortium for Frontotemporal Lobar Denegeration. *Acta Neuropathol.* 114:5-22, 2007.

Cannon A., Baker M, Boeve B., Josephs K., Knopman D., Petersen R., Parisi J., Dickson D., Adamson J., Snowden J., Neary D., Mann D., Hutton M., Pickering-Brown S.M. CHMP2B mutations are not a common cause of frontotemporal lobar degeneration. *Neuroscience Lett.* 398: 83-84, 2006

Cruts M., Gijselinck I., van der Zee J., Engelborghs S., Wils H., Pirici D, Rademarkers R., Vanderberghe R., Dermaut B., Martin J.J., van Duijn C., Peeters K., Sciot R., Santens P., De Pooter T., Mattheijssens M., Van den Broeck M., M Cuij I., Vennekens K., De Deyn P.P., Kumar-Singh S., Van Broeckhoven C. Null mutations in progranulin cause ubiquitin-positive frontotemporal dementia linked to chromosome 17q21. *Nature*. 442:920-924, 2006.

Daniel R., He Z, Carmichael K.P., Halper J., Bateman A. Cellular localization of gene expression for progranulin. *J. Histochem. Cytochem*. 48:999-1009, 2000.

Davies R.R., Kipps C.M., Mitchell J., Kril J.J., Halliday G.M., Hodges J.R. Progression in frontotemporal dementia. *Arch. Neurol*. 63:1627-1631, 2006.

Finch N., Baker M., Crook R., Swanson K., Kuntz K., Surtees R., Bisceglio G., Rovelet-Lecrux A., Boeve B., Petersen C., Dickson D.W., Younkin S.G., Deramecourt V., Crook J., Graff-Radford N.R., Rademakers R. Plasma progranulin levels predict progranulin mutation status in frontotemporal dementia patients and asymptomatic family members. *Brain 132:583-591,* 2009.

Foster N.L., Heidebrink J.L., Clark C.M., Jagust W.J., Arnold S.E., Barbas N.R., DeCarli C.S., Turner R.S., Koeppe R.A:, Higdon R., Minoshima S. FDG-PET improves accuracy in distinguishing frontotemporal dementia and Alzheimer's disease. *Brain* 130:2616-2635, 2007.

Goedert M., Spillantini M.G., Cairns N.J., Crowther R.A. Tau proteins of Alzheimer paired helical filaments: abnormal phosphorylation of all six brain isoforms. *Neuron* 8:159-168, 1992.

Graham A. Epidemiology of frontotemporal dementia. In: JR Hodges (Ed.), *Frontotemporal dementia syndromes*. Cambridge University Press, UK, 2007, pp. 25-37.

Grossman M., Libon D.J., Forman M.S., Massimo L., Wood E., Moore P., Anderson C., Farmer J., Chatterjee A., Clark C.M., Colsett H.B., Hurtig H.I., Lee V.M.-Y., Trojanowski J.Q. Distinct antemortem profiles in patients with pathologically defined frontotemporal dementia. *Arch. Neurol*. 64:1601-1609, 2007.

Harvey R.J., Skelton-Robinson M., Rossor M.N. The prevalence and causes of dementia in people under the age of 65 years. J. *Neurol. Neurosurg. Psychiatry* 74:1206-1209, 2003.

Hornberger M., Piguet O., Kipps C., Hodges J.R. Executive function in progressive and nonprogressive behavioral variant frontotemporal dementia. *Neurology* 71: 1481-1488, 2008.

Hornberger M., Shelley B.P., Kipps C.M., Piguet O., Hodges J.R. Can progressive and non-progressive behavioral variant frontotemporal dementia be distinguished at presentation? *J. Neurol. Neurosurg. Psychiatry* 80:591-593, 2009.

Hu W.T., Mandrekar J.N., Parisi J.E., Knopman D.S., Boeve F., Petersen R.C., Hutton M., Dickson D.W., Josephs K.A. Clinical features of pathologic subtypes of behavioral-variant frontotemporal dementia. *Arch. Neurol*. 64:1611-1616, 2007.

Kamphorst H.S.W., Rosso S.M., Azmani A., Masdjedi R., de Koning I., Maat-Kievit J.A., Anar B., Kaat L.D., Dooijes D., Rozemuller J.M., Bronner I.F., Rizzu P., van Siete J.C. Distinct genetic forms of frontotemporal dementia. *Neurology* 71:1220-1226, 2008.

Kertesz A., Davidson W., Fox H., Frontal behavioral inventory: diagnostic criteria for frontal lobe dementia. *Can. J. Neurol. Sci.* 24:29-36, 1997

Kimonis V.E., Fulchiero E., Vesa J., Watts G. VCP disease associated with myopathy, Paget disease of bone and frontotemporal dementia: review of a unique disorder. *Biochim. Biophys. Acta* 1782:744-748, 2008.

Kipps C.M., Knibb J.A., Hodges J.R. Clinical presentation of frontotemporal dementia. In: JR Hodges (Ed.), *Frontotemporal dementia syndromes*. Cambridge University Press, UK, 2007, pp. 38-79.

Knopman D.S., Petersen R.C., Edland S.D., Cha R.H., Rocca W.A. The incidence of frontotemporal lobe degeneration in Rochester, Minnesota, 1990 through 1994. *Neurology* 62:506-508, 2004.

Lam Y.S.P., Fong S. Y.Y., Yiu G.C., Wing Y.K. Fahr's disease: a differential diagnosis on frontal lobe syndrome. *Hong Kong Med. J.* 13:75-77, 2007.

Le Ber I., Camuzat A., Mannequin D., Pasquier F., Guedj E., Rovelet-Lecrux A., Hahn-Barma V., van der Zee J., Clot F., Bakchine S., Puel M., Ghanim M., Lacomblez L., Mikol J., Deramecourt V., Lejeune P., de la Sayette V., Belliard S., Vercelletto M., Meyrignac C., van Broeckhoven C., Lambert J.C., Verpillat P., Campion D., Habert M.O:, Dubois B., Brice A. Phenotype variability in progranulin mutation carriers: a clinical, neuropsychological, imaging and genetic study. *Brain* 131:732-746, 2008.

Lein C., Bonifati V. Dissecting the complexity of frontotemporal dementia. *Neurology* 69:129-130, 2007.

Mackenzie I.R., Neumann M., Bigio E.H., Cairns N.J., Alafuzoff I., Kril J., Kovasc G.G., Ghetti B., Halliday G., Holm I.E., Ince P.G., Kamphorst W., Revesz T., Rozemuller J.M., Kumar-Singh S., Akiyama H., Baborie A., Spina S., Dickson D.W., Trojanowski J.Q., Mann D.M.A. Nomenclature for neuropathological subtypes of frontotemporal lobar degeneration: consensus recommendations. *Acta Neuropathol.* 117:15-18, 2009.

Madry H., Prudlo J., Grgic A., Freyschmidt J. Nasu-Nakola disease (PLOSL): report of five cases and review of the literature. *Clin. Orthop. Relat. Res.* 454:262-269, 2007.

Mendez M.F., Perryman K.M. Neuropsychiatric features of frontotemporal dementia: evaluation of consensus criteria and review. *J. Neuropsychiatry Clin. Neurosci.* 14:424-429, 2002.

Mendez NF, McMurtray A, Frontotemporal-like phenotypes associated with presenilin-1 mutations. *Am. J. Alzheimer's Dis. Other Demen.* 21:281-286, 2006.

Milan G., Lamenza F., Iavarone A., Galeone F., Lorè E., De Falco C., Sorrentino P., Postiglione A. Behavioural assessment in the differential diagnosis of frontotemporal dementia. *Acta Neurol. Scand.* 117:260-265, 2008.

Momeni P., Schymick J., Jain S., Cookson M.R., Cairns N.J., Greggio E., Greenway M.J., Berger S., Pickeirng-Brown S., Chio A., Fung H.C., Holtzman D.M., Huey E.D., Wassermann E.M., Adamson J., Hutton M.L., Rogaeva E., George-Hyslop P., Rothstein J.D., Hardiman O., Grafman J., Singleton A., Hardy J., Traynor B.J.. Analysis of IFT74 as a candidate gene for chromosome 9p-linked ALS-FTD. *BMC Neurol.* 6:44, 2006.

Morita M., Al Chalabi A., Andersen P.M., Hosler B., Sapp P., Englund E., Mitchell J.E., Habgood J.J., de Belloroche J., Xi J, Jongjaroenprasert W., Horvitz H.R., Gunnarson L.G., Brown R.H. Jr. A locus on chromosome 9p confers susceptibility to ALS and frontotemporal dementia. *Neurology* 66:839-844, 2006.

Neary D., Snowden J., Mann D. Frontotemporal dementia. *Lancet Neurology* 4: 771-780, 2005.

Neary D., Snowden J.S., Gustafson L. et al. Frontotemporal lobe degeneration: a consensus on clinical diagnostic criteria. *Neurology* 51:1546-1554, 1998.

Neumann M., Sampathu D.M., Kwong L.K., Truax A.C., Micsenyi M.C., Chou T.T., Bruce J., Schuck T., Grossman M., Clark C.M., McCluskey L.F., Miller B.L., Masliah E., Mackenzie I.R., Feldman H., Feiden W., Kretzschmar H.A., Trojanowski J.Q., Lee V.M. Ubiquinated TDP-43 in frontotemporal lobar degeneration and amyotrophic lateral sclerosis. *Science* 314:130-133, 2006.

Novelli V., Milan G., Calabria A., Malovini A., Viviani Anselmi C., Roncarati R., Lamenza F., Condorelli G.L., Postiglione A., Puca A.A. A genome-wide linkage of familial frontotemporal dementia. *Dement. Geriatr. Cogn. Disord.* 26 (S1): 27, 2008.

Pickering-Brown S.M., Rollinson S., Du Plessis D., Morrison K.E., Varma A., Richardson A.M.T., neary D., Snowden J.S., Mann D.M.A. Frequency and clinical characteristics of progranulin mutation carriers in the Manchester frontotemporal lobar degeneration cohort: comparison with patients with MAPT and no known mutations. Brain 131:721-731, 2008

Piguet O., Hornberger M., Shelley B.P., Kipps C.M., Hodges J.R. Sensitivty of current criteria for the diagnosis of behavioral variant frontotemporal dementia. *Neurology* 72:732-737, 2009.

Pijnenburg Y.A.L., Mulder J.L., van Swieten J.C., Uitdehaag B.M.J., Stevens M.S., Scheltens P., Jonker C. Diagnostic accuracy of Consensus Diagnostic Criteria for frontotemporal Dementia in a Memory Clinic Population. *Dement. Geriatr. Cogn. Disord.* 25:157-164, 2008.

Postiglione A., Milan G., Pappatà S., De Falco C., Gallotta G., Sorrentino P., Schiattarella V., Striano S. Frontotemporal dementia presenting as Geschwind's sindrome. *Neurocase* 14:264-270, 2008

Ratnavalli E., Brayne C., Dawson K., Hodges J.R. The prevalence of frontotemporal dementia. *Neurology* 58:1615-1621, 2002.

Rohrer J.D:, Ahsan R.L., Isaacs A.M., Nielsen J.E., Ostergaard L., Scahill R., Warren J.D:, Rossor M.N., Fox N.C., Johannsen P., the FReJA consortium Presymptomatic generalized brain atrophy in frontotemporal dementia caused by CHMP2B mutation. *Dement. Geriatr. Cogn. Disord.* 27:182-186, 2009.

Rosso S.M., Kaat L.D. Frontotemporal dementia in the Netherlands: patients characteristics and prevalence estimates from a population-based study. *Brain* 126:2016-2022, 2003.

Skibinski G, Parkinson NJ, Brown JM, Chakrabarti L, Lloyd SL, Hummerich H, Nielsen JE, Hodges J.R., Spillantini M.G., Thusgaard T., Brandner S., Brun A., Rossor M.N., Gade A., Johannsen P., Sorensen S.A., Gydesen S., Fisher E.M., Collinge J. Mutations in the endosomal ESCRTIII-complex subunit CHMP2B in frontotemporal dementia. *Nature genet.* 37:806-808, 2005.

Srinivasan R., Davidson Y., Gibbons L., Payton A., Richardson A.M., Varma A., Julien C., Stopford C., Thompson J., Horan M.A., Pendleton N., Pickering-Brown S.M., Neary D., Snowden J.S., Mann D.M. The apolipoprotein E epsilon 4 allele selectively increases the risk of frontotemporal lobar degeneration in males. *J. Neurol. Neurosurg. Psychiatry* 77:154-158, 2006.

Tang-Wai D., Lewis P., Boeve B., Hutton M., Golde T., Baker M., Hardy J., Michels V., Ivnik R., Jack C., Petersen R. Familial frontotemporal dementia associated with a novel presenilin-1 mutation. *Dement. Geriatr. Cogn. Disord.* 14:13-21, 2002.

Tuleja E., Chermann J.F., Sereni C., Hart G., Sereni D. Kluver Bucy sindrome, unusual consequence of excessive rapid correction of sever hyponatremia. *Press Med.* 37:975-979, 2008.

Varrone A., Pappatà S., Caracò C., Soricelli A., Milan G., Quarantelli M., Alfano B., Postiglione A., Salvatore S. Voxel-based comparison of rCBF in frontotemporal dementia and Alzheimer's Disease highligths the involvement of different cortical networks. *Europ. J. of Nuclear Med.* 29:1447-1454, 2002.

Vrieze E., Pieters G. De Clerambault's syndrome. A case report and a review of the literature on the difference between primary and secondary erotomania. *Tijdschr Psychiatry* 49: 845-849, 2007.

Watts G.D., Wymer J., Kovach M.J., Mehta S.G., Mumm S., Darvish D., Pestronk A., Whyte M.P., Kimonis V.E. Inclusion body myopathy associated with Paget disease of bone and frontotemporal dementia is caused by mutant valosin-containing protein. *Nature Genet.* 36:377-381, 2004.

Weder N.D., Aziz R., Wilkins K., Tampi R.R. Frontotemporal dementias.A review. *Ann. General Psychiatry* 6:15-23, 2007.

Whitwell J.L:, Jack C.R., Boeve B.F., Senjem M.L:, Baker M., Rademakers R., Ivnik R.J., Knopman D.S., Wszolek Z.K., Petersen R.C., Josephs K.A. Voxel-based morphometry patterns of atrophy in FTLD with mutations in MAPT or PGRN. *Neurology* 72:813-820, 2009

Zekanovski C., Golan M.P., Krzysko K.A., Lipczynska-Lojkowska W., Filipek S., Kowalska A., Rossa G., Peplonska B., Styczynska M., Maruszak A., Religa D., Wender M., Kulczycki J., Barcikowska M., Kuznicki J. Two novel presenilin 1 gene mutations connected with frontotemporal dementia-like clinical phenotype: genetic and bioinformatic assessment. *Exp. Neurol.* 200: 82-88, 2006.

In: Alzheimer's Disease and Dementia (Vol. 4)
Editor: Miao-Kun Sun ISBN:978-1-60876-152-4

Chapter XII

Cognitive Impairment in Schizophrenia

Verity C Leeson and Eileen M Joyce
UCL Institute of Neurology, Queen Square, London WC1N 3BG

Abstract

Since the first description of the disorder, schizophrenia has been characterised not only by psychosis but also by cognitive dysfunction. Although essentially a disorder of young people, the cognitive impairment of schizophrenia was initially thought to resemble that of the neurodegenerative dementias, arising at the onset of psychosis and deteriorating over the course of the illness. Current evidence, however, suggests that a neurodevelopmental process affects intellectual function during childhood and adolescence prior to the onset of the clinical syndrome, and that once psychosis is manifest, cognition is essentially static. The strongest evidence is for a generalised impairment reflected in reduced IQ and deficits across a wide range of cognitive domains. Additionally, there is some evidence that specific functions may be more relevant than others, being differentially or disproportionately impaired. Of particular importance are verbal memory and information processing speed. Studies of the longitudinal trajectory of cognitive impairment both during development and following the onset of psychosis, suggest that this reflects the underlying pathophysiology of the disorder and is of such a significant degree that it contributes to poor clinical outcome. As a consequence, the possibility of cognitive remediation, pharmacologically or psychologically, is an increasing area of research interest.

Introduction

In 1896 Emil Kraepelin provided the first detailed account of a psychiatric disorder that remains one of the main causes of disability in the world (Murray and Lopez, 1997), affecting around one in two hundred of the world population (Saha et al., 2005). He described a psychotic disorder, termed 'dementia praecox' or premature dementia, which he believed was organic in nature, distinct from disorders of mood and characterised by progressive cognitive decline (Adityanjee et al., 2002). A decade later, in 1908, Eugen Bleuler proposed a new name suggesting that dementia praecox was inappropriate because symptoms did not always first appear in young adults and the disorder did not invariably result in deterioration (Black and Boffeli, 1989). Bleuler instead recommended using the term 'schizophrenia', meaning splitting of mind and implying a more psychodynamic aetiology.

However, whilst Bleuler's 'schizophrenia' has replaced Kraepelin's 'dementia praecox' in the naming of the disorder, the concept of core cognitive dysfunction has not been abandoned. Indeed, in recent years, the development of sophisticated neuropsychological assessment and neuroimaging techniques has reasserted the importance of cognition in our understanding of schizophrenia. Early neuroscientific studies revealed brain morphological abnormalities with computed tomography (CT) (Johnstone et al., 1976; Weinberger et al., 1979) and information processing deficits which were implicated as the basis from which psychotic symptoms emerged (Broen and Storms, 1967; Hemsley, 1977; Frith, 1979). In addition, although advances in treatment throughout the latter part of the 20th century resulted in reasonable success in ameliorating the positive symptoms of schizophrenia, such as delusions and hallucinations (Hegarty et al., 1994), it soon became evident that concomitant recovery of independent living or social functioning was often not achieved (Velligan et al., 1997).

Recent reviews of relevant literature suggest that cognitive deficits are good predictors of residual dysfunction across many domains of social, occupational and independent living activities (Green, 1996; Green et al., 2000; Green et al., 2004). For example, Gold et al. (2002), in a study of established schizophrenia, found that, out of a wide variety of measures, IQ had the highest correlation with total hours worked over the subsequent twelve months. Leeson et al. (2009a) also found that IQ predicted levels of social functioning four years later, this time in a large group of patients followed from illness onset. The discovery of the relationship between cognition and clinical outcome has recently led to the hypothesis that cognitive-enhancing treatments may be necessary for improvement of function in schizophrenia (Cohen and Insel, 2008).

Prevalence and Course of Cognitive Impairments in Schizophrenia

Schizophrenia is a disease of considerable heterogeneity with no single psychotic symptom evident in all cases. By contrast, there is increasing evidence that cognitive impairment is present in the majority of individuals with schizophrenia and this characteristic may be more prevalent than most symptoms. Descriptions of schizophrenia in both DSM-IV-TR and ICD-10 diagnostic manuals include several references to cognitive impairment. For example, the description of schizophrenia in DSM-IV-TR states that the characteristics of schizophrenia "involve a range of *cognitive* and emotional dysfunctions that include perception, inferential thinking, language and communication, behavioral monitoring, affect, fluency and production of thought and speech, hedonic capacity, volition and drive, and attention". On direct cognitive testing, one large study found 73% of their schizophrenia patients to be clinically impaired on at least two tests from a comprehensive neuropsychological assessment covering verbal ability, psychomotor skill, cognitive flexibility, attention, learning, retention and motor skills (Palmer et al., 1997). Similarly, Gold (2008), commenting on the performance of nearly 600 schizophrenia patients on the Repeatable Battery for the Assessment of Neuropsychological Status (RBANS) in a study by Wilk et al. (2004), suggested that if criteria of scoring one standard deviation below normal are employed, this would correctly identify 80% of patients. Although the diagnostic criteria of schizophrenia currently do not include the requirement of cognitive impairment, future inclusion has been widely debated on the basis of such findings (Keefe and Fenton, 2007).

MacCabe (2008) argues that the poorer neuropsychological performance in patients when compared to controls in case-control studies can be interpreted as being due to any combination of at least seven mechanisms including: 1. direct, causal risk factors for schizophrenia; 2. factors involved in the etiology of schizophrenia but not causal themselves; 3. early symptoms of the disorder itself, which predate the onset of psychotic symptoms; 4. core symptoms of the disorder that arise concurrently with the onset of psychotic symptoms; 5. a consequence of the symptoms of schizophrenia, such as auditory hallucinations, agitation, or apathy; 6. the adverse effects of drug treatment for schizophrenia; and 7. the effect of the chronically impoverished social and occupational environment of many patients with schizophrenia.

There are several pertinent findings that shed light on these possible explanations. For example, many studies have demonstrated that cognitive deficits can be observed from illness onset, suggesting that these occur in concert with or predate psychotic symptoms. In particular, two studies involving large samples of first-episode patients revealed pronounced performance impairment on many neuropsychological tests assessing a wide range of cognitive domains (Mohamed et al., 1999; Bilder et al., 2000). Bilder et al. (2000) reported an average deficit in patients relative to control subjects of 1.5 standard deviations. Mohamed et al. (1999) found deficits of a slightly more modest magnitude but, importantly, demonstrated equivalent levels in patients whether they were naive to antipsychotic medication or not. Thus in these studies of cognition at illness onset, the deficits could not be ascribed to the effects of medication or to institutionalisation (Bilder et al., 1992).

There is good evidence to suggest that patients with schizophrenia not only underperform on cognitive tests when compared to healthy controls, matched on age, sex, socioeconomic status or parental education level, but also demonstrate current cognitive functioning that has declined from their own premorbid level. Thus, while schizophrenia patients may be found who perform within the normal range on cognitive tests, it is likely that these patients have suffered a decrement in their cognitive functions. Tests of irregular word reading such as the Wechsler Test of Adult Reading (Wechsler, 2001) and the National Adult Reading Test (Nelson and Willison, 1991) are widely used to estimate premorbid IQ, as word reading ability is generally well maintained in the face of more widespread intellectual decline (Crawford et al., 1998). In the general population, IQ scores estimated from a single irregular word reading test closely approximate full scale IQ scores calculated using batteries including a range of diverse tests, for example the Wechsler Adult Intelligence Test (Wechsler, 1997). This is not so in schizophrenia populations. For example, Crawford et al. (1992) reported significantly higher estimated premorbid IQ than current IQ in patients and studies which have categorised schizophrenia patients according to premorbid and current IQ suggest that 40-50% undergo a decline in IQ by at least 10 points (Weickert et al., 2000; Joyce et al., 2005; Badcock et al., 2005; Kremen et al., 2008). In keeping with these findings, studies which have matched schizophrenia patients and healthy controls on measures of estimated premorbid IQ almost unequivocally report poorer performance in the patient group when compared on neuropsychological test performance (e.g. Hutton et al., 1998; Keefe et al., 2005).

One of the criticisms of using a verbal test such as word reading, to estimate premorbid IQ in schizophrenia is that the discrepancy between this and IQ derived from a range of different cognitive functions may not so much reflect a decline in general cognitive function as a selective preservation of verbal skills. In support of this, NART IQ has been found to deviate from measures of full scale IQ actually obtained years before the onset of psychosis (Russell et al., 2000). A further study (Kremen et al., 2001) matched schizophrenia patients and controls on current IQ and found evidence for significantly higher verbal IQ and lower performance IQ in the patients consistent with their higher premorbid IQ estimated with a reading test. This superior verbal IQ may have underpinned the finding of better irregular word reading in the patients.

This difficulty of interpretation, inherent in studies using tests administered after psychosis onset to estimate premorbid function, is avoided in population based cohort studies. These utilise cognitive test scores from large scale studies of young populations and link them to medical records to determine which subjects went on to develop schizophrenia. These studies allow examination of true premorbid performance of individuals with schizophrenia against that of their non-psychotic peers. One such study that examined cognitive performance at the time of conscription to the Swedish military as a predictor of a subsequent diagnosis of schizophrenia (David et al., 1997) reported that conscripts scoring in the lowest IQ band were nine times more likely to be diagnosed later with schizophrenia than those falling within the highest IQ band. Other studies have examined cognitive function at even earlier time points and have similarly demonstrated a distinction between those who became psychotic many years later and those that did not. Furthermore, these studies, by examining cognitive function longitudinally, have been able to provide important information about the trajectory of cognitive development in those children destined to develop schizophrenia. For example, using data from the MRC child developmental study conducted in the UK, Jones et al. (1994) reported a relationship between cognitive function, assessed at ages eight, 11 and 15, and later schizophrenia; with poor performance on non-verbal tests being the best predictor. In the USA, the Philadelphia birth cohort study (Cannon et al., 2000) investigated the likelihood of later developing schizophrenia in children grouped into quartiles based on IQ assessment at ages four and seven. They reported a 30 to 60% increase in schizophrenia risk per unit decrease in ability category, such that an individual at age four scoring in the deficient range was over five times more likely to develop schizophrenia than one scoring in the high average to superior range. These results remained significant after controlling for the influence of socio-economic factors on outcome. A meta-analytic review (Woodberry et al., 2008) of studies reporting psychometric measures of intelligence in individuals who later went on to develop schizophrenia, compared to those that did not, found consistent evidence for underperformance in the affected individuals. Thus, whereas populations of healthy individuals have an average IQ of 100, Woodberry et al. found the average to be under 95 in the population who later developed schizophrenia, confirming an earlier review (Aylward et al., 1984). Thus the evidence that generalised intellectual impairment predates the onset of overt psychotic symptoms by several years is striking.

The finding that cognitive deficits predate symptom onset, often by a decade or more, seems to rule out the possibility that poor performance on cognitive tests is purely secondary to symptoms of the illness, medication effects or other factors relating to chronic illness and institutionalisation such as poor social and occupational environment. It also suggests that cognitive impairment does not arise *de novo* at the onset of psychosis. This type of methodology also avoids the possibility of selection bias inherent in studies that recruit participants who are already unwell. The latter may describe findings unrepresentative of schizophrenia as a whole, for example because they contain those with higher levels of functioning or those who are in closer contact with services. However, a limitation of cohort studies is that measures of cognition are restricted to those covered by the intelligence and aptitude tests employed for testing the cohort rather than those specifically designed to measure cognition in schizophrenia. Thus some cognitive domains may be underrepresented.

In addition to findings of attenuated cognitive function in children and adolescents who later develop schizophrenia, there is some evidence that this also deteriorates further, prior to illness onset. Data from a birth cohort study (Kremen et al., 1998), examining IQ at age four confirmed that low intellectual function in childhood predicts later schizophrenia. However, it additionally found that decline in intellectual functioning from age four to seven was a substantial predictor of illness, with those demonstrating the largest IQ decline being seven times more likely to later develop schizophrenia. A further longitudinal study of premorbid functioning (Fuller et al., 2002) reported that decline in scholastic performance between the ages of 13 and 16 was related to later onset of schizophrenia. These findings, as well as the observation that estimated premorbid IQ is higher than current IQ in a substantial proportion of patients, suggests that intellectual impairment may be a reflection of the neuropathological processes giving rise to schizophrenia, i.e. a causal risk factor, rather than a relevant but indirect aetiological agent and that, in some, intellectual decline during adolescence may be an early indication of the emerging clinical syndrome.

By contrast, the majority of studies examining the trajectory of cognitive function following onset of schizophrenia do not find evidence for further cognitive decline during the course of the illness. Cross sectional studies have examined individuals with varying length of illness on a single occasion, and have drawn inferences about the course of cognition based on the relationship between chronicity and neuropsychological test performance. Comparing patients with varying lengths of illness in this way, studies have reported equivalent levels of impairment in patients across illness duration (Hyde et al., 1994; Mockler et al., 1997) or cognitive function which changes at the same rate as healthy matched controls (Eyler Zorrilla et al., 2000).

In order to examine changes in cognition across illness duration more directly, longitudinal studies have employed repeated assessment following the onset of psychosis over certain periods of time. These studies can be confounded by attrition but, since changes are being charted in the same individuals, they allow more confident conclusions to be made about the relationship between performance and length of illness. Most longitudinal studies indicate that the course of cognition in schizophrenia is relatively static (see Rund, 1998; Kurtz, 2005). However, the follow-up period in these studies is frequently short, with some of the longest to date examining the same individuals over five to ten years (Wadington and Youssef, 1996; Gold et al., 1999; Heaton et al., 2001; Hoff et al., 2005). Further, those studies with the longest follow-up period have reported data on relatively small numbers of patients, limiting the power to detect changes. Indeed, due to either limited cohort size or short follow-up period, it remains possible that existing studies have failed to detect declining cognition if it occurs at a sufficiently slow rate.

A further issue is that of "normal" change over repeated test occasions, occurring because of practice effects or healthy aging. For example, a recent review of longitudinal studies of cognition in schizophrenia (Szoke et al., 2008) reported evidence for improvement in memory tests with shorter test–retest intervals. Memory measures are among the most susceptible to the effects of practice and the test–retest interval has a substantial influence on the magnitude of the practice effect. It is essential to model such changes in a matched group of healthy controls as practice effects may mask deterioration over the course of the illness and, conversely, typical age related cognitive decline could be ascribed to illness factors in the absence of control data. A number of longitudinal studies have not included a matched group of healthy controls, limiting the conclusions that can be drawn from these studies. Nevertheless, most studies to date converge on the finding that deterioration in excess of that predicted by normal aging does not occur over five to ten years of illness.

The exception to this are studies reporting change in cognitive function in older institutionalised patients with schizophrenia. Longitudinal studies of groups falling into this category report accelerated decline after age 65 (Rajji and Mulsant, 2008). For example, Harvey et al. (1999) examined over 300 schizophrenia patients, aged 65 or more, over a 30 month period. They reported that approximately 30% of the patients who had baseline scores in the less impaired range manifested a worsening of a clinical dementia rating score, changing from that of mild impairment to moderate or severe. In contrast, only 7% of the sample with lower scores at baseline appeared to improve in their cognitive functioning. This suggests that at least a subset of patients in this category worsened during a relatively short period of time and that this was not simply due to test-retest inconsistency (which would predict a similar number improving as declining). Incorporating elements of both a cross-sectional and longitudinal design, Friedman et al. (2001) compared poor outcome schizophrenia patients aged between 20 and 80 to healthy controls and patients with dementia of the Alzheimer's type over six years. Results revealed that the risk of a one or more point decline on the clinical dementia rating scale was minimal for schizophrenia patients under 65 years of age but beyond 65, the probability increased to 37.5%, and between the ages 75 and 80, it was 100%. Percent risk of decline was uniformly 80–90% across all age ranges in the dementia patients and was negligible across all age ranges in the healthy controls.

These studies of elderly schizophrenia patients mainly comprise individuals that were institutionalised and had a poor outcome. The lack of studies examining community dwelling elderly patients with schizophrenia makes it difficult to determine whether this finding of cognitive decline is common to all schizophrenia patients over age 65 or restricted to those that are most unwell. Two such studies of community dwelling elderly schizophrenia patients (Heaton et al., 2001; Palmer et al., 2003) both found no evidence of decline over three years, suggesting that the finding may not generalise. Also relevant are studies of late onset schizophrenia. The majority of patients with schizophrenia have an onset in late adolescence to early adulthood, but some patients develop schizophrenia after the age of 50. A recent review (Rajji and Mulsant, 2008) reported that comparing typical early-onset schizophrenia patients during their later life and late-onset schizophrenia patients of a comparable age returns no difference in terms of their cognitive profiles. The difference in duration of illness in these two groups, yet equivalent levels of cognitive functioning, implies that any decline occurring in geriatric patients with schizophrenia does not develop after a critical number of years of illness but rather at a certain age.

Heterogeneity and Specific Domains of Dysfunction

As outlined above, the evidence for cognitive impairment in individuals with schizophrenia is robust. There seems little doubt that groups of patients with schizophrenia underperform compared to groups of healthy controls, matched in terms of age, sex and socio-economic factors. Nevertheless, underperformance as a group does not necessarily equate to homogeneity of functioning and it is possible that patients may demonstrate different cognitive profiles, with some individuals potentially being unimpaired.

Efforts to define subgroups of patients by cognitive and related clinical phenomena have often utilised cluster analyses to derive subgroups of patients with different abilities and impairments (Heinrichs and Awad, 1993; Goldstein and Shemansky, 1995; Hill et al., 2002). These studies have generally reported clusters reflecting more discrete impairments although the exact nature of the cognitive impairments has varied from study to study. However, all have reported a large cluster of patients with generalised cognitive impairment. In keeping with this, having divided schizophrenia patients into preserved, deteriorated or consistently low IQ based on the difference between estimated premorbid and current IQ measures, Weickert et al. (2000) demonstrated that these groups evinced different profiles of current neuropsychological test performance. Notably, the preserved IQ group did not show impairment on all cognitive domains, only on tests of attention or higher order executive function; a finding that has been replicated (Kremen et al., 2008). Moreover, Wilk et al. (2005) demonstrated that, even when schizophrenia patients are one-to-one matched with healthy controls on full scale WAIS IQ, examination of performance on the subtests that are used to calculate full scale IQ reveals underperformance on those requiring speeded visual processing and memory. This suggests that, even in patients who may appear cognitively intact, subtle deficits remain and that cognitive impairment is a core feature of schizophrenia, being common to all patients.

It has been suggested that individual variation in performance across cognitive domains may be meaningful, with different cognitive deficits having different neurobiological substrates. In line with this suggestion is evidence that first degree relatives of patients with schizophrenia show deficits on some cognitive domains found to be impaired in schizophrenia but not others (Thompson et al., 2005; Skelley et al., 2008; Ceaser et al., 2008). This suggests that only some cognitive deficits found in individuals with schizophrenia are involved in genetic risk for schizophrenia and these may qualitatively differ from those cognitive domains that are impaired in patients but not first degree relatives. The following section reviews some of the most prominent domains of cognition that have been investigated and reported to be disproportionately or selectively attenuated in schizophrenia.

Executive Functions

One such proposed impairment is in executive function, also more recently labelled "cognitive control", reflecting abnormal frontostriatal processing. The executive system controls and manages other cognitive functions using a range of processes such as attention, working memory and inhibition for the planning, execution and monitoring of goal directed operations. Deficits in executive function have long been considered to be one of the hallmark cognitive characteristics of schizophrenia and numerous studies have demonstrated underperformance of patients with schizophrenia on tasks designed to measure this (Kerns et al., 2008). Cognitive batteries, as described in the previous section, frequently contain measures of executive function and, thus, impairment in this domain of functioning within the context of a generalised deficit is well documented. However, some studies have reported disproportionately poor performance on executive tasks (Elliott et al., 1995; Evans et al., 1997; Chan et al., 2006). Shallice et al. (1991) examined five patients with schizophrenia using case study approach to carry out detailed assessments and concluded that, 'all chronic schizophrenics have problems with processes tapped by "frontal" tests and that some schizophrenics have, in addition, a more widespread cognitive impairment'. Further, Kremen et al. (2001) examined performance on a number of neuropsychological measures in schizophrenia patients and healthy controls matched on current IQ and categorised them as either low-average or average IQ. The patients underperformed on a number of cognitive domains compared to controls in the same IQ subgroup. However, only the domain of executive function was poorer in schizophrenia patients in both IQ subgroups.

Possibly the most well known test of executive control is the Wisconsin card sort test in which a subject is required to sort cards according to rules that they need to deduce and that change from time to time. Performance on this task requires the use of many executive processes, including maintaining a task goal or rule, dynamically adjusting performance after error feedback, generating rules to guide performance, inhibiting of previously reinforced responses, and developing a strategy. Patients with schizophrenia have been observed to perform to a similar degree to that seen in patients with frontal-lobe lesions on this task (Pantelis et al., 1999). A review of studies examining the Wisconsin card sort test in schizophrenia (Laws, 1999) found substantial evidence that patients perform more poorly than controls. However, the effect size for Wechsler Adult Intelligence Scale IQ scores, taken from the same studies, was greater than any from the Wisconsin card sort test, suggesting that deficits were not selective and could be explained as a result of general intellectual deficits. Thus, despite some studies reporting specific or disproportionate dysfunction of executive processes in schizophrenia, much of the evidence may still be commensurate with more generalised dysfunction (Braver et al., 1999). In keeping with this, whilst Warrington et al.

(1986) reported that significant IQ decrements do not occur in many cases of frontal lobe injury in adults, poor performance on tests such as the Wisconsin card sort test correlates with lower IQ in schizophrenia patients (Goldstein et al., 1996).

Recently, schizophrenia patient and healthy control performance on a neuropsychological test battery has been compared using modelling to determine any differences in the relationship between domains of cognition (Dickinson et al., 2008). In both patients and controls, performance across many cognitive domains, including one represented by measures of executive function, was explained by a higher order, common ability factor. These findings were reported in the context of poorer performance in the schizophrenia patients than the controls and suggest that specific deficits observed in schizophrenia are operating via general ability. However, the study did report evidence for some direct illness effects on the domains of verbal memory and processing speed, suggesting that additional selective deficits may occur in these cognitive domains, not solely mediated by general ability.

Episodic Long-Term Memory

The ability to successfully remember a prior event or thought is the outcome of a complex set of episodic memory processes that occur at different times and include encoding, storage and retrieval. The obvious relevance of this cognitive domain to schizophrenia is the way in which it influences our understanding of the world and personal relationships. A meta-analysis of neuropsychological test performance in schizophrenia (Heinrichs and Zakzanis, 1998) reported evidence of deficits in all cognitive domains examined over the 204 studies reviewed but found the largest effect size for memory functions. They reported evidence for impairment in both verbal and non-verbal memory although verbal memory deficits were more consistent. A further meta-analysis (Aleman et al., 1999) attempted to characterise the memory deficits in schizophrenia by individually examining the various specific measures of memory in 70 studies of schizophrenia. The findings suggested impairment in all long-term memory measures including free recall, cued recall, and recognition of verbal and non-verbal material.

Reporting on their findings of evidence for a direct effect of diagnosis on verbal memory and processing speed in an hierarchical factor analysis, Dickinson et al. (2008) concluded that these aspects of cognitive functioning may be "more specifically implicated in schizophrenia than other cognitive domains". In line with their findings on verbal memory, a number of studies have demonstrated selective impairment in the domain of memory. For example, Bilder et al. (2000) reported that, although many of their first episode cohort demonstrated both memory and executive impairment, memory deficits were observed in a subset of otherwise neuropsychologically normal patients. Further, a recent study of patients with first-episode schizophrenia (Leeson et al., 2009b) has demonstrated that, despite evidence of impairment in all cognitive domains measured, retention in verbal memory is independent of other cognitive measures including IQ, executive function and even verbal learning.

Whilst performance on tasks demanding long-term memory processes is poorer in schizophrenia patients than healthy controls, memory processes also require cognitive control, making it difficult to separate the contribution of different cognitive domains to impaired performance. Under many circumstances, long-term memory encoding and retrieval entails executive processes that affect the ability to plan, initiate strategies, and inhibit distractions. For example, the most effective encoding of word lists requires strategies such as categorising or mentalising items and this aspect of word list learning has been reported to be impaired in patients with schizophrenia. Kristian Hill et al. (2004) examined first episode schizophrenia patients using the California verbal learning task; a task that allows the use of categorisation to facilitate encoding and later retrieval. They reported a strong relationship between the employment of semantic organizational strategies and reduced learning capacity, implicating prefrontal dysfunction as a contributor to memory deficits in schizophrenia.

A further aspect of memory that is of interest in schizophrenia (Ragland et al., 2009) is that of reinforcement learning. Many problem-solving tasks entail a process in which each successive step is informed by the results of the immediately previous strategic effort. If, however, the ability to detect failure is reduced, the likelihood of developing a successful trial and error strategy will be limited. A failure of reinforcement learning could explain deficient performance observed in the Wisconsin card sort task where patients fail to shift attention from a previously learned response. A variant of this task, the ID/ED attentional set shifting task which allows the component processes of the Wisconsin card sort task to be decomposed, has provided support for this notion. Schizophrenia patients fail to reach criterion on reversals of relatively simple rules not requiring the consideration of multiple stimulus dimensions (Elliott et al., 1995) and, in the case of schizophrenia patients with longer illness duration, this is at levels worse than those observed in patients with frontal lobe lesions (Pantelis et al., 1999).

Working Memory

In addition to reporting deficits in all aspects of long-term memory, the review by Aleman et al. (1999) also found evidence for poor digit span, indicating that working memory is impaired. Working memory refers to a cognitive system involved in the maintenance and manipulation of information over a short period of time, serving as a temporary workspace. Working memory is responsible for operations include rehearsal of phonological or visuospatial data as well as complex procedures such as planning, problem solving, and reasoning. Moreover, the contents of working memory are thought to be ''buffered,'' such that they are protected from interference due to either distracting information or decay over time (Baddeley, 2003). Thus, this aspect of functioning can be seen as both a mnemonic and executive process.

Findings of impairment in relevant cognitive domains may be explained by working memory deficits. For example Huddy et al. (2007) examined eye movement during a computerised Tower of London Task, assessing planning, in first-episode schizophrenia patients. Compared to healthy controls, patients made more planning errors and decision times were longer. However, the patients showed the same gaze biases as controls prior to making a response, using appropriate fixation strategies to plan and elaborate solutions but with increased duration of long gaze periods towards the screen. This suggested that the patients had difficulty in encoding the essential features of the stimulus array and is compatible with slowing of working memory consolidation.

Lee and Park (2005) reviewed studies that specifically examined working memory in schizophrenia. Measures considered to tap working memory included visual and verbal tasks requiring maintenance of information in memory such as number span and verbal list learning, as well as those that also required manipulation of the information such as letter number sequencing where subjects are given a list such as Q1B83J2 and required to place the numbers in numerical order and then the letters in alphabetical order. Working memory deficits were evident in all included studies, but the extent of the working memory deficit was unrelated to the length of delay involved in the task, implicating a deficit in encoding or retrieval rather than storage. Again, this suggests that those higher order executive processes responsible for generating a search strategy underpinned poor performance rather than a failure of memory processes *per se*. However, a recent review (Forbes et al., 2008) attempted to delineate the different types of working memory in schizophrenia in order to determine whether deficits were limited to certain domains. They examined visuospatial, phonological and executive working memory, in keeping with the fractionation in Baddeley's model of working memory (Baddeley, 2003). Although the study confirmed the presence of working memory deficits in schizophrenia, these did not appear to be restricted to a particular aspect of working memory.

Processing Speed

Processing speed refers to the speed at which cognitive operations can be executed. Driven by some notable findings, this cognitive process has recently become a focus of interest in the schizophrenia literature. As previously outlined, when schizophrenia patients and controls are one-to one matched for full scale IQ, controls show better performance on subtests dependent on processing speed (Wilk et al., 2005). Also, Dickinson et al. (2008) have reported evidence that deficits in processing speed observed in patients with schizophrenia were not wholly mediated via general ability, suggesting that this might represent an independent deficit.

The digit symbol substitution task, a subtest of the Wechsler Adult Intelligence Scale (Wechsler, 1997) is commonly used as a measure of processing speed. This simple pencil and paper task requires subjects to use a key to match as many digits as possible with their corresponding symbols in two minutes. Two studies reviewing the literature (Henry and Crawford, 2005; Dickinson et al., 2007) showed that deficits on the digit symbol substitution task were robust and substantial. Notably, the effect size in both these meta-analytic reviews were larger for digit symbol than for other cognitive functions including those that have received much more attention such as memory and executive function. Dickinson (2008) argues that, rather than taking this finding of disproportionately poor performance on digit symbol tasks as evidence of a discrete cognitive impairment, it should be considered a central feature of the general cognitive impairment observed in schizophrenia. This explanation is certainly plausible given how fundamental speeded processing is in completing a wide range of cognitive tasks.

It does appear that the digit symbol substitution, whether reflecting a specific and selective impairment or simply tapping something central to the general cognitive deficit of schizophrenia, is particularly sensitive, even when compared to other tasks designed to measure processing speed. Dickinson et al. (2007) found a smaller effect size than for digit symbol substitution on both the trail making test part A, where subjects are required to draw a line to connect randomly arranged numbers into a consecutive order, and the Stroop task, where subjects are required to name the colour of the ink of a word which is incongruent with the required response. These tasks may be operationally simpler or involve different subprocesses than the digit symbol task. The difference in strength of effect between tasks seems to demonstrate that the concept of processing speed may be too simplistic and the deficit lies in a particular aspect of speeded processing or alternatively, an interaction between this domain of functioning and another.

Conclusions

With evidence from hundreds of studies, cognitive impairment is now widely recognised as an important and reliable feature of schizophrenia. The weight of current evidence suggests that the cognitive impairment in schizophrenia is expressed before clinical onset of the disorder, deteriorates further at the time of psychosis development and then remains stable, at least over the early years of the illness. Whilst evidence of linear decline with increasing age and chronicity has not been reported, there may be further cognitive deterioration in excess of normal aging in patients after the age of 65, at least in those most severely affected. With respect to the exact nature of the deficit, while there is certainly underperformance in a range of cognitive domains in schizophrenia, giving rise to a general impairment, whether there are more specific areas of dysfunction over and above this is not clear. The interdependence of various cognitive domains means that multiple functions operate in concert during most real life situations. This is also reflected in neuropsychological test design, rendering the task of concluding exactly what deficient processes underpin poor observed performance very difficult. Joyce and Huddy (2004) argue that, to better understand cognitive abnormalities in psychotic disorders, we need to use experimental approaches that allow task performance to be broken down into more basic cognitive processes than currently is the case in many studies. This objective is particularly necessary given the importance now placed on cognition in schizophrenia.

The development of both psychological (McGurk et al., 2007; Wykes, 2008) and pharmacological (Marder and Fenton, 2004; Carter, 2005) interventions aimed at remediation of cognitive deficits is already in progress. Thus, the need for a clear and accurate understanding of which cognitive functions are impaired and or remain intact, and how these are related to clinical outcome and social function is evident. Already, a large scale initiative is in place with the goal of identifying cognitive measurement approaches that may be implemented in efforts to develop treatments for impaired cognition in schizophrenia (Carter and Barch, 2007). The current focus on cognition is also evident in the fact that the identification of important genes in schizophrenia is increasingly looking to cognition as an intermediate phenotype of the disorder (Owen et al., 2007).

References

Adityanjee, A., Aderibigbe, Y.A., Theodoridis, D., Vieweg, V.R. Dementia praecox to schizophrenia: The first 100 years. *Psychiatr Clin Neurosci* 53: 437-448, 2002.

Aleman, A., Hijman, R., de Haan, E.H.F., Kahn, R.S. Memory Impairment in Schizophrenia: A Meta-Analysis. *Am J Psychiatr* 156: 1358-1366, 1999.

Aylward, E., Walker, E., Bettes, B. Intelligence in schizophrenia: meta-analysis of the research. *Schizophr Bull* 10: 430-459, 1984.

Badcock, J.C., Dragovic, M., Waters, F.A.V., Jablensky, A. Dimensions of intelligence in schizophrenia: evidence from patients with preserved, deteriorated and compromised intellect. *J Psychiatr Res* 39: 11-19, 2005.

Baddeley, A. Working memory: looking back and looking forward. *Nat Rev Neurosci* 4: 829-839, 2003.

Bilder, R.M., Goldman, R.S., Robinson, D., Reiter, G., Bell, L., Bates, J.A., Pappadopulos, E., Willson, D.F., Alvir, J.M., Woerner, M.G., Geisler, S., Kane, J.M., Lieberman, J.A. Neuropsychology of First-Episode Schizophrenia: Initial Characterization and Clinical Correlates. *Am J Psychiatr* 157: 549-559, 2000.

Bilder, R.M., Turkel, E., Lipschutz-Borch, L., Lieberman JA Antipsychotic medication effects on neuropsychological functions. *Psychopharmacol Bull* 28: 353-366, 1992.

Black, D.W., Boffeli, T.J. Simple schizophrenia: past, present, and future. *Am J Psychiatr* 146: 1267-1273, 1989.

Braver, T.S., Barch, D.M., Cohen, J.D. Cognition and control in schizophrenia: a computational model of dopamine and prefrontal function. *Biol Psychiatr* 46: 312-328, 1999.

Broen, W.E., Storms, L.H. A theory of response interference in schizophrenia. *Progress in Experimental Personality Research* 4: 269-312, 1967.

Cannon, T.D., Bearden, C.E., Hollister, J.M., Rosso, I.M., Sanchez, L.E., Hadley, T. Childhood Cognitive Functioning in Schizophrenia Patients and Their Unaffected Siblings: A Prospective Cohort Study. *Schizophr Bull* 26: 379-393, 2000.

Carter, C.S. Applying New Approaches From Cognitive Neuroscience to Enhance Drug Development for the Treatment of Impaired Cognition in Schizophrenia. *Schizophr Bull* 31: 810-815, 2005.

Carter, C.S., Barch, D.M. Cognitive Neuroscience-Based Approaches to Measuring and Improving Treatment Effects on Cognition in Schizophrenia: The CNTRICS Initiative. *Schizophr Bull* 33: 1131-1137, 2007.

Ceaser, A.E., Goldberg, T.E., Egan, M.F., McMahon, R.P., Weinberger, D.R., Gold, J.M. Set-Shifting Ability and Schizophrenia: A Marker of Clinical Illness or an Intermediate Phenotype? *Biol Psychiatr* 64: 782-788, 2008.

Chan, R.C.K., Chen, E.Y.H., Law, C.W. Specific executive dysfunction in patients with first-episode medication-naive schizophrenia. *Schizophr Res* 82: 51-64, 2006.

Cohen, J.D., Insel, T.R. Cognitive Neuroscience and Schizophrenia: Translational Research in Need of a Translator. *Biol Psychiatr* 64: 2-3, 2008.

Crawford, J.R., Besson, J.A., Bremner, M., Ebmeier, K.P., Cochrane, R.H., Kirkwood, K. Estimation of premorbid intelligence in schizophrenia. *Br J Psychiatr* 161: 69-74, 1992.

Crawford, J.R., Parker, D.M., Besson, J.A. Estimation of premorbid intelligence in organic conditions. *Br J Psychiatr* 153: 178-181, 1998.

David, A.S., Malmberg, S., Brandt, L., Allebeck, P., Lewis, G. IQ and risk for schizophrenia: a population-based cohort study. *Psychol Med* 27: 1311-1323, 1997.

Dickinson, D. Digit symbol coding and general cognitive ability in schizophrenia: worth another look? *Br J Psychiatr* 193: 354-356, 2008.

Dickinson, D., Ragland, J.D., Gold, J.M., Gur, R.C. General and Specific Cognitive Deficits in Schizophrenia: Goliath Defeats David? *Biol Psychiatr* 64: 823-827, 2008.

Dickinson, D., Ramsey, M.E., Gold, J.M. Overlooking the Obvious: A Meta-analytic Comparison of Digit Symbol Coding Tasks and Other Cognitive Measures in Schizophrenia. *Arch Gen Psychiatr* 64: 532-542, 2007.

Elliott, R., McKenna, P.J., Robbins, T.W., Sahakian, B.J. Neuropsychological evidence for frontostriatal dysfunction in schizophrenia. *Psychol Med* 25: 619-630, 1995.

Evans, J.J., Chua, S.E., McKenna, P.J., WILSONWilson, B.A. Assessment of the dysexecutive syndrome in schizophrenia. *Psychol Med* 27: 635-646, 1997.

Eyler Zorrilla, L.T., Heaton, R.K., McAdams, L.A., Zisook, S., Harris, M.J., Jeste, D.V. Cross-Sectional Study of Older Outpatients Withwith Schizophrenia and Healthy Comparison Subjects: No Differences in Age-Related Cognitive Decline. *Am J Psychiatr* 157: 1324-1326, 2000.

Forbes, N., Carrick, L., McIntosh, A., Lawrie, S. Working memory in schizophrenia: a meta-analysis. *Psychol Med* 39; 889-905epub ahead of print:, 2009 8.

Friedman, J.I., Harvey, P.D., Coleman, T., Moriarty, P.J., Bowie, C., Parrella, M., White, L., Adler, D., Davis, K.L. Six-Year Follow-Up Study of Cognitive and Functional Status Across the Lifespan in Schizophrenia: A Comparison With Alzheimer's Disease and Normal Aging. *Am J Psychiatr* 158: 1441-1448, 2001.

Frith, C.D. Consciousness, information processing and schizophrenia. *Br J Psychiatr* 134: 225-235, 1979.

Fuller, R., Nopoulos, P., Arndt, S., O'Leary, D., Ho, B.C., Andreasen, N.C. Longitudinal Assessment of Premorbid Cognitive Functioning in Patients With Schizophrenia Through Examination of Standardized Scholastic Test Performance. *Am J Psychiatr* 159: 1183-1189, 2002.

Gold, J.M. Is cognitive impairment in schizophrenia ready for diagnostic prime time? *World Psychiatr* 7: 32-33, 2008.

Gold, J.M., Goldberg, R.W., McNary, S.W., Dixon, L.B., Lehman, A.F. Cognitive Correlates of Job Tenure Among Patients With Severe Mental Illness. *Am J Psychiatr* 159: 1395-1402, 2002.

Gold, S., Arndt, S., Nopoulos, P., O'Leary, D.S., Andreasen, N.C. Longitudinal Study of Cognitive Function in First-Episode and Recent-Onset Schizophrenia. *Am J Psychiatr* 156: 1342-1348, 1999.

Goldstein, G., Beers, S.R., Shemansky, W.J. Neuropsychological differences between schizophrenic patients with heterogeneous Wisconsin Card Sorting Test performance. *Schizophr Res* 21: 13-18, 1996.

Goldstein, G., Shemansky, W.J. Influences on cognitive heterogeneity in schizophrenia. *Schizophr Res* 18: 59-69, 1995.

Green, M.F. What are the functional consequences of neurocognitive deficits in schizophrenia? *Am J Psychiatr* 153: 321-330, 1996.

Green, M.F., Kern, R.S., Heaton, R.K. Longitudinal studies of cognition and functional outcome in schizophrenia: implications for MATRICS. *Schizophr Res* 72: 41-51, 2004.

Green, M.F., Kern, R.S., Braff, D.L., Mintz, J. Neurocognitive Deficits and Functional Outcome in Schizophrenia: Are We Measuring the "Right Stuff"? *Schizophr Bull* 26: 119-136, 2000.

Harvey, P.D., Silverman, J.M., Mohs, R.C., Parrella, M., White, L., Powchik, P., Davidson, M., Davis, K.L. Cognitive decline in late-life schizophrenia: a longitudinal study of geriatric chronically hospitalized patients. *Biol Psychiatr* 45: 32-40, 1999.

Heaton, R.K., Gladsjo, J.A., Palmer, B.W., Kuck, J., Marcotte, T.D., Jeste, D.V. Stability and Course of Neuropsychological Deficits in Schizophrenia. *Arch Gen Psychiatr* 58: 24-32, 2001.

Hegarty, J.D., Baldessarini, R.J., Tohen, M., Waternaux, C., Oepen, G. One hundred years of schizophrenia: a meta-analysis of the outcome literature. *Am J Psychiatr* 151: 1409-1416, 1994.

Heinrichs, R.W., Zakzanis, K.K. Neurocognitive deficit in schizophrenia: A quantitative review of the evidence. *Neuropsychology* 12: 426-445, 1998.

Heinrichs, R.W., Awad, A.G. Neurocognitive subtypes of chronic schizophrenia. *Schizophr Res* 9: 49-58, 1993.

Hemsley, D.R. What have cognitive deficits to do with schizophrenic symptoms? *Br J Psychiatr* 130: 167-173, 1977.

Henry, J.D., Crawford, J.R. A meta-analytic review of verbal fluency deficits in schizophrenia relative to other neurocognitive deficits. *Cognit Neuropsychiatry* 10: 1-33, 2005.

Hill, S.K., Ragland, J.D., Gur, R.C., Gur, R.E. Neuropsychological profiles delineate distinct profiles of schizophrenia, an interaction between memory and executive function, and uneven distribution of clinical subtypes. *J Clin Exp Neuropsychol* 24: 765-780, 2002.

Hoff, A.L., Svetina, C., Shields, G., Stewart, J., DeLisi, L.E. Ten year longitudinal study of neuropsychological functioning subsequent to a first episode of schizophrenia. *Schizophr Res* 78: 27-34, 2005.

Huddy, V., Hodgson, T.L., Kapasi, M., Mutsatsa, S.H., Harrison, I., Barnes, T.R., Joyce, E.M. Gaze strategies during planning in first-episode psychosis. *J Abnorm Psychol* 116: 589-598, 2007.

Hutton, S.B., Puri, B.K., Duncan, L.J., Robbins, T.W., Barnes, T.R.E., Joyce, E.M. Executive function in first-episode schizophrenia. *Psychol Med* 28: 463-473, 1998.

Hyde, T.M., Nawroz, S., Goldberg, T.E., Bigelow, L.B., Strong, D., Ostrem, J.L., Weinberger, D.R., Kleinman, J.E. Is there cognitive decline in schizophrenia? A cross-sectional study. *Br J Psychiatr* 164: 494-500, 1994.

Johnstone, E.C., Crow, T.J., Frith, C.D., Husband, J., Kreel, L. Cerebral ventricular size and cognitive impairment in chronic schizophrenia. *Lancet* 2: 924-926, 1976.

Jones, P., Murray, R., Jones, P., Rodgers, B., Marmot, M. Child developmental risk factors for adult schizophrenia in the British 1946 birth cohort. *The Lancet* 344: 1398-1402, 1994.

Joyce, E.M., Huddy, V. Defining the cognitive impairment in schizophrenia. *Psychol Med* 34: 1151-1155, 2004.

Joyce, E.M., Hutton, S.B., Mutsatsa, S.H., Barnes, T.R.E. Cognitive heterogeneity in first-episode schizophrenia. *Br J Psychiatr* 187: 516-522, 2005.

Keefe, R.S.E., Eesley, C.E., Poe, M.P. Defining a cognitive function decrement in schizophrenia. *Biol Psychiatr* 57: 688-691, 2005.

Keefe, R.S.E., Fenton, W.S. How Should DSM-V Criteria for Schizophrenia Include Cognitive Impairment? *Schizophr Bull* 33: 912-920, 2007.

Kerns, J.G., Nuechterlein, K.H., Braver, T.S., Barch, D.M. Executive Functioning Component Mechanisms and Schizophrenia. *Biol Psychiatr* 64: 26-33, 2008.

Kremen, W.S., Buka, S.L., Seidman, L.J., Goldstein, J.M., Koren, D., Tsuang, M.T. IQ Decline Duringduring Childhood and Adult Psychotic Symptoms in a Community Sample: A 19-Year Longitudinal Study. *Am J Psychiatr* 155: 672-677, 1998.

Kremen, W.S., Seidman, L.J., Faraone, S.V., Tsuang, M.T. IQ decline in cross-sectional studies of schizophrenia: Methodology and interpretation. *Psychiatry Res* 158: 181-194, 2008.

Kremen, W.S., Seidman, L.J., Faraone, S.V., Tsuang, M.T. Intelligence quotient and neuropsychological profiles in patients with schizophrenia and in normal volunteers. *Biol Psychiatr* 50: 453-462, 2001.

Kristian Hill, S., Beers, S.R., Kmiec, J.A., Keshavan, M.S., Sweeney, J.A. Impairment of verbal memory and learning in antipsychotic-naive patients with first-episode schizophrenia. *Schizophr Res* 68: 127-136, 2004.

Kurtz, M.M. Neurocognitive impairment across the lifespan in schizophrenia: an update. *Schizophr Res* 74: 15-26, 2005.

Laws, K.R. A meta-analytic review of Wisconsin Card Sort studies in schizophrenia: general intellectual deficit in disguise? *Cognit Neuropsychiatry* 4: 1-30, 1999.

Lee, J., Park, S. Working Memory Impairments in Schizophrenia: A Meta-Analysis. *J Abnorm Psychol* 114: 599-611, 2005.

Leeson, V.C., Barnes, T.R.E., Hutton, S.B., Ron, M.A., Joyce, E.M. IQ as a predictor of functional outcome in schizophrenia: A longitudinal, four-year study of first-episode psychosis. *Schizophr Res* 107: 55-60, 2009a.

Leeson, V.C., Robbins, T.W., Franklin, C., Harrison, M., Harrison, I., Ron, M.A., Barnes, T.R.E., Joyce, E.M. Dissociation of Long Term Verbal Memory and Fronto-Executive Impairment in First-Episode Psychosis. *Psychol Med* , 2009b.

MacCabe, J.H. Population-based Cohort Studies on Premorbid Cognitive Function in Schizophrenia. *Epidemiol Rev* 30: 77-83, 2008.

Marder, S.R., Fenton, W. Measurement and Treatment Research to Improve Cognition in Schizophrenia: NIMH MATRICS initiative to support the development of agents for improving cognition in schizophrenia. *Schizophr Res* 72: 5-9, 2004.

McGurk, S.R., Twamley, E.W., Sitzer, D.I., McHugo, G.J., Mueser, K.T. A Meta-Analysis of Cognitive Remediation in Schizophrenia. *Am J Psychiatr* 164: 1791-1802, 2007.

Mockler, D., Riordan, J., Sharma, T. Memory and intellectual deficits do not decline with age in schizophrenia. *Schizophr Res* 26: 1-7, 1997.

Mohamed, S., Paulsen, J.S., O'Leary, D., Arndt, S., Andreasen, N. Generalized Cognitive Deficits in Schizophrenia: A Study of First-Episode Patients. *Arch Gen Psychiatr* 56: 749-754, 1999.

Murray, C.J., Lopez, A.D. Global mortality, disability, and the contribution of risk factors: Global Burden of Disease Study. *The Lancet* 349: 1436-1442, 1997.

Nelson,H.E. & Willison,J.R. (1991) The Revised National Adult Reading Test-Test Manual. Windsor: NFER-Nelson.

Owen, M.J., Craddock, N., Jablensky, A. The Genetic Deconstruction of Psychosis. *Schizophr Bull* 33: 905-911, 2007.

Palmer, B.W., Bondi, M.W., Twamley, E.W., Thal, L., Golshan, S., Jeste, D.V. Are Late-Onset Schizophrenia Spectrum Disorders Neurodegenerative Conditions? Annual Rates of Change on Two Dementia Measures. *J Neuropsychiatry Clin Neurosci* 15: 45-52, 2003.

Palmer, B.W., Heaton, R.K., Paulsen, J.S., Kuck, J., Braff, D.L., Harris, M.J., Zisook, S., Jeste, D.V. Is it possible to be schizophrenic yet neuropsychologically normal? *Neuropsychology* 11: 437-446, 1997.

Pantelis, C., Barber, F.Z., Barnes, T.R.E., Nelson, H.E., Owen, A.M., Robbins, T.W. Comparison of set-shifting ability in patients with chronic schizophrenia and frontal lobe damage. *Schizophr Res* 37: 251-270, 1999.

Ragland, J.D., Cools, R., Frank, M., Pizzagalli, D.A., Preston, A., Ranganath, C., Wagner, A.D. CNTRICS Final Task Selection: Long-Term Memory. *Schizophr Bull* 35: 197-212, 2009.

Rajji, T.K., Mulsant, B.H. Nature and course of cognitive function in late-life schizophrenia: A systematic review. *Schizophr Res* 102: 122-140, 2008.

Rund, B.R. A Review of Longitudinal Studies of Cognitive Functions in Schizophrenia Patients. *Schizophr Bull* 24: 425-435, 1998.

Russell, A.J., Munro, J., Jones, P., Hayward, P., Hemsley, D.R., Murray, R.M. The National Adult Reading Test as a measure of premorbid IQ in schizophrenia. *Br J Clin Psychol* 39: 297-305, 2000.

Saha, S., Chant, D., Welham, J., McGrath, J. A Systematic Review of the Prevalence of Schizophrenia. *PLoS Medicine* 2: e141, 2005.

Shallice, T., Burgess, P., Frith, C.D. Can the neuropsychological case-study approach be applied to schizophrenia? *Psychol Med* 21: 661-673, 1991.

Skelley, S.L., Goldberg, T.E., Egan, M.F., Weinberger, D.R., Gold, J.M. Verbal and visual memory: Characterizing the clinical and intermediate phenotype in schizophrenia. *Schizophr Res* 105: 78-85, 2008.

Szoke, A., Trandafir, A., Dupont, M.E., Meary, A., Schurhoff, F., Leboyer, M. Longitudinal studies of cognition in schizophrenia: meta-analysis. *Br J Psychiatr* 192: 248-257, 2008.

Thompson, J.L., Watson, J.R., Steinhauer, S.R., Goldstein, G., Pogue-Geile, M.F. Indicators of Genetic Liability to Schizophrenia: A Sibling Study of Neuropsychological Performance. *Schizophr Bull* 31: 85-96, 2005.

Velligan, D.I., Mahurin, R.K., Diamond, P.L., Hazleton, B.C., Eckert, S.L., Miller, A.L. The functional significance of symptomatology and cognitive function in schizophrenia. *Schizophr Res* 25: 21-31, 1997.

Wadington, J.L., Youssef, H.A. Cognitive dysfunction in chronic schizophrenia followed prospectively over 10 years and its longitudinal relationship to the emergence of tardive dyskinesia. *Psychol Med* 26: 681-688, 1996.

Warrington, E.K., James, M., Maciejewski, C. The WAIS as a lateralizing and localizing diagnostic instrument: a study of 656 patients with unilateral cerebral lesions. *Neuropsychologia* 24: 223-239, 1986.

Wechsler,D. (1997) Wechsler Adult Intelligence Scale-3rd Edition (WAIS-3). San Antonio, TX: Harcourt Assessment.

Wechsler,D. (2001) The Wechsler Test of Adult Reading (WTAR). San Antonio, TX: The Psychological Corporation.

Weickert, T.W., Goldberg, T.E., Gold, J.M., Bigelow, L.B., Egan, M.F., Weinberger, D.R. Cognitive Impairments in Patients Withwith Schizophrenia Displaying Preserved and Compromised Intellect. *Arch Gen Psychiatr* 57: 907-913, 2000.

Weinberger, D.R., Torrey, E.F., Neophytides, A.N., Wyatt, R.J. Structural abnormalities in the cerebral cortex of chronic schizophrenic patients. *Arch Gen Psychiatr* 36: 935-939, 1979.

Wilk, C.M., Gold, J.M., McMahon, R.P., Humber, K., Iannone, V.N., Buchanan, R.W. No, it is not possible to be schizophrenic yet neuropsychologically normal. *Neuropsychology* 19: 778-786, 2005.

Wilk, C.M., Gold, J.M., Humber, K., Dickerson, F., Fenton, W.S., Buchanan, R.W. Brief cognitive assessment in schizophrenia: normative data for the Repeatable Battery for the Assessment of Neuropsychological Status. *Schizophr Res* 70: 175-186, 2004.

Woodberry, K.A., Giuliano, A.J., Seidman, L.J. Premorbid IQ in Schizophrenia: A Meta-Analytic Review. *Am J Psychiatr* 165: 579-587, 2008.

Wykes, T. Review: Cognitive remediation improves cognitive functioning in schizophrenia. *Evid Based Ment Health* 11: 117, 2008.

INDEX

4

4-hydroxynonenal, 203, 216

A

Aβ, v, viii, 40, 41, 50, 67, 68, 69, 70, 71, 72, 73, 74, 75, 76, 77, 78, 79, 85, 86, 87, 90, 91, 92, 93, 94, 95, 96, 97, 98, 99, 100, 101, 102, 199, 202, 203, 204, 205, 206, 209
A1c, 128
AA, 58, 86, 214
AAA, 244, 248
AAV, 97
abnormalities, 117, 217, 238, 264, 274, 280
academic, 102
accuracy, 232, 233, 255, 257, 259, 261
ACE, 38, 45, 49, 56, 58, 59, 60, 61
acetate, 58
acetylation, 207, 208, 210, 213, 214
acetylcholine, 69, 78, 193, 221, 236
acid, 42, 43, 61, 68, 95, 115, 125, 127, 129, 139, 147, 164, 176, 196, 200, 202, 206, 210, 212, 216, 247
acidic, viii, 48, 57, 58, 185, 187, 190
acidification, 195
acromegaly, 117
actin, 199, 200, 201, 208, 212, 214, 215
action potential, 72
activated receptors, 167
activation, 22, 33, 41, 44, 49, 51, 54, 60, 65, 67, 69, 71, 72, 78, 79, 89, 91, 96, 100, 108, 121, 137, 138, 139, 165, 166, 168, 169, 171, 172, 173, 177, 178, 179, 180, 182, 183, 184, 186, 188, 189, 190, 191, 203, 217, 248
activators, 48
acute, viii, 72, 74, 76, 81, 91, 145, 146, 149, 153, 161, 164, 165, 173, 178, 211, 212
Adams, 23, 30, 56, 57
adenosine triphosphate, 178
adenovirus, 95, 96, 106, 112
adhesion, 55, 58, 59, 201
adipocyte, 55
administration, 49, 53, 60, 71, 75, 76, 79, 87, 91, 92, 93, 96, 97, 98, 103, 105, 112, 119, 123, 138, 141, 173, 184, 199, 202, 205, 209, 214, 224
adolescence, 263, 267, 269
adolescents, 267
ADP, 206
adult, 10, 21, 42, 44, 47, 56, 121, 138, 201, 277
adulthood, 158, 269
adults, 10, 11, 12, 13, 14, 15, 16, 22, 23, 24, 26, 28, 29, 30, 32, 33, 155, 199, 264, 271
advanced glycation end products, 42, 184
adverse event, 89, 92, 94, 99
aetiology, 212, 264
affective experience, 13
African American, 148, 159
age, 10, 11, 13, 14, 15, 16, 29, 31, 33, 39, 40, 41, 42, 61, 62, 70, 87, 88, 96, 97, 98, 100, 104, 108, 114, 116, 117, 120, 121, 122, 128, 132, 133, 134, 137, 142, 148, 149, 152, 155, 159, 162, 168, 174, 178, 181, 188, 190, 193, 194, 195, 201, 206, 223, 225, 226, 227, 229, 245, 247, 248, 252, 253, 255, 259, 265, 266, 267, 268, 269, 274, 278
ageing, 154, 180, 227, 231
agent, viii, 52, 53, 119, 120, 121, 122, 123, 137, 139, 163, 173, 199, 205, 267

agents, vii, viii, 50, 52, 97, 114, 117, 118, 120, 121, 122, 123, 124, 128, 136, 137, 138, 167, 174, 180, 181, 187, 188, 191, 208, 214, 278
age-related macular degeneration, 193
AGEs, 42
aggregates, 48, 53, 64, 68, 101, 109, 114, 119, 125, 129, 132, 186, 202, 210
aggregation, 48, 49, 58, 59, 86, 95, 101, 105, 111, 167, 174, 177, 178, 186, 188, 203, 205, 210, 247
aging, 9, 10, 11, 12, 13, 15, 22, 27, 30, 31, 32, 34, 35, 42, 44, 51, 59, 87, 88, 99, 112, 117, 124, 140, 141, 162, 168, 174, 178, 180, 182, 188, 194, 195, 217, 268, 274
aging process, 11, 22, 117, 180
agnosia, 246, 254
agonist, 60, 72, 81, 122, 152, 153
aid, 28, 167
akinesia, 246
alkaline phosphatase, 130, 131
allele, 56, 147, 148, 149, 150, 152, 153, 154, 155, 156, 157, 158, 159, 164, 211, 261
alleles, 147, 148, 150, 153, 173
alpha, 55, 57, 62
ALS, 164, 260
alternative, 17, 54, 92, 95, 98, 114, 118, 120, 122, 124, 128, 138, 149, 200, 221, 224
alters, 70, 78, 103, 104, 177, 183, 211
amelioration, 208, 210
amino, 61, 68, 93, 95, 115, 120, 125, 129, 132, 139, 147, 164, 186, 195, 200, 201, 247
amino acid, 61, 68, 93, 95, 115, 120, 125, 129, 132, 147, 164, 186, 200, 201, 247
amino acids, 93, 115, 120, 129, 132, 186, 201
amnesia, 31, 236, 254
AMPA, 73, 79
amplitude, 70
amygdala, 10, 11, 12, 15, 17, 22, 26, 27, 28, 31, 33, 34, 35, 224, 229, 231, 236
Amyloid, v, 37, 56, 59, 61, 63, 64, 67, 79, 80, 81, 82, 88, 103, 106, 107, 111, 112, 114, 115, 116, 119, 139, 140, 142, 150, 157, 175, 176, 178, 179, 180, 181, 183, 193, 195, 196, 205, 209, 211, 212, 216
amyloid angiopathy, 62, 80, 86, 110, 111, 214
amyloid beta, 57, 58, 59, 60, 61, 62, 63, 64, 65, 79, 80, 81, 82, 103, 104, 108, 110, 111, 141, 161, 167, 175, 177, 182, 183, 193, 196, 199, 210, 211, 212, 213, 215, 216
amyloid deposits, 61, 62, 91, 109, 112, 149, 178, 179, 184, 193, 203
amyloid fibril formation, 104, 212
amyloid fibrils, 56, 58, 95, 203, 211, 215
amyloid plaques, vii, 11, 47, 49, 58, 68, 76, 90, 103, 105, 150, 152, 174, 187, 188, 199, 203, 206
amyloid precursor protein, 38, 55, 58, 61, 67, 68, 79, 80, 81, 82, 86, 102, 108, 109, 110, 112, 139, 140, 141, 142, 146, 164, 168, 181, 184, 185, 186, 194, 195, 212, 216, 217, 244, 248
Amyloid Precursor Protein (APP), 37, 81, 114, 115
amyloid β, vii, 200
amyloidosis, 39, 40, 60, 82, 183, 201, 202, 212, 214, 215
amyotrophic lateral sclerosis, 164, 208, 215, 261
anaerobic, 136
analog, 205
angiopoietin, 172
Angiotensin, 38, 49, 59, 61
angiotensin converting enzyme, 38, 45, 55, 56, 63
angiotensin II, 63
angiotensin-converting enzyme (ACE), 57, 59, 62
animal models, 33, 51, 69, 85, 114, 118, 123, 137
animal studies, 46, 168
animals, 46, 54, 69, 70, 76, 114, 117, 118, 121, 133, 134, 137, 138, 167, 168, 173, 187, 202, 203, 209
antagonist, 69, 70, 71, 122
anti-apoptotic, 199, 200, 208, 213, 215
Antibodies, v, 52, 85, 90, 106, 108
antibody, 54, 60, 64, 85, 87, 88, 89, 90, 91, 92, 93, 94, 95, 96, 97, 98, 99, 100, 101, 102, 103, 104, 105, 107, 109, 110, 111, 115, 120, 129, 167, 170, 177, 184, 193, 200, 201, 204, 205, 211, 214
anticholinergic, 236
antidepressant, 52
antigen, 86, 87, 96, 97, 103, 165, 178, 190
antigen presenting cells, 96, 190
anti-inflammatory agents, 161, 167, 174, 180
antioxidant, 121, 123, 213, 216
antipsychotic, 265, 278
antipsychotics, 257
antisense, 137, 138
anus, 87
apathy, 252, 253, 265
APC, 190
aphasia, 243, 244, 245, 246, 252, 253
APO, 193, 244
APOE, viii, 42, 145, 146, 147, 148, 149, 150, 151, 152, 153, 154, 155, 156, 157, 158, 159, 168, 176, 183, 248, 252
Apolipoprotein E (Apo E), v, 38, 41, 60, 145, 146, 154, 155, 156, 157, 158, 159, 181

apoptosis, 139, 152, 172, 173, 186, 187, 188, 189, 191, 195, 196, 200, 203, 206, 208, 209, 212, 213, 214, 215, 216, 217
apoptotic, 43, 61, 176, 181, 191, 200, 201, 206, 210, 214, 215
APP, v, vii, 37, 38, 39, 40, 41, 47, 49, 50, 53, 54, 61, 63, 67, 68, 69, 70, 73, 74, 76, 78, 79, 81, 86, 87, 88, 91, 93, 95, 96, 97, 98, 100, 107, 109, 110, 112, 113, 114, 115, 116, 117, 118, 119, 120, 121, 122, 123, 124, 126, 136, 137, 138, 140, 141, 142, 145, 146, 164, 166, 168, 170, 175, 178, 184, 185, 186, 187, 188, 189, 190, 192, 196, 200, 201, 202, 205, 206, 209, 215, 217, 244, 248
application, 88, 100, 229, 241, 251, 255, 257
apraxia, 246, 251, 253
aptitude, 267
arachidonic acid, 196
arginine, 146, 147
argument, 122
Arizona, 161
arousal, 13, 16, 17, 22, 23, 24, 25, 26, 28, 29, 30, 32, 34
arrest, 216
arteries, 168
asbestos, 163
asparagines, 126, 132, 135
assessment, 55, 79, 80, 223, 224, 225, 257, 260, 262, 264, 265, 266, 267, 280
astrocyte, 42, 45, 53, 56, 60, 156, 166
astrocytes, vii, 37, 38, 40, 41, 42, 43, 44, 45, 46, 47, 55, 56, 57, 60, 62, 64, 65, 82, 147, 151, 157, 168, 174, 178, 179, 182, 196, 203, 209, 213
astrogliosis, 42, 98
asymmetry, 34, 247
asymptomatic, 252, 253, 256, 259
atherosclerosis, 157, 163, 168, 175, 182, 183
atomic force, 107
atomic force microscopy, 107
ATP, 186
ATPase, 244, 248
atrophy, 34, 152, 157, 194, 225, 227, 228, 229, 230, 231, 234, 235, 236, 237, 238, 239, 240, 247, 251, 255, 256, 261, 262
attacks, 30
auditory domain, 32
auditory hallucinations, 265
autoantibodies, 92, 190
autobiographical memory, 253
autocrine, 41
autoimmune, 89, 163, 164
autoimmunity, 92, 98, 185
autophagic vacuoles, 126, 188, 195
autophagy, 188, 189, 217
autopsy, 77, 90, 102, 119, 132, 165, 169, 225, 253
autosomal dominant, 146, 164, 202, 245, 253, 256
availability, 165
awareness, 28
axon, 109, 141
axonal, 58, 152, 188, 189, 247
axons, 46, 135, 189, 248
Aβ, vii, 37, 38, 39, 40, 41, 42, 43, 44, 45, 46, 47, 48, 49, 50, 51, 52, 53, 54, 67, 68, 69, 70, 71, 73, 74, 75, 76, 79, 186, 188, 189, 195, 199, 200, 201, 202, 203, 204, 205, 206, 208

B

B cell, 85, 93, 95, 102
bacteria, 125, 163
bacterial, 43, 44, 203
barrier, vii, 37, 38, 47, 50, 56, 57, 59, 61, 63, 65, 69, 80, 82, 86, 92, 104, 121, 164, 176, 177
barriers, 65, 197
basal forebrain, 193, 224
basal ganglia, 12, 221, 229, 232, 234, 238, 247
basement membrane, 58
batteries, 265, 270
battery, 89, 271
BBB, 37, 38, 43, 50, 51, 52, 54, 86, 92, 100, 101
behavior, 208, 246
behavioral change, 238, 246
behavioral disorders, viii
behavioral effects, 11
behavioural disorders, 254
behaviours, 251
Belgium, 251
beneficial effect, 9, 22, 28, 91, 95, 96, 98, 122, 209
benefits, 25, 29, 90, 153
bias, 17, 23, 28, 245, 247, 267
binding, 41, 42, 43, 44, 45, 51, 52, 55, 62, 86, 93, 95, 102, 105, 117, 119, 129, 136, 137, 138, 147, 150, 151, 158, 164, 166, 176, 178, 199, 200, 201, 204, 205, 208, 232, 238, 244, 245, 247, 249
bioactive compounds, 163
biochemistry, 116, 118, 124, 132
biological activity, 89, 216
biological markers, 175
biological responses, 153
biomarker, 128, 141, 172
biomarkers, 132, 163, 240, 257

biosynthesis, 140, 214, 217
birefringence, 204
birth, 10, 250, 266, 267, 277
blocks, 72, 81, 139, 188, 233
blood, vii, 37, 38, 40, 41, 47, 49, 50, 51, 53, 55, 56, 57, 62, 63, 65, 69, 80, 82, 86, 87, 92, 97, 101, 104, 121, 163, 164, 169, 170, 172, 176, 177, 180, 181, 197, 201, 205, 246
Blood Brain Barrier, 38, 50
blood pressure, 49, 246
blood vessels, 41, 87, 201
blood-brain barrier, 47, 56, 57, 63, 65, 69, 80, 82, 86, 92, 104, 164, 177
blurring, 168
body language, 13
bolus, 72
bone marrow transplant, 40, 41, 52, 53
borderline, 251
Boston, 9, 85, 88
bovine, 194
brain injury, 33, 76, 149, 150, 154, 155, 156, 201, 209
brain size, 136
brain stem, 192
brain structure, 11
Brazil, 56
breakdown, 11, 162, 192
breast cancer, 122, 207, 215
buffer, 72, 116, 127, 129
burn, 215
bypass, 149

C

Ca^{2+}, 143
Caenorhabditis elegans, 115
calcification, 254
calcium, 141, 196, 200, 206, 212
calnexin, 126, 133
calreticulin, 126, 128, 130
Canada, 135, 142
cancer, 162, 163, 211, 214
cancer cells, 211, 215
candidates, 98, 172
capillary, 52
caps, 200
carbohydrates, 128, 134, 135, 140, 187
carboxyl, 50, 194, 195, 199, 200, 202, 206, 217
carcinoma, 212
cardiac operations, 159
cardiopulmonary, 149
cardiopulmonary bypass, 149
Caribbean, 87, 107, 148, 156, 159
case study, 270
caspase, 187, 191, 196, 197, 200, 206, 210, 213, 217
caspase-dependent, 191, 196
caspases, 109, 141, 190, 192, 210
cast, 222
catabolic, 60
catabolism, 65, 82, 191
catalysis, 126
Cathepsin B, 45, 49, 55, 62, 187, 192, 194, 195, 196
Cathepsins, v, 185, 189, 192
Caucasian, 148
Caucasian population, 148
causal relationship, 231
CBS, 258
cDNA, 62, 97, 108, 139, 142
ceiling effect, 17, 231
cell, 46, 47, 49, 53, 56, 61, 62, 63, 68, 74, 78, 80, 81, 85, 93, 94, 95, 96, 98, 101, 102, 106, 114, 116, 118, 121, 124, 125, 126, 128, 132, 135, 137, 142, 147, 151, 156, 164, 165, 171, 172, 176, 187, 188, 189, 190, 193, 200, 201, 202, 203, 206, 207, 209, 210, 212, 213, 214, 221, 225, 238, 248
cell adhesion, 172, 201
cell culture, 49, 137, 202, 203, 210, 214
cell death, 114, 121, 187, 193, 201, 206
cell differentiation, 95
cell growth, 207
cell invasion, 62, 189
cell line, 47, 56, 137, 172, 203, 212
cell surface, 47, 68, 74, 78, 80
central nervous system, 39, 68, 86, 90, 103, 107, 145, 146, 153, 157, 159, 175, 179, 186, 200, 201, 214, 224, 247
centromeric, 247
cerebellum, 63
cerebral amyloid angiopathy, 62, 80, 86, 110, 111
cerebral amyloidosis, 39
cerebral cortex, 48, 158, 175, 212, 280
cerebral hemisphere, 254
cerebral hemorrhage, 202, 214
cerebral hypoperfusion, 176
cerebral ischemia, 192, 196, 201, 214
cerebrospinal fluid, 65, 81, 86, 88, 141, 147, 157, 173, 197, 200, 210, 216, 225
cerebrovascular, 48, 162, 167, 176
certification, 162
cervix, 211

CFA, 86, 87, 88, 94
c-Fos, 206
channel blocker, 69, 71
channels, 73, 128, 130, 131
chaperones, 125, 126, 128, 133, 135, 139, 140, 186, 194
Chaperones, 125, 128, 132, 134, ,
cheese, 125
chelates, 51
chemoattractant, 165, 172
chemokine, 41, 96, 171, 173, 178, 190
chemokine synthesis, 178
chemokines, 41, 44, 47, 60, 165, 170, 213
chemotherapeutic agent, 52
chemotherapy, 211
chicks, 141
child development, 266
childhood, 263, 267
children, 266, 267
cholera, 97, 108
cholesterol, 43, 50, 147, 148, 151, 164, 168, 174, 203, 210, 215
cholesterol-lowering drugs, 50
cholinergic, 145, 146, 150, 153, 221, 224
cholinesterase, 114, 123
chromaffin cells, 190, 194
Chromatin, 207, 210, 211, 213
chromatography, 116, 130, 131
chromosome, 116, 147, 201, 243, 244, 245, 247, 248, 249, 258, 259, 260
chronic illness, 267
chronic stress, 149
cingulated, 256
circulation, 51, 53
classes, 170
classical, 44, 95, 137, 164, 165, 180, 219, 221, 223, 227, 243, 245, 256
cleavage, 38, 45, 48, 50, 51, 68, 69, 74, 86, 98, 110, 116, 120, 151, 164, 187, 190, 192, 201, 206, 216
clinical approach, 250
clinical diagnosis, 86, 162, 172, 251, 254
clinical presentation, 245, 250
clinical symptoms, 232, 252
clinical syndrome, 249, 252, 263, 267
clinical trial, vii, 41, 53, 85, 87, 89, 90, 92, 99, 102, 114, 118, 119, 120, 121, 122, 123, 124, 128, 137, 152, 153, 161, 164, 167, 174, 205
clinical trials, vii, 41, 53, 85, 87, 89, 90, 92, 102, 114, 118, 121, 123, 124, 128, 137, 161, 164, 167, 174, 205
clinically significant, 224
clinician, 31
cloning, 139, 213
clustering, 229
clusters, 227, 229, 269
CNS, 51, 52, 64, 86, 90, 99, 101, 104, 146, 147, 150, 153, 159, 176, 177, 186, 187, 189, 193, 196, 200, 201, 205, 208, 211
cocaine, 213
Cochrane, 275
codes, 247
coding, 96, 148, 276
cognition, 33, 91, 96, 111, 139, 149, 153, 155, 159, 239, 263, 264, 265, 267, 268, 270, 271, 274, 277, 278, 279
cognitive ability, vii, 276
cognitive deficits, 61, 91, 97, 98, 112, 139, 149, 184, 220, 223, 224, 264, 265, 267, 269, 274, 277
cognitive development, 266
cognitive domains, 219, 220, 231, 263, 265, 267, 269, 270, 271, 272, 274
cognitive dysfunction, 11, 190, 221, 228, 236, 241, 263, 264
cognitive flexibility, 224, 265
cognitive function, 69, 76, 89, 90, 92, 106, 110, 114, 117, 118, 119, 122, 123, 128, 132, 138, 139, 140, 149, 164, 167, 171, 208, 224, 234, 236, 238, 265, 266, 267, 268, 269, 270, 271, 273, 274, 278, 279, 280
cognitive impairment, 22, 27, 30, 33, 34, 93, 97, 155, 156, 159, 173, 178, 208, 220, 223, 227, 234, 235, 236, 237, 239, 240, 263, 264, 267, 269, 270, 273, 274, 276, 277, 278
cognitive performance, 89, 99, 220, 238, 266
cognitive process, 11, 273, 274
cognitive profile, 231, 269
cognitive system, 272
cognitive tasks, 273
cognitive test, 264, 265, 266, 267
cohort, 159, 241, 248, 252, 253, 255, 256, 261, 266, 267, 268, 271, 276, 277
collagen, 42, 58
Columbia, 185
coma, 149, 158
communication, 201, 264
communities, 148
community, 82, 156, 157, 245, 268
complement, 42, 44, 109, 161, 164, 165, 166, 168, 175, 180, 183, 186, 211, 221
complement pathway, 165, 180

complex systems, 239
complexity, 28, 29, 223, 245, 256, 260
complications, 70, 248
components, 17, 44, 76, 137, 138, 161, 163, 164, 165, 169, 171, 187
compounds, 163, 188, 201, 205, 257
comprehension, 232, 246, 252, 253, 254
computed tomography, 264
concentration, 50, 68, 86, 92, 93, 202, 204, 205, 227, 228, 230
conduction, 135
confabulation, 222
configuration, 125
conflict, 192
conflict of interest, 192
conformational stability, 152
Congo red, 204
connectivity, 11, 15, 17, 22, 26, 29, 34, 79, 151
consciousness, 162
consensus, 14, 23, 27, 132, 135, 245, 250, 258, 260
conservation, 125
consolidation, 26, 32, 33, 213, 272
construction, 28
consumption, 123
contamination, 136
continuity, 23, 24
control, 15, 25, 33, 39, 44, 46, 47, 62, 69, 87, 94, 148, 150, 161, 165, 166, 167, 170, 174, 186, 206, 209, 220, 224, 229, 230, 239, 252, 265, 268, 270, 271, 275
control group, 206, 220, 229, 230
conversion, 57, 68, 190
copper, 203
correlation, 17, 115, 119, 120, 122, 132, 169, 208, 225, 230, 231, 264
correlations, 55, 225, 231
cortex, 87, 88, 90, 140, 156, 171, 180, 206, 215, 223, 234, 255, 256
cortical neurons, 49, 81, 155, 212
corticobasal degeneration, 244, 249, 254
corticotropin, 81
cortisol, 76, 80, 117
covariate, 255
covering, 225, 265
COX-2, 166, 171
$cPLA_2$, 170
C-reactive protein, 169
creativity, 251
cross-sectional, 268, 277, 278
cross-sectional study, 277
CRP, 169
CSF, 69, 86, 88, 89, 92, 95, 96, 98, 103, 107, 119, 120, 127, 128, 129, 130, 131, 132, 156, 157, 163, 173, 175, 200, 202, 203, 204
C-terminal, 68, 91, 95, 97, 103, 147, 151, 152, 164
C-terminus, 90
cues, 24, 234
culture, 67, 73, 74, 76, 78, 157, 167, 202
curcumin, 174, 176
cycling, 72, 74, 79
cyclooxygenase, 166, 167
cysteine, 49, 56, 146, 187, 188, 194, 197, 200, 247
cysteine proteases, 56, 197
cytochrome, 213
cytokine, 96, 101, 168, 171, 174, 183, 190
cytokines, 40, 41, 44, 60, 94, 95, 163, 165, 170, 174, 175, 182, 186, 203, 213
cytopathology, 47
cytoplasm, 151, 155, 208, 247
cytoskeleton, 125
cytosol, 46, 124, 125, 151, 152, 187
cytosolic, 121, 126, 134, 136, 142, 170, 204
cytotoxic, 52, 89, 178, 186
cytotoxicity, 49, 59, 98, 108, 111, 210

D

daily living, 27, 139, 223, 251
data set, 171, 238
de novo, 211, 224, 267
death, 86, 109, 115, 122, 133, 141, 154, 162, 176, 186, 187, 190, 191, 196, 197, 248, 250, 251, 253
decay, 26, 272
decisions, 227
declarative memory, 32, 34, 219, 221, 222, 224, 230, 231, 233
deep brain stimulation, 237
defects, 46, 117, 126, 256
defense, 203
deficiency, 42, 44, 45, 56, 58, 64, 80
deficit, 11, 17, 25, 33, 34, 122, 220, 221, 222, 232, 237, 253, 265, 270, 273, 274, 277, 278
deficits, 22, 25, 26, 33, 46, 61, 91, 96, 97, 98, 105, 108, 112, 139, 142, 149, 155, 184, 190, 202, 212, 219, 220, 221, 222, 223, 224, 232, 233, 234, 236, 237, 238, 240, 241, 251, 254, 263, 264, 265, 267, 269, 270, 271, 272, 273, 274, 277, 278
definition, 213
degenerate, 231

degradation, vii, 37, 38, 40, 41, 42, 45, 46, 48, 49, 51, 52, 60, 61, 65, 69, 74, 100, 138, 152, 188, 189, 213, 248
degrading, vii, 37, 38, 41, 45, 46, 47, 52, 54, 55, 56, 57, 58, 59, 60, 61, 62, 64, 65, 187, 188
delivery, 56, 96, 98, 99, 151
delusion, 254
delusions, 264
dementia, vii, viii, 11, 30, 31, 33, 57, 61, 63, 64, 76, 80, 85, 86, 90, 113, 114, 116, 118, 119, 124, 132, 138, 139, 140, 141, 145, 146, 150, 152, 153, 154, 156, 159, 162, 164, 168, 174, 176, 178, 179, 180, 185, 186, 188, 189, 191, 195, 219, 220, 221, 222, 223, 225, 226, 229, 234, 235, 236, 237, 238, 239, 240, 243, 244, 245, 246, 248, 249, 251, 253, 254, 258, 259, 260, 261, 262, 263, 264, 268
demyelinating disease, 189, 192
demyelination, 195
dendrites, 73, 76, 208, 248
dendritic cell, 95, 194
density, 58, 80, 139, 146, 147, 168, 176, 213, 227, 229, 232
dentate gyrus, 69, 82
depolarization, 72
depolymerization, 212
deposition, 11, 40, 41, 45, 47, 49, 50, 52, 54, 55, 56, 57, 58, 59, 60, 64, 67, 76, 77, 80, 87, 88, 89, 90, 94, 95, 96, 97, 99, 101, 102, 103, 109, 112, 113, 114, 117, 132, 149, 150, 154, 156, 157, 158, 168, 169, 179, 181, 184, 189, 190, 202, 203, 205, 206, 211, 212
deposits, 39, 40, 51, 53, 54, 61, 62, 70, 81, 86, 91, 100, 101, 102, 109, 111, 112, 126, 128, 149, 150, 166, 178, 179, 184, 193, 201, 203, 205, 210
depressed, 71
depression, 81, 174, 237, 253
deprivation, 200, 214
deregulation, 150
derivatives, 93, 99, 111
destruction, 163, 187, 224
detection, 33, 225, 227, 240
developed nations, 162
dexamethasone, 59
diabetes, 145, 146, 152, 153, 154, 155, 158
diabetes mellitus, 155
diagnostic criteria, 245, 259, 260, 265
Diamond, 55, 62, 108, 141, 279
diet, 123, 168
dietary, 147, 180, 206, 215, 246
differential diagnosis, 228, 251, 257, 260
differentiation, 55, 95, 240
diffusion, 52, 256, 258
diffusion tensor imaging, 256, 258
digestion, 141
dimer, 107
dimeric, 46, 97
direct observation, 102, 210
disability, 263, 279
disaster, 10
Discovery, 137, 154
discriminatory, 251
discs, 148
disease model, 177
disease progression, 27, 40, 51, 68, 85, 87, 154, 155, 164, 175, 222, 251
diseases, 187, 188, 189, 191, 244
disinhibition, 243, 245, 252, 253
disorder, vii, 38, 102, 176, 237, 245, 246, 252, 253, 256, 259, 263, 264, 265, 274
disposition, 65
dissociation, 31, 89, 204, 233, 236
distracters, 232
distribution, 11, 27, 80, 148, 225, 277
disulfide, 124, 142, 200, 216
DNA, 55, 92, 95, 96, 97, 100, 102, 104, 105, 106, 108, 109, 111, 172, 179, 194, 200, 206, 207, 244, 245, 247, 248, 249
DNA repair, 172
doctors, 162
dogs, 99, 102
donors, 169
dopamine, 221, 224, 232, 236, 238, 240, 275
dopaminergic, 219, 224, 232, 233, 236, 238, 239
dorsolateral prefrontal cortex, 232, 233
dosage, 233
dosing, 90, 93, 99
Down syndrome, 199, 200, 201, 213
downregulating, 54
down-regulation, 98, 172, 176, 182, 207
Drosophila, 115, 208, 216
drug delivery, 64
drug discovery, 167, 194
drug targets, 189
drug treatment, 183, 265
drugs, 50, 52, 72, 114, 118, 121, 124, 137, 138, 167, 196
DSM, 264, 278
DSM-IV, 264
duplication, 116

duration, 17, 25, 124, 148, 247, 252, 253, 267, 269, 272
dynamin, 74, 75, 80, 81, 195
dysgraphia, 246
dyskinesia, 280
dyslexia, 246
dysregulation, 208
Dysregulation, 192

E

E. coli, 87, 94, 97, 108
earthquake, 31
eating, 251, 253
echolalia, 251
ecological, 28, 223
EEG, 68, 70, 72
EEG activity, 70, 72
elaboration, 9, 10, 14, 26
elderly, 30, 32, 113, 117, 118, 122, 123, 124, 126, 127, 132, 135, 137, 138, 145, 146, 156, 157, 158, 162, 176, 179, 185, 186, 237, 268
elderly population, 186
electrodes, 70
electroencephalography, 70
electron, 55, 74, 125, 155, 204
electron microscopy, 74
electrons, 125
electrophoresis, 159
ELISA, 252
embryo, 118, 136
embryonic development, 117
emission, 77, 220, 244, 245, 254
emotion, vii, 9, 10, 11, 12, 13, 14, 16, 17, 22, 24, 25, 26, 27, 28, 30, 31, 32, 33, 34, 35
emotional, 9, 10, 11, 12, 13, 14, 15, 16, 17, 22, 23, 24, 25, 26, 27, 28, 29, 30, 31, 32, 33, 246, 251, 253, 254, 264
emotional bias, 24
emotional experience, 10, 13, 32
emotional information, 10, 11, 12, 13, 15, 22, 26, 27, 28, 30, 32, 33
emotional memory, 9, 10, 11, 12, 13, 14, 15, 16, 17, 22, 24, 25, 26, 27, 28, 29, 31, 32, 33
emotional responses, 15, 22
emotional stimuli, 23, 28, 29, 31
emotional valence, 14, 22
emotions, 10, 13, 16, 17, 30, 34
empathy, 246, 251
employment, 272
encephalitis, 104, 108, 254
encephalomyelitis, 195
encoding, 22, 24, 25, 29, 60, 95, 106, 221, 222, 231, 240, 248, 250, 254, 271, 272, 273
endocytosis, 38, 49, 56, 67, 68, 74, 75, 76, 78, 80, 81, 201
endoplasmic reticulum, 46, 68, 74, 114, 139, 140, 143
endothelial cell, 51, 52, 54, 169, 176, 183
endothelial cells, 51, 52, 54, 169, 183
Endothelin, 38, 48, 57, 58
endothelin-1, 65
endothelium, 48, 176
energy, 125, 146, 153
England, 31
enlargement, 248
entorhinal cortex, 69
environment, 187, 247, 265, 267
environmental factors, 145, 146, 188
enzymatic, 136, 152
enzymatic activity, 136
enzymes, vii, 37, 38, 41, 45, 48, 49, 52, 54, 57, 61, 64, 124, 136, 152, 165, 186, 187, 189, 192, 195
epidemic, 162
epidemiologic studies, 180
epidemiology, 161
epidermis, 140
epigenetic, 207, 208, 209
epilepsy, 80, 189, 191, 254
episodic memory, 252, 271
epitope, 85, 92, 93, 95, 97, 102, 105, 108, 109, 120, 129, 142, 177
epitopes, 90, 93, 102, 115, 118
equilibrium, 37, 38, 205, 208
erythrocytes, 43, 62
Escherichia coli, 107
ester, 216
estradiol, 141
estrogen, 122, 124, 139, 143
Estrogen, 122
estrogens, 140
ethnicity, 155
etiology, 113, 118, 124, 126, 135, 145, 146, 153, 164, 265
eukaryotes, 125
eukaryotic cell, 125
evaporation, 94
event-related potentials, 9
evolution, 179, 219, 220, 221, 223, 229, 231
exaggeration, 247

excretion, 128
execution, 270
executive function, 221, 238, 251, 254, 269, 270, 271, 273, 277
executive functions, 221, 251, 254
executive processes, 270, 272, 273
exocytosis, 71, 72, 73, 74, 78
experimental allergic encephalomyelitis, 195
experimental design, 171
exposure, 17, 150, 187, 191, 233
extracellular matrix, 47
eye movement, 272

F

face recognition, 222
facial expression, 16, 22, 30
factor analysis, 271
failurc, vii, 15, 41, 86, 119, 120, 121, 122, 132, 137, 161, 167, 248, 272, 273
false negative, 222
false positive, 222
familial, vii, 39, 57, 80, 86, 156, 158, 193, 212, 214, 216, 248, 250, 251, 256, 258, 261
family, 42, 46, 47, 50, 51, 55, 64, 76, 115, 125, 126, 134, 147, 181, 202, 248, 250, 252, 254, 256, 259
family history, 256
family members, 55, 76, 259
Fas, 193, 200, 201
fats, 168
fatty acids, 55, 174
FBI, 244, 257
FDG, 77, 259
feedback, 71, 79, 169, 270
females, 172
fetal, 42
fibers, 201
fibrillar, 39, 42, 46, 47, 48, 56, 59, 60, 68, 99, 105, 106, 111, 165, 202, 204
fibrils, 65, 97, 98, 101, 199, 202, 203, 204, 209, 210, 215, 217
fibrin, 48
fibroblasts, 191, 196, 217
fibronectin, 194
filament, 158, 200, 244, 249, 250
Finland, 148
firms, 120
first degree relative, 269
fish, 72
fixation, 272
flow, 119
fluctuations, 77
fluid, 49, 65, 68, 72, 80, 81, 86, 88, 90, 141, 148, 157, 159, 173, 197, 200, 210, 211, 216, 225
fluorescence, 61
fMRI, 9, 17, 21, 29, 34, 220, 232, 238, 240
focusing, 15, 77
folding, 125, 214, 248
food, 72, 153, 180, 253
forgetting, 10, 25, 222, 223
Fox, 89, 103, 104, 105, 239, 258, 259, 261
fractionation, 55, 273
fractures, 248
fragmentation, 200
free energy, 125
free radical, 196
free recall, 219, 222, 271
frontal cortex, 54, 165, 171, 206, 255, 256
frontal lobe, 220, 230, 256, 259, 260, 270, 272, 279
frontotemporal dementia, 244, 245, 246, 248, 249, 258, 259, 260, 261, 262
frontotemporal lobar degeneration, 244, 257, 258, 261
FTD, 243, 244, 245, 246, 249, 254, 260
FTLD, 243, 244, 245, 247, 248, 249, 250, 251, 253, 254, 255, 256, 257, 258, 262
fuel, 164
functional analysis, 31
functional imaging, 80
functional magnetic resonance imaging, 9, 35
functional MRI, 21
funding, 114
funds, 217
fungal, 43, 61
fusiform, 231
fusion, 72

G

G8, 129
GABA, 71, 82
Gamma, 139
ganglia, 12, 221, 229, 232, 234, 238, 247
GDNF, 172
gel, 128, 159
gender, 227, 245
gene, 39, 42, 49, 52, 54, 61, 63, 64, 76, 85, 95, 96, 110, 114, 116, 117, 137, 140, 145, 146, 147, 152, 161, 163, 164, 166, 170, 173, 176, 179, 181, 183,

200, 201, 202, 207, 212, 213, 214, 215, 243, 247, 248, 253, 254, 256, 258, 259, 260, 262
gene expression, 63, 64, 152, 161, 163, 170, 173, 179, 181, 183, 207, 215, 259
gene therapy, 52, 54
gene transfer, 61, 63
generation, 39, 41, 48, 67, 70, 73, 74, 76, 80, 92, 95, 96, 97, 99, 102, 186, 187, 188, 189, 190, 194, 195, 203, 211
genes, 40, 86, 111, 143, 145, 146, 168, 170, 172, 173, 176, 181, 196, 202, 206, 207, 208, 215, 250, 274
genetic code, 125
genetic defect, 250, 256
genetic disease, 244
genetic factors, 148, 181
genetic mutations, 145, 146, 164, 243, 251, 256
genetics, viii, 125, 145, 146, 150, 153, 154, 175, 211
genome, 171, 176, 261
genomics, 64
genotype, 148, 154, 155, 157, 158, 173, 176, 183, 248, 252
genotypes, 148, 152, 153, 154, 158, 179, 247
geriatric, 140, 269, 277
GFAP, 38, 166, 168
GFP, 137
gift, 88
Ginkgo biloba, 121, 139, 142
glasses, 224
glatiramer acetate, 58
GlaxoSmithKline, 92, 145
glial, 42, 55, 96, 159, 166, 168, 172, 175, 180, 238
Glial, 57, 253
glial cells, 55
glial fibrillary acidic protein (GFAP), 42, 166
glioma, 207, 213
gliosis, 86, 98, 249, 250
glucagon, 136
glucose, 58, 150, 152, 153, 169, 184, 200, 214
glucose metabolism, 152, 153
glutamate, 68, 71, 72, 82, 193
glutamate decarboxylase, 82
glutamatergic, 71
glutamic acid, 202
glutamine, 202
glutathione, 124, 125, 136
Glycation, 38, 50, 164, 179
glycine, 127, 129
glycogen, 108
glycogen synthase kinase, 108
glycoprotein, 46, 61, 65,115, 140, 171, 180, 197,247
glycosylated, 91, 126, 128, 129, 135, 139
glycosylation, 126, 129, 132, 135, 137, 142
GM-CSF, 95, 96, 103
goal setting, 251
goals, 14, 16, 28
G-protein, 71, 136, 137
grading, 31
grafts, 81
grain, 244, 249
grants, 29, 66, 192
granule cells, 82
granulocyte, 172
gray matter, 219, 221, 223, 225, 227, 228, 229, 230, 231, 235, 237
grey matter, 30, 255
groups, 11, 14, 23, 28, 29, 40, 53, 69, 90, 91, 96, 102, 119, 120, 124, 136, 148, 170, 199, 201, 204, 206, 227, 229, 233, 256, 258, 268, 269
growth, 41, 68, 115, 116, 117, 118, 120, 139, 158, 171, 172, 193, 207, 247
growth factor, 41, 115, 116, 117, 118, 120, 158, 171, 172, 193, 247
guanine, 138
guidelines, 257
gyri, 231
gyrus, 11, 46

H

H1, 256
H_2, 256
half-life, 80
hallucinations, 219, 220, 221, 223, 229, 231, 237, 239, 240, 251, 264, 265
handling, 190
haplotype, 258
haplotypes, 252, 256
harmful effects, 189
Harvard, 37, 85
HDL, 43, 146, 147, 148
head injury, 149, 150, 156, 157, 158, 159
head trauma, 149, 158, 247
healing, 163
health, 65, 152
heart disease, 162
heat, 87, 94, 97, 203
heat shock protein, 203
heaths, 118, 135
hedonic, 264

helix, 211
hematomas, 91
heme, 203
heme oxygenase, 203
hemoglobin, 128
hemorrhages, 110,111
hepatocyte, 136, 155
herpes, 86, 96, 254
herpes simplex, 86, 96
heterogeneity, 264, 276, 278
heterogeneous, 225, 276
heterozygotes, 148
Higgs, 60
high density lipoprotein, 55, 141, 168, 213
high risk, 172, 248
high temperature, 125
high-density lipoprotein, 146, 147
hip, 248
hippocampal, 10, 12, 15, 26, 31, 46, 47, 48, 56, 63, 70, 71, 74, 80, 82, 91, 98, 103, 105, 142, 147, 157, 171, 176, 188, 195, 196, 202, 215, 216, 217, 219, 221, 224, 225, 226, 227, 228, 229, 230, 231, 234, 235, 236, 238, 256, 257
hippocampus, 10, 11, 12, 27, 42, 46, 48, 53, 54, 55, 59, 64, 69, 70, 71, 72, 74, 76, 81, 87, 88, 98, 165, 170, 173, 181, 192, 193, 212, 214, 222, 225, 226, 227, 228, 229, 230, 231, 233, 234, 236, 256
Hispanics, 148, 156, 159
histological, 253, 256
histone, 200, 207, 208, 211, 212, 213, 214, 217
Histone deacetylase, 211, 216
histopathology, 244, 249, 252, 254, 256
HIV, 52, 146, 151, 164
HIV-1, 146, 151
HLA, 61, 102, 165, 180
Holland, 251
homeostasis, 49, 150, 172
homogeneity, 269
homolog, 44
Hong Kong, 260
hormone, 76, 120, 122, 126, 142, 159
hormones, 10, 117
horses, 237
hospital, 24, 132, 140
hospitalized, 277
host, 43, 58, 95, 163
HSP, 125
human, 33, 35, 39, 40, 42, 45, 46, 47, 48, 49, 51, 53, 54, 55, 56, 57, 59, 61, 62, 63, 69, 77, 79, 80, 85, 86, 88, 89, 90, 92, 96, 98, 99, 102, 107, 109, 110, 111, 114, 117, 119, 123, 127, 129, 139, 141, 142, 146, 147, 150, 151, 155, 156, 159, 161, 163, 164, 165, 166, 167, 169, 170, 171, 173, 177, 178, 179, 181, 182, 183, 186, 188, 191, 206, 207, 210, 211, 212, 213, 215, 216, 238
human behavior, 33
human brain, 35, 48, 49, 79, 80, 171, 177, 182, 183, 238
human immunodeficiency virus, 146, 164
human leukocyte antigen, 86
human subjects, 170
humans, 32, 42, 67, 69, 70, 76, 77, 78, 87, 89, 92, 93, 108, 118, 119, 121, 125, 147, 154, 164, 168, 172, 179
Huntington's disease, 152, 195, 200, 208, 211, 212
hybrid, 213
hydrolases, 187
hydrolysis, 101, 128
hydrophobic, 50, 114, 116, 126, 128, 151, 202
hydroxyl, 203, 211
hygiene, 246
hyperactivity, 180
hyperemia, 203, 215
hyperinsulinemia, 154
hyperlipoproteinemia, 147
hyperphosphorylation, 151, 159
hyperthyroidism, 117
hyponatremia, 262
hypoperfusion, 169, 256
hypothesis, 9, 15, 41, 86, 105, 132, 136, 149, 152, 158, 161, 164, 165, 167, 168, 188, 191, 203, 221, 222, 237, 264
hysterectomy, 143

I

IB, 60
ibuprofen, 121
ICAM, 169, 171, 172, 173
ICD, 264
ice, 94, 206
id, 42, 49, 231, 233
identification, 12, 17, 22, 136, 157, 161, 168, 170, 188, 196, 223, 243, 247, 257, 274
idiopathic, 235
IFA, 87
IFN, 86, 94, 96, 171
IGF, 120
IGF-1, 120
IgG, 90, 99, 104, 171

IL-1, 41, 63, 106, 168, 171, 172, 173, 180
IL-10, 106
IL-15, 171
IL-2, 171, 172
IL-4, 63, 95, 96, 103, 168, 174, 180
IL-6, 165, 173, 174
IL-8, 172, 173
image analysis, 227
images, 11, 23, 225, 227, 255
imaging, 9, 35, 53, 66, 77, 80, 137, 219, 220, 221, 227, 234, 235, 244, 254, 256, 260
immune activation, 167
immune cells, 40, 53, 186
immune response, 44, 52, 87, 90, 92, 93, 94, 95, 96, 99, 102, 103, 105, 106, 108, 109, 110, 111, 165, 183, 190, 193
immune system, 87, 95, 163, 165, 175
immunity, 111
immunization, 41, 52, 53, 56, 62, 87, 88, 89, 90, 91, 92, 93, 94, 97, 98, 99, 100, 101, 102, 103, 104, 105, 106, 107, 108, 109, 110, 111, 140, 142, 170, 178, 180, 193, 205, 211
immunocytochemistry, 55
immunogen, 85, 87, 93, 110
immunogenicity, 89, 103, 110
immunoglobulin, 86, 92, 106, 110, 111, 170, 171, 172
immunoglobulin G, 111
immunoglobulins, 92, 104
immunohistochemical, 39, 40, 63, 183, 245
immunohistochemistry, 254
immunological, 64, 165, 171, 183
immunomodulatory, 53
immunoprecipitation, 129, 204
immunoreactivity, 44, 47, 87, 151, 159, 180
immunotherapy, 54, 55, 85, 86, 87, 88, 89, 92, 98, 99, 100, 101, 102, 103, 105, 106, 107, 108, 109, 110, 111, 112, 170, 179, 181, 182, 184, 192, 194, 205, 210
impairments, viii, 27, 141, 222, 232, 238, 252, 255, 257, 269
implementation, 13
implicit memory, 233
impulsivity, 237
in situ, 42, 63, 64, 65
in vitro, 41, 42, 47, 49, 50, 56, 58, 62, 64, 65, 69, 73, 74, 86, 93, 98, 101, 108, 111, 121, 136, 150, 159, 165, 168, 179, 180, 182, 194, 202, 204, 208, 210, 212, 215, 217
in vivo, 41, 42, 44, 45, 48, 49, 53, 55, 58, 70, 71, 73, 74, 76, 80, 86, 96, 101, 103, 106, 108, 109, 150, 163, 180, 190, 201, 208, 210, 213, 214, 216, 225
inactive, 47, 48, 187
incidence, 96, 98, 121, 122, 146, 148, 162, 245, 257, 260
inclusion, 149, 151, 188, 235, 247, 248, 249, 250, 253, 257, 265
inclusion bodies, 188, 247
incubation, 204
indication, 123, 170, 267
indirect effect, 9, 12, 26, 27, 117
indomethacin, 59
inducible protein, 171
induction, 59, 82, 94, 152, 188, 193
industry, 114
inertia, 251
infection, 64
infections, 123, 163
infectious, 162
infectious diseases, 162
inferences, 267
inflammation, 60, 61, 62, 86, 88, 93, 98, 108, 155, 161, 162, 163, 164, 165, 166, 167, 168, 169, 170, 173, 174, 175, 177, 178, 179, 181, 183, 186, 208, 247
inflammatory, 40, 41, 44, 47, 50, 60, 94, 95, 106, 138, 161, 162, 163, 164, 165, 166, 167, 168, 169, 170, 172, 173, 174, 175, 176, 180, 181, 182, 183, 186, 201, 203, 205, 211, 213, 217
inflammatory cells, 47
inflammatory mediators, 170, 173
inflammatory response, 60, 161, 163, 168, 173, 201, 211, 213
information processing, 263, 264, 276
infusions, 53, 98
ingestion, 153
inheritance, 147, 190, 245, 253, 256
inherited, 148
inhibition, 59, 60, 71, 74, 75, 98, 120, 138, 170, 183, 200, 207, 209, 211, 270
inhibitor, viii, 46, 49, 58, 59, 65, 73, 120, 121, 123, 139, 188, 190, 199, 207, 211, 212
inhibitors, 52, 71, 73, 114, 121, 167, 174, 186, 187, 188, 189, 191, 192, 193, 194, 196, 208, 216, 257
inhibitory, 121, 123
initiation, 149, 185
injection, 46, 54, 72, 88, 90, 91, 93, 110, 138, 170
injections, 89, 94, 119
injuries, 189, 201

injury, 76, 124, 148, 149, 150, 156, 157, 158, 159, 188, 193, 201, 209, 271
innate immunity, 61
inoculation, 106
inositol, 136
insecticide, 137
insertion, 49
insight, 246, 251, 254
inspection, 225, 229
instability, 152, 158, 192
institutionalisation, 265, 267
institutionalization, 251
insulin, 45, 46, 56, 58, 62, 64, 120, 139, 152, 158, 159, 171, 176
insulin resistance, 159
insulin sensitivity, 152
insulin signaling, 176
insulin-like growth factor, 158
insults, 149, 187, 203
integration, 11
integrin, 44, 60
integrins, 42
integrity, 11, 27, 35, 222, 231
intellect, 275
intellectual functioning, 267
intelligence, 266, 267, 275, 276
interaction, 14, 74, 101, 145, 146, 153, 168, 177, 180, 211, 274, 277
interactions, 10, 12, 16, 27, 35, 44, 51, 150, 210
interdependence, 274
interference, 138, 200, 272, 275
interferon, 86, 94, 170, 173, 179, 193
interleukin, 105, 165, 171, 179, 181
interleukin-1, 179
Interleukin-1, 182
interleukin-8, 171
internalization, 44, 74, 76, 79
interstitial, 68, 80, 81
interval, 25, 223, 229, 268
intervention, 57, 110
intracerebral, 40, 50, 51, 53, 55, 77, 146, 149, 154, 235
intracerebral hemorrhage, 146, 149
intracranial, 77, 184, 227, 254
intraperitoneal, 88
intravenous, 86, 110
intrinsic, 79, 126
invasive, 77
Investigations, 13
investment, 121
involution, 223
ions, 50, 203
IP, 173
IP-10, 173
ipsilateral, 70
IQ, 263, 264, 265, 266, 267, 269, 270, 271, 273, 276, 278, 279, 280
IQ scores, 265, 270
irritability, 253, 254
ischemia, 65, 77, 178, 187, 192, 196, 201, 209, 214
ischemic, 196, 197, 217
ischemic brain injury, 217
isoforms, 63, 142, 147, 150, 152, 177, 247, 259
isolation, 76, 80
isozyme, 142
Italy, 243, 251
IVIg, 86, 92

J

JAK2, 103
JAMA, 139, 140, 175
Japan, 148
Japanese, 148
Jordan, v, 110, 113, 156, 236
judge, vii
Jun, 203, 206, 236
Jung, 181

K

kernel, 227
ketogenic, 153
ketones, 153
kidney, 55
kinase, 180, 203
kinetics, 71
King, 212, 237, 258
Kirchhoff, 63
knockout, 46, 56, 115, 151, 152, 191, 201, 209, 214
Kobe, 31

L

labeling, 12, 155
labor, 225
laboratory studies, 17, 25
Langerhans cells, 97

language, 13, 232, 243, 245, 246, 250, 251, 252, 254, 264
language impairment, 243, 245, 250
late-onset, vii, 56, 145, 152, 154, 155, 156, 158, 176, 201, 216, 245, 269
late-onset AD, vii, 145, 152
later life, 150, 269
LDL, 50, 51, 60, 63, 76, 82, 146, 147, 157
learning, 26, 46, 61, 76, 87, 96, 99, 101, 105, 107, 108, 141, 203, 208, 211, 212, 220, 221, 222, 223, 229, 230, 231, 232, 233, 235, 236, 239, 240, 265, 271, 272, 273, 278
learning behavior, 208
learning process, 221
learning task, 231, 272
lectin, 129
left hemisphere, 254
lentiviral, 54
lesions, 169, 221, 256, 270, 272, 280
leucocyte, 178
leukocyte, 86, 163
levodopa, 225, 233, 234
Lewy bodies, 225, 235, 236, 240
liberal, 17, 23
life expectancy, 85, 86, 246
life experiences, 10, 16
lifespan, 10, 188, 278
lifetime, 14, 77, 187
ligand, 42, 166, 180, 183
ligands, 43, 51, 86, 98, 139, 214
likelihood, 10, 25, 266, 272
limbic system, 11, 231
limitation, 267
linear, 274
linkage, 156, 261
lipid, 86, 94, 108, 121, 145, 146, 147, 148, 150, 151, 153, 157, 187, 203
lipid peroxidation, 203
lipopolysaccharide, 42, 173
lipoprotein, 43, 55, 58, 60, 63, 80, 81, 146, 147, 148, 176, 213
lipoproteins, 42, 43, 148, 156, 157, 168
liver, 46, 51, 62, 63, 115, 120, 128, 133, 137, 138, 139, 141, 147, 151, 153, 155, 156, 214
liver failure, 214
liver transplant, 147, 156
L-lactide, 86, 94
localised, 248
localization, 55, 58, 59, 69, 76, 152, 155, 190, 229, 259
location, 34, 43, 45, 68, 70, 205, 233, 255
locus, 39, 148, 248, 260
London, 35, 263, 272
longevity, 123, 181
longitudinal studies, 223, 247, 267, 277, 268
llong-term memory, 271, 272
long-term potentiation, 86, 105, 107, 139, 178, 194, 202, 216
long-term retention, 222
low molecular weight, 205, 210
low-density, 51, 63, 146, 147, 169
low-density lipoprotein, 51, 63, 146, 147, 169
low-density lipoprotein receptor, 51, 63, 169
low-intensity, 22
LPS, 38, 42, 44, 47, 61, 173
LRP1, 43, 51, 52, 53, 54, 76
LTP, 86, 91, 97, 98, 210
luciferase, 137
lumen, 68, 126, 134
luminal, 51, 52
lymph, 69
lymphocyte, 161, 177
lymphocytes, 163, 165
lysine, 93, 132
lysosomal enzymes, 187, 189
lysosome, 74, 193
lysosomes, 49, 187, 196

M

M1, 69, 78, 80, 81
mAb, 111
machinery, 76, 78
macrophage, 41, 60, 61, 64, 96, 172
macrophage inflammatory protein, 172
macrophages, 40, 42, 44, 47, 52, 163, 165, 168, 177, 217
macular degeneration, 193
magnetic, 219, 220, 221, 227, 234, 235, 244
magnetic resonance, 9, 35, 219, 220, 221, 227, 234, 235, 244
magnetic resonance imaging, 9, 35, 86, 89, 219, 220, 221, 227, 234, 235, 244
MAI, 145
maintenance, 16, 48, 148, 172, 272, 273
major histocompatibility complex, 140, 165
malaria, 43, 62, 123
males, 172, 261
malignancy, 177
Mammalian, 64

mammalian cells, 125
manipulation, 27, 72, 85, 153, 209, 221, 232, 272, 273
MAPK, 171
mapping, 79, 151, 235
MARCO, 38, 42, 43
market, 122
marriage, 250
marrow, 53, 60, 63
mask, 268
Massachusetts, 37
matrix, 38, 45, 47, 55, 56, 57, 62, 65, 117
matrix metalloproteinase, 45, 56, 62, 65
matrix protein, 55, 117
Mb, 247
MCI, 9, 17, 21, 22, 23, 27, 28, 29, 173, 174, 220
MCP, 38, 41, 47, 165, 166, 171, 173, 177
MCP-1, 38, 41, 47, 166, 173, 177
measurement, 170, 274
measures, 17, 30, 72, 77, 90, 104, 222, 223, 225, 232, 233, 251, 264, 266, 267, 268, 269, 270, 271
media, 69, 73, 202, 203
median, 148, 246, 255
mediation, 27
mediators, 65, 170, 173
medication, 232, 237, 265, 267, 275
medications, 232
melt, 125
membranes, 46, 136, 151, 211
memory capacity, 232
memory deficits, 62, 101, 104, 108, 142, 203, 212, 219, 221, 222, 223, 224, 227, 232, 234, 271, 272, 273
memory formation, 202, 214
memory loss, 52, 62, 86, 91, 107, 108, 141, 222, 231
memory performance, 30, 230, 237
memory processes, 9, 10, 26, 271, 273
men, 88, 254
meningoencephalitis, 53, 85, 89, 92, 102, 109, 119, 167, 172
menopause, 122
mental representation, 28
mental state, 9, 21
Merck, 90, 120
mesenchymal stem cells, 54, 60
meta-analysis, 11, 33, 58, 155, 174, 222, 223, 232, 233, 237, 239, 240, 271, 275, 276, 277, 279
metabolic, 67, 77, 117, 118, 138, 150, 152, 202, 231, 232, 255
metabolic disturbances, 150
metabolic dysfunction, 152
metabolic syndrome, 117
metabolism, 43, 59, 70, 80, 126, 145, 146, 152, 153, 158, 168, 170, 173, 178, 181, 187, 196, 212, 216, 231, 255
metabolites, 214
metabolizing, 152
metabotropic glutamate receptors, 68, 71, 193
metal ions, 50
metalloproteinase, 49, 50, 55, 65
metalloproteinases, 45, 47, 56, 63, 65, 82
metals, 203
methylene, 123
MHC, 171
mice, 39, 40, 41, 42, 44, 45, 46, 47, 48, 49, 51, 52, 53, 54, 55, 56, 57, 58, 59, 60, 61, 62, 63, 64, 69, 70, 71, 72, 73, 74, 75, 76, 78, 80, 81, 85, 87, 88, 90, 91, 93, 94, 95, 96, 97, 98, 100, 101, 102, 103, 104, 107, 108, 109, 110, 111, 112, 114, 117, 119, 124, 138, 139, 140, 141, 142, 147, 150, 151, 152, 155, 159, 161, 163, 166, 167, 169, 170, 173, 175, 178, 179, 181, 182, 183, 184, 191, 193, 194, 201, 205, 206, 209, 210, 211, 212, 215, 217
microarray, 172, 179, 180
microbial, 43, 163
microcirculation, 201
microdialysis, 70, 71, 72, 74, 77, 80
microglial cells, 44, 53, 100, 192
microhemorrhages, 91, 94, 96, 102, 109
microinjection, 191
microparticles, 94, 97, 110
microscope, 204
microscopy, 74, 107
microsomes, 120, 128, 129, 133, 142
microtubule, vii, 151, 244, 247
microvascular, 215
Mild Cognitive Impairment (MCI), 22, 27, 30, 34, 155, 159, 173, 178, 220, 223, 227, 234, 235, 236, 237, 239, 240
military, 266
Mini-Mental State Examination, 173
Minnesota, 113, 260
minority, 253
MIP, 172, 173
mirror, 233
misfolded, 186
misfolding, 112, 210
Missouri, 67
mitochondria, 151, 152, 182

mitochondrial, 50, 58, 152, 153, 158, 173, 181, 194, 210, 213, 214, 215
mitochondrial membrane, 213, 215
mitogen, 183, 203
mitogen-activated protein kinase, 183, 203
mitogenesis, 152
mixing, 205
MMP, 38, 45, 47, 50, 55, 62
MMP-2, 47
MMP-9, 45, 47, 50, 55, 62
MMPs, 45, 47
MMSE, 9, 17, 21, 225, 231
MND, 244, 245, 246, 248, 249, 252, 254, 256
mnemonic processes, 10, 15, 16
mobility, 179
modality, 26, 45, 52, 53, 54
model system, 70, 166, 176
modeling, 206
models, vii, 12, 13, 33, 34, 39, 40, 42, 45, 48, 49, 51, 52, 59, 67, 69, 76, 85, 87, 95, 102, 114, 117, 118, 120, 122, 123, 124, 128, 136, 137, 138, 153, 161, 163, 165, 166, 169, 170, 177, 208, 210, 212, 228, 236
modulation, 10, 15, 26, 27, 56, 69, 78, 101, 103, 105, 181, 236
molecular mechanisms, 196, 207
molecular weight, 70, 125, 127, 129, 205, 206, 210
molecules, 70, 72, 76, 170, 172, 174, 186, 190, 200
money, 114
monkeys, 87, 88, 99, 105, 179
monoclonal, 62, 90, 97, 98, 100, 101, 105, 107, 111, 115, 129, 177, 204
monoclonal antibodies, 62, 97, 100, 105, 107, 111
monoclonal antibody, 91, 97, 98, 101, 107, 111, 115, 129, 177, 204
monocyte, 53, 65, 165, 172, 184
monocyte chemoattractant protein, 165, 172
monocyte chemotactic protein, 184
monocytes, 38, 54, 62, 175
monomeric, 46, 60, 68, 91
monomers, 97, 98, 202
mononuclear cells, 172, 180
monosaccharide, 134
mood, 264
morphine, 136
morphological, 212, 213, 239, 264
morphological abnormalities, 264
morphology, 54, 98, 103, 165, 204
mortality, 41, 149, 162, 279
mosaic, 180
motivation, 28
motor function, 208, 222, 230, 236
motor neuron disease, 152, 244, 246, 248, 254
motor skills, 265
motor system, 224
mouse, 39, 41, 42, 44, 45, 46, 51, 52, 53, 56, 58, 59, 60, 62, 64, 67, 69, 76, 80, 87, 88, 95, 98, 102, 103, 104, 105, 106, 107, 108, 109, 110, 111, 112, 114, 118, 119, 121, 124, 151, 153, 154, 156, 166, 175, 177, 182, 183, 184, 186, 192, 193, 196, 206, 208, 210, 211, 212, 215, 217
mouse model, 39, 41, 42, 45, 46, 52, 53, 56, 58, 59, 60, 67, 69, 76, 80, 87, 88, 102, 103, 104, 105, 106, 108, 109, 111, 112, 114, 118, 119, 121, 153, 154, 156, 175, 177, 184, 193, 196, 206, 208, 210, 211, 212
movement, 140, 187, 220, 228, 237, 241
movement disorders, 220, 228, 241
MRI, 21, 34, 86, 89, 104, 136, 220, 221, 223, 227, 229, 230, 238, 244, 251, 254, 255, 256
mRNA, 46, 47, 48, 49, 155
multidrug resistance, 52
multiple sclerosis, 56, 164, 165
murine model, 195
muscle, 46, 57, 248, 254
muscle cells, 57
muscle weakness, 248
mutant, 39, 80, 96, 117, 166, 194, 248, 262
mutants, 216
mutation, 39, 117, 125, 126, 193, 201, 202, 212, 214, 243, 247, 248, 249, 250, 252, 253, 254, 256, 259, 260, 261
mutations, 86, 116, 145, 146, 164, 166, 174, 201, 202, 214, 215, 243, 247, 248, 249, 251, 253, 254, 255, 256, 258, 260, 261, 262
myelin, 118, 135, 189, 192, 194, 216
myeloid, 40
myocardial infarction, 148
myopathy, 244, 248, 259, 262

N

N-acety, 134
naming, 246, 252, 264
narratives, 24
NART, 266
National Academy of Sciences, 30
National Adult Reading Test, 265, 279
National Institutes of Health, 83, 192
natural, 10, 88, 92, 163, 187

necrosis, 47, 50, 56, 165, 171, 189
negative experiences, 14
negativity, 17, 23
neglect, 251
neocortex, 46, 113, 114
neonatal, 44, 47, 55, 59, 104, 115
nerve, 81, 118, 135, 151, 191
nerve regeneration, 151
nervous system, 145, 153, 171
Netherlands, 245, 261
network, 17, 82, 204, 237
neural mechanisms, 29, 31, 32
neural systems, 29, 224
neuritic plaques, 86, 164, 175, 179
neuritis, 225
neurobiological, 28, 146, 269
neurobiology, 112
neuroblastoma, 210
neurodegeneration, 40, 54, 59, 61, 151, 155, 177, 178, 182, 184, 185, 186, 188, 189, 190, 191, 192, 194, 195, 196, 206, 208, 216, 224, 248
neurodegenerative, viii, 29, 65, 86, 103, 112, 126, 152, 159, 161, 164, 176, 182, 185, 186, 187, 188, 189, 191, 194, 196, 201, 208, 211, 220, 243, 245, 250, 256, 263
neurodegenerative dementia, 263
neurodegenerative disease, viii, 29, 112, 126, 159, 161, 182, 185, 186, 187, 189, 191, 194, 201, 243, 245
neurodegenerative diseases, viii, 112, 126, 161, 182, 185, 186, 187, 189, 191, 194, 243, 245
neurodegenerative disorders, 65, 103, 152, 188, 196, 208
neurofibrillary tangles, vii, 11, 86, 150, 151, 152, 161, 164, 165, 174, 175, 188, 201
neuroimaging, 10, 14, 15, 29, 232, 244, 264
neuroimaging techniques, 264
neuroinflammation, viii, 59, 63, 96, 110, 161, 164, 174, 180, 257
neurologic disorders, 189, 190
neurological deficit, 150
neurological disease, 171, 174, 183
neurological disorder, 102
neurologist, 250
neuron death, 109, 141
neuronal apoptosis, 186, 206, 216
neuronal cells, 151
neuronal death, 86, 186, 187, 190, 191, 196, 197
neuronal degeneration, 64, 203, 208
neuronal loss, 86, 90, 185, 190, 206, 208, 249, 250
neurons, 38, 39, 46, 48, 54, 55, 56, 67, 68, 72, 73, 78, 79, 92, 103, 117, 133, 138, 147, 151, 157, 159, 164, 166, 168, 169, 170, 181, 188, 189, 190, 193, 195, 196, 200, 201, 202, 209, 214, 216, 217, 247, 253
neuropathic pain, 193
neuropathological, 89, 149, 208, 219, 225, 235, 248, 256, 258, 260, 267
neuropathology, 29, 50, 103, 139, 143, 150, 157, 166, 174, 177, 184, 245, 248
neuroprotection, 159
neuroprotective, 62, 195, 209
neuropsychological assessment, 264, 265
neuropsychological tests, 220, 257, 265
neuropsychology, 31, 240
neuroscience, 30
neurotoxic, 46, 93, 151, 165, 187, 188, 189, 202
neurotoxic effect, 188
neurotoxicity, 44, 64, 65, 81, 101, 104, 105, 146, 152, 153, 164, 166, 168, 169, 178, 182, 188, 202, 209, 212, 213, 215, 216
neurotoxins, 214
neurotransmission, 72, 193, 194
neurotransmitter, 72, 74, 187
neurotrophic, 172, 176, 192, 201
neutrophils, 59, 161, 163, 175
New York, 30, 32, 33, 140, 199, 217
newspapers, 224
Newton, 74, 81
NFT, 86
Nielsen, 40, 42, 62, 261
nigrostriatal, 232
NIH, 66, 217
nitric oxide, 59, 165, 179, 182, 209
Nixon, 56, 106, 140, 186, 187, 188, 189, 190, 193, 196, 217
NMDA, 69, 73, 78, 79, 81, 114, 123, 196, 210
NMDA receptors, 73, 78, 210
NO, 165
non-human, 85, 87, 88, 99, 102, 107
non-human primates, 85, 87, 88, 99, 102
non-steroidal anti-inflammatory drugs, 50
nontoxic, 111, 203, 211
normal, 11, 12, 13, 17, 27, 31, 32, 40, 46, 47, 49, 51, 53, 55, 70, 72, 77, 87, 99, 114, 115, 117, 118, 119, 121, 125, 127, 128, 129, 132, 135, 143, 145, 146, 150, 152, 153, 155, 166, 180, 182, 188, 189, 195, 202, 205, 210, 212, 213, 214, 221, 224, 227, 230, 231, 232, 251, 255, 265, 268, 271, 274, 278, 279, 280

normal aging, 11, 31, 32, 51, 87, 99, 182, 268, 274
normal development, 115, 117
normalization, 225, 227
North America, 251
North Carolina, 145
NSAIDs, 121, 183
N-terminal, 62, 91, 93, 95, 98, 99, 105, 107, 126, 147, 151, 188, 195, 203
nuclear, 126, 136, 167, 208, 244, 248, 249
nucleation, 200
nuclei, 206, 224
nucleus, 201, 213, 221, 229, 237, 247
nutrition, 200

O

observations, 101, 120, 124, 132, 137, 149
occlusion, 169
occupational, 264, 265, 267
ODN, 86, 95
older adults, 10, 11, 12, 13, 14, 15, 16, 22, 23, 24, 26, 28, 29, 30, 32, 33
olfactory nerve, 151
oligodeoxynucleotides, 86, 95, 111
oligomer, 97, 107
oligomeric, 46, 60, 63, 68, 97, 104, 109, 142, 165
oligomerization, 92, 97, 109, 202
oligomers, 46, 61, 68, 82, 85, 95, 97, 98, 101, 106, 107, 108, 110, 112, 115, 119, 139, 164, 176, 202, 214, 216
oligosaccharide, 129, 134
Omega-3, 174, 176
omission, 222
Oncogene, 139, 214, 215
onion, 135
on-line, 221
operator, 225
oral, 94, 97, 105, 110, 246
organ, 52, 87, 133
organelles, 81, 126, 187, 188
organic, 264, 276
organism, 117, 135, 163
osmotic, 98, 138
OST, 134, 135, 142
ovariectomized, 122
ovary, 136
overproduction, 86
oxidants, 174
oxidation, 124, 136, 140, 203, 211
oxidative, 150, 164, 168, 169, 173, 179, 187, 189, 191, 195, 196, 199, 203, 206, 209, 212, 214, 215, 216
oxidative damage, 179, 203, 215
oxidative stress, 150, 164, 168, 169, 173, 187, 189, 191, 195, 196, 199, 203, 206, 209, 214, 215, 216
oxide, 59, 165, 179, 182, 209
oxygen, 125, 169, 182, 200, 214

P

P300, 17
Paget's disease, 244, 248
pain, 193, 248
parenchyma, 50, 51, 60
parenchymal, 44, 51, 62, 98, 112, 169, 183, 184, 256
parietal cortex, 256
parietal lobe, 11, 27, 171, 255
parietal lobes, 11, 27, 255
Paris, 63
Parkinson, 234, 235, 236, 239, 240, 244, 261
Parkinson's, vi, viii, 152, 164, 187, 200, 208, 219, 220, 224, 225, 227, 234, 235, 236, 237, 238, 239, 240, 241
Parkinson's disease (PD) viii, 152, 164, 187, 200, 208, 219, 220, 224, 225, 227, 234, 235, 236, 237, 238, 239, 240, 241
parkinsonism, 236, 237, 239, 244, 245, 249, 251, 253, 258
particles, 148, 156
passive, vii, 17, 22, 53, 69, 85, 90, 91, 92, 97, 98, 100, 101, 102, 103, 107, 110, 170, 180, 195, 222
patents, 113
pathogenesis, vii, viii, 38, 40, 44, 57, 67, 68, 79, 86, 104, 108, 152, 158, 159, 176, 186, 187, 189, 190, 191, 196, 205, 212, 256, 257
pathogenic, vii, viii, 48, 50, 61, 87, 164, 176, 214, 215, 252, 254
pathogens, 43, 61, 163
pathological aging, 11
pathology, 11, 12, 13, 17, 27, 39, 40, 41, 42, 44, 46, 51, 54, 58, 60, 61, 63, 64, 69, 76, 77, 80, 81, 82, 87, 90, 91, 93, 96, 102, 103, 104, 108, 109, 110, 111, 140, 156, 161, 164, 166, 168, 171, 173, 175, 182, 186, 190, 193, 194, 202, 206, 212, 235, 237, 246, 249
pathophysiology, 199, 263
pathways, vii, 37, 38, 39, 42, 50, 51, 54, 59, 67, 69, 76, 138, 177, 188, 196, 200, 201, 248
PCA, 171

PCR, 47, 171
PDGF, 172
PDI, 125, 126, 133
pedigree, 250, 252
peer, 123
peer review, 123
peers, 266
penetrance, 253
peptidase, 50, 128, 171
peptide, vii, 37, 42, 44, 50, 55, 57, 59, 60, 61, 62, 63, 65, 68, 74, 80, 82, 85, 86, 87, 88, 89, 90, 92, 93, 94, 95, 96, 97, 98, 100, 101, 102, 103, 104, 105, 106, 107, 108, 109, 110, 111, 112, 115, 126, 128, 129, 132, 140, 141, 142, 150, 154, 158, 161, 163, 164, 166, 167, 168, 170, 175, 177, 178, 179, 181, 183, 185, 186, 187, 188, 189, 190, 194, 200, 202, 205, 209, 211, 212, 215, 216
perception, 12, 17, 114, 264
perfusion, 72, 255, 256, 258
Peripheral, 53, 54, 101, 104, 169, 177, 210, 211, 212
peripheral blood mononuclear cell, 172
permeabilization, 203
permit, 22, 70
peroxidation, 203
peroxisomes, 46, 62, 146, 151
personal hygiene, 246
personal relationship, 271
personality, 247, 250, 252, 253, 254
personality traits, 247
PET, 17, 77, 219, 220, 231, 232, 233, 240, 244, 254, 255, 257, 259
PG, 60, 61
P-glycoprotein, 52, 56, 65, 80
PGRN, 243, 244, 247, 249, 251, 253, 254, 255, 256, 257, 262
pH, 48, 58, 127, 129
phage, 92, 95, 98, 105, 107
phagocytic, 44, 52, 56, 90, 91, 168
phagocytosis, 38, 41, 44, 45, 49, 52, 53, 54, 60, 61, 64, 89, 100, 109, 166, 167, 168, 170, 182, 186, 217
pharmaceutical, 90, 92, 114, 120
pharmaceutical companies, 90, 92
pharmaceutical industry, 114
pharmacological, 72, 85, 87, 174, 219, 274
pharmacological treatment, 72, 85, 87, 174, 219
pharmacology, 64
pharmacotherapy, 108
phenolic, 176
phenotype, 41, 109, 211, 213, 225, 246, 252, 258, 262, 274, 279
phenotypes, 115, 182, 208, 210, 245, 253, 260
phenylbutyrate, 211, 215
pheochromocytoma, 212
Philadelphia, 266
phonological, 272, 273
phosphate, 134
phosphoinositides, 200
phospholipase C, 136, 138, 142
phospholipids, 148
phosphorylation, 108, 151, 259
Phosphorylation, 154
photon, 245, 254
photoreceptor, 208
physicians, 162, 255
physiological, 118, 120, 136, 204, 205, 221
physiology, 188
Pick's bodies, 247
pig, 55,61, 79, 188, 191
pilot study, 87, 132, 155, 239
pioglitazone, 153, 155
pituitary tumors, 117
placebo, 89, 90, 106, 114, 119, 121, 122, 123, 124, 139, 140, 175
planning, 221, 251, 270, 272, 277
plaque, 41, 46, 47, 53, 54, 56, 59, 61, 62, 63, 65, 68, 69, 70, 80, 85, 87, 88, 89, 90, 91, 93, 94, 95, 98, 99, 101, 103, 105, 108, 109, 110, 114, 117, 119, 121, 122, 124, 127, 128, 132, 138, 150, 165, 166, 167, 168, 169, 170, 173, 175, 180, 181, 184, 208
plasma, 46, 48, 50, 51, 53, 63, 67, 68, 72, 74, 76, 78, 88, 90, 99, 101, 104, 111, 126, 135, 136, 137, 145, 146, 147, 152, 153, 163, 172, 177, 181, 199, 200, 201, 204, 205, 209, 210, 211, 212, 213, 215, 216, 252, 257
plasma levels, 76
plasma membrane, 46, 48, 67, 68, 72, 74, 76, 78, 126, 135, 136, 137
plasmid, 136
plasminogen, 38, 48, 59, 60, 61, 64
plasticity, 79, 82, 97, 98, 106, 107, 111, 142, 152, 188, 208, 213, 216
platelet, 172, 178, 217
platelet derived growth factor, 172
platelets, 62, 169, 176
play, vii, 40, 43, 44, 46, 47, 48, 49, 50, 51, 53, 63, 80, 185, 187, 188, 191, 201, 204, 205
pneumonia, 162
polarization, 61

polarized light, 204
polyglutamine, 208, 216
polymerase, 206
polymerization, 208
polymers, 201
polymorphism, viii, 145, 146, 156, 158, 159, 189
polypeptides, 86, 88, 142, 186
polyunsaturated fatty acid, 206, 210
pools, 76
poor, 119, 138, 149, 155, 166, 190, 231, 251, 254, 263, 266, 267, 268, 270, 271, 272, 273, 274
poor performance, 266, 267, 270, 271, 273
population, 113, 122, 148, 149, 154, 158, 162, 186, 245, 250, 257, 261, 263, 265, 266, 276
pore, 126, 132, 203
pores, 214
positive correlation, 93, 173, 206
positive feedback, 169
positive macrophages, 177
positron emission tomography, 77, 254
posterior cingulated, 256
posterior cortex, 256
postmenopausal women, 122, 140, 143
postmortem, 46, 49, 161, 165, 169, 183
postsynaptic, 69, 72, 78, 79
power, 124, 222, 241, 268
PPARγ, 152
praxis, 252
preclinical, 85, 87, 89, 90, 123, 235
prediction, 12, 132, 181
predictors, 15, 150, 158, 179, 223, 264
pre-existing, 90, 93, 99
preference, 26, 253
prefrontal cortex, 28, 34, 99, 221, 232, 233
premature death, 61
presenilin 1, 116, 248, 254, 262
Presenilin 2, 244
pressure, 49, 246
presynaptic, 69, 71, 72, 73, 78, 193
prevention, 88, 99, 107, 120, 121, 179
preventive, 167
primates, 51, 85, 87, 99, 111, 112, 197
priming, 12, 32, 33, 93, 94
priming paradigm, 33
principal component analysis, 171
prion diseases, 152
private, 114
probability, 25, 268
probe, 22, 72
problem-solving, 272
problem-solving task, 272
procedural memory, 234
prodrome, 178
production, 37, 38, 56, 57, 69, 70, 73, 74, 75, 78, 80, 81, 93, 94, 95, 97, 98, 101, 107, 109, 114, 117, 118, 120, 165, 166, 168, 172, 173, 186, 187, 188, 189, 190, 191, 194, 196, 201, 203, 209, 215, 264
prognosis, 246, 257
program, 29, 121, 225, 227
progranulin gene, 243, 247, 258
progressive neurodegenerative disorder, 186
progressive supranuclear palsy, 239, 244, 249, 254
proinflammatory, 165, 172, 192
pro-inflammatory, 40, 41, 44, 94, 176, 201, 203, 205
prokaryotes, 126
prokaryotic, 126
proliferation, 80, 94, 168, 182, 213, 248
promoter, 39, 114, 117, 137, 148, 156, 159, 166
propagation, 72, 118
property, 121
prostaglandin, 166, 179
prostate, 132
protease inhibitors, 52, 188, 191, 193, 194
proteases, 57, 60, 69, 115, 186, 187, 188, 189, 190, 193, 194, 195, 196
protection, 103, 152
protective factors, 180
protective role, 41, 150, 201
protein disulfide isomerase, 136, 139, 140, 142
protein family, 140
protein folding, 214, 248
protein misfolding, 112, 210
protein oxidation, 203
protein synthesis, 172
proteins, 49, 50, 51, 55, 62, 65, 74, 111, 113, 114, 116, 118, 124, 125, 126, 127, 128, 129, 133, 135, 136, 137, 139, 140, 141, 142, 148, 151, 157, 159, 166, 167, 168, 172, 175, 181, 186, 187, 188, 189, 191, 192, 194, 202, 203, 207, 247, 248, 250, 259
Proteins, 115, 124, 125, 126, 127, 134, 136
proteolysis, 61, 64, 99, 152, 192, 206
proteolytic enzyme, 45, 192
proteomics, 163, 170
prototype, 93
pruning, 109, 117, 138, 141
PSEN1, 38, 39
pseudo, 125
Pseudomonas, 86, 95
PSP, 244, 249, 254
psychiatric disorder, 263

psychiatric hospitals, 245
psychological distress, 76, 82
psychosis, 263, 266, 267, 274, 277, 278
psychotic, 254, 263, 264, 265, 266, 274
psychotic symptoms, 264, 265, 267
public funding, 114
pumps, 54
purification, 135, 142, 196
pyramidal, 48, 49, 251, 254

Q

quality of life, 224, 257
questionnaires, 224

R

R&D, 145
racial groups, 148
radiological, 258
RAGE, 43, 50, 51, 54, 57, 65, 104, 164, 169, 177, 180, 184
rain, 11, 98, 180
range, 22, 23, 28, 46, 132, 149, 164, 167, 168, 171, 174, 204, 227, 255, 263, 264, 265, 266, 268, 270, 273, 274
RANTES, 171, 172
ras, 215
rat, 42, 46, 47, 55, 56, 57, 58, 60, 62, 63, 65, 82, 98, 137, 138, 141, 142, 148, 155, 193, 194, 196
rating scale, 219, 225, 230, 268
ratings, 17, 33
rats, 47, 55, 111, 141, 155, 168, 174, 180
RB, 80
reaction time, 220, 232, 233
reactive oxygen, 44, 56, 60, 165, 181, 186, 203, 213
reactive oxygen species, 44, 56, 60, 165, 181, 186, 203, 213
reactive oxygen species (ROS), 186
reactivity, 108
reading, 77, 252, 253, 265, 266
reagent, 136
reagents, 128, 137, 142, 165
real time, 171
reality, 32
reasoning, 232, 272
recall, 14, 16, 17, 23, 24, 25, 219, 221, 222, 223, 231, 234, 253, 271
recall information, 24
recalling, 224
receptors, vii, 37, 38, 41, 42, 43, 44, 45, 50, 52, 53, 54, 55, 57, 58, 60, 61, 63, 68, 69, 71, 72, 73, 78, 80, 100, 137, 138, 147, 157, 164, 167, 171, 193, 210, 232
recognition, 9, 17, 21, 22, 23, 24, 25, 30, 34, 61, 93, 110, 126, 219, 221, 222, 223, 231, 234, 271
recognition test, 222, 223
recollection, 23, 233
reconstruction, 34, 250
recovery, viii, 70, 72, 145, 146, 149, 150, 151, 153, 156, 264
recruiting, 29
recycling, 68, 72, 74, 76, 78, 81
red wine, 123
redox, 172
refining, 254
reflection, 267
reflexes, 246, 252, 254
refractory, 236
regeneration, 151, 212
regional, 35, 143, 159, 225, 227
Registry, 222
regular, 46, 47, 246
regulation, 49, 59, 61, 65, 75, 78, 98, 152, 172, 176, 181, 182, 185, 189, 192, 193, 200, 207, 215, 239, 246, 247
regulators, 187, 212
rehabilitation, 156
reinforcement, 221, 272
reinforcement learning, 272
relationship, vii, 62, 65, 67, 69, 70, 71, 80, 124, 149, 179, 193, 216, 231, 233, 236, 238, 243, 251, 264, 266, 267, 271, 272, 280
relatives, 157, 270
relevance, 29, 54, 65, 223, 224, 231, 271
reliability, 225
religiosity, 254
remediation, 263, 274, 280
remodeling, 47, 213
remodelling, 211
repair, 145, 146, 148, 151, 152, 153, 172, 247
reperfusion, 196
repetitions, 233
replication, 12, 27, 173
reproduction, 246
reservoir, 51, 117
residues, 45, 93, 95, 108, 147, 188, 200
resistance, 52, 159, 182, 213
resolution, 132

resources, 15
respiratory, 248
responsiveness, 153
retention, 25, 34, 222, 236, 265, 271
retention interval, 25
reticulum, 45, 46, 68, 74, 114, 139, 140, 143
returns, 269
Reynolds, 142, 186, 196
rheumatoid arthritis, 163
ribose, 206
right hemisphere, 254
rigidity, 246, 251
risk, 49, 58, 76, 77, 82, 93, 122, 146, 148, 149, 150, 153, 154, 156, 157, 158, 159, 172, 182, 189, 190, 211, 245, 247, 248, 252, 261, 265, 266, 267, 268, 270, 276, 277, 279
risk factors, 148, 149, 157, 190, 245, 247, 248, 265, 277, 279
risks, 154
RNA, 170, 200
RNAi, 143
rodent, 42, 110, 123, 165
rofecoxib, 175
ROI, 220, 225, 226, 227, 229, 231
ROS, 186
rosiglitazone, 152, 153, 158, 159
Royal Society, 35
Russia, 123

S

safety, 87, 89, 92, 96, 99, 103, 109, 143
sales, 121
salt, 123
sample, 156, 204, 220, 222, 223, 225, 229, 230, 231, 233, 268
sampling, 70
saturated fat, 123
Scandinavia, 30, 34
scavenger, 42, 51, 55, 56, 57, 58, 59, 60, 61, 64, 214
Schiff, 110
schizophrenia, viii, 33, 237, 263, 264, 265, 266, 267, 268, 269, 270, 271, 272, 273, 274, 275, 276, 277, 278, 279, 280
schizophrenic patients, 276, 280
Schwann cells, 135
sclerosis, 257
scores, 122, 132, 221, 222, 229, 231, 265, 268
SD, 65, 243, 245, 246, 252, 253, 254, 256
SDS, 116, 128, 131
search, 24, 118, 125, 196, 273
secrete, 132
secretion, 59, 65, 74, 82, 97, 116, 117, 120, 128, 188, 200, 215
seed, 68
segmentation, 225, 227
seizures, 70, 71, 74
selectivity, 231
Self, 213
self-awareness, 28
self-care, 251
self-report, 223
SEM, 71, 73, 75
semantic, 10, 30, 222, 223, 243, 245, 246, 252, 272
semantic information, 222
semantic relatedness, 30
senescence, 192
senile, 30, 39, 40, 42, 44, 57, 61, 62, 63, 64, 80, 104, 161, 179, 180, 185, 190, 192, 201, 245
senile dementia, 57, 61, 63, 64, 180
senile plaques, 40, 42, 44, 80, 104, 179, 185, 190, 192, 201
senility, 162
sensation, 26
sensitivity, 152, 257
sensory systems, 28
sentences, 252
separation, 187
September 11, 30
sequencing, 273
series, 15, 24, 101, 113, 114, 149, 169, 171, 172, 258
serine, 48
serotonin, 257
serum, 87, 89, 91, 174, 203
services, 267
severity, 17, 27, 101, 150, 169, 199, 206, 208, 227, 231, 232, 233
sex, 155, 225, 265, 269
sexual behaviour, 254
shares, 50
sharing, 247
shock, 203
short period, 24, 90, 207, 268, 272
short-term memory, 34
shoulder, 248
side effects, 89, 92, 98, 167
signal peptide, 126, 200, 205
signal transduction, 121, 141, 174
signaling, 41, 51, 64, 78, 145, 146, 153, 158, 171, 173, 176, 181, 214

signaling pathways, 78, 171
signals, 34
signs, 89, 116, 224, 246, 251
similarity, 23
sites, 40, 41, 45, 48, 50, 54, 81, 115, 120, 126, 147, 148, 204, 205
skills, 10, 29, 118, 223, 233, 246, 265, 266
skin, 13, 97
smoothing, 227
social cognition, 34
social skills, 246
social withdrawal, 251
socioeconomic, 257, 265
SOD, 215
sodium, 49, 69, 71, 73, 207, 211
sodium butyrate, 207, 211
solubility, 93, 119, 121, 163
solvent, 94
somatosensory, 215
sorting, 79, 81
South Carolina, 185, 192
Spain, 219
spatial, 15, 46, 52, 55, 56, 97, 99, 142, 196, 223, 225, 233, 239, 251
spatial array, 15
spatial learning, 52, 56, 97, 196
spatial location, 233
spatial memory, 55, 142
specialized cells, 163
species, 44, 56, 60, 68, 79, 87, 99, 109, 142, 165, 180, 181, 182, 186, 203, 213
specific knowledge, 233
specificity, 32, 55, 63, 257
SPECT, 156, 245, 254, 256, 257
spectrum, 148, 181
speculation, 86
speech, 246, 252, 264
speed, 118, 233, 271, 273, 274
spinal anesthesia, 132
spine, 81, 98
sporadic, vii, 56, 57, 80, 113, 114, 116, 117, 118, 119, 121, 155, 158, 174, 176, 182, 201, 235, 249, 250
sprouting, 194, 208
stability, 79, 152
stabilization, 85, 102
stages, 13, 29, 90, 99, 100, 114, 181, 212, 219, 221, 223, 224, 229, 234, 235
standard deviation, 220, 230, 265
standards, 116, 130, 131
statins, 167, 174, 181
statistical analysis, 255
statistics, 162
stem cells, 63
stereotypical, 77
steroid, 50, 126, 141
steroid hormone, 50, 126
stimulant, 232
stimulus, 14, 16, 22, 24, 28, 29, 200, 233, 253, 272
storage, 25, 232, 271, 273
strategies, 13, 15, 85, 89, 92, 95, 98, 102, 110, 153, 186, 272, 277
strength, 11, 221, 274
stress, 10, 22, 76, 80, 81, 121, 149, 150, 164, 168, 169, 170, 172, 173, 187, 189, 191, 193, 195, 196, 199, 203, 206, 209, 210, 214, 215, 216
stressors, 76, 178
striatum, 213, 233, 240
stroke, 162, 164, 211
strokes, 122
stromal, 171
structural defect, 117
subgroups, 229, 240, 269, 270
subjective, 30
substantia nigra, 180, 247
substitution, 202, 273
substrates, 187, 191, 213, 232, 233, 235, 269
suffering, 102, 113, 150
sugars, 134
sulfur, 136
Sun, ii, iii, v, vii, 61, 62, 80, 112, 161, 195
superoxide, 203
superoxide dismutase, 203
suppression, 60, 70, 188, 191, 192, 201
suppressor, 178
surgery, 132, 149, 159, 224
surgical, 150, 224
survival, 46, 47, 54, 90, 125, 154, 163, 179, 188, 201, 208, 215, 217, 246, 251
surviving, 117
survivors, 155
susceptibility, viii, 60, 145, 146, 148, 150, 152, 153, 157, 176, 188, 260
susceptibility genes, 145, 146
Sweden, 257
switching, 94
symbols, 253, 273
sympathy, 246
symptoms, 86, 114, 116, 156, 162, 221, 232, 246, 247, 251, 253, 254, 255, 257, 264, 265, 267, 277

synapse, 74, 170
synapses, 117, 133, 135, 138, 176, 208
synaptic plasticity, 79, 82, 97, 98, 106, 107, 111, 142, 188, 208
synaptic strength, 221
synaptic transmission, 67, 69, 71, 72, 74, 76, 78, 79
synaptic vesicles, 72, 74
synaptogenesis, 152
synaptophysin, 74
synchronous, 70, 155
syndrome, 116, 117, 118, 210, 235, 253, 254, 256, 260, 262, 276
synthesis, 116, 118, 120, 126, 127, 128, 134, 135, 147, 172, 178, 191, 194, 207
systemic immune response, 190
systems, 34, 121, 125, 137, 138, 182, 213, 221, 224, 233, 239, 240

T

T cell, 53, 88, 89, 92, 93, 96, 97, 102, 108, 109, 112, 165, 171, 183, 193, 194
T cells, 89, 165, 171, 183
tandem repeats, 95, 106, 247
tangles, 12, 109, 123, 161, 165
TAR, 244, 247, 248, 249
tardive dyskinesia, 280
targets, 57, 64, 79, 157, 164, 167, 189, 257
task demands, 22, 23, 27
task difficulty, 231
task force, 237
task performance, 14, 274
tau, vii, 86, 89, 90, 96, 102, 108, 109, 151, 153, 159, 192, 193, 243, 244, 246, 247, 249, 251, 253, 256, 257, 258
tau mutation, 243, 247
tau pathology, 109
T-cell, 94, 96, 171
technology, 29
telephone, 253
temperature, 133
temporal, viii, 31, 32, 46, 77, 79, 81, 156, 174, 221, 222, 223, 224, 230, 231, 240, 243, 244, 245, 247, 251, 254, 255, 256
temporal lobe, 31, 32, 77, 81, 221, 230, 231, 240, 243, 244, 245, 247, 251, 254, 255
terminals, 71
terrorist, 30
terrorist attack, 30
test items, 23
test scores, 266
testis, 46
tetanus, 71, 72, 86, 96
Tetanus, 72
TGF, 64, 117, 166, 168, 184
TGFβ, 38, 41
thalamus, 11, 12
therapeutic agents, viii, 114, 117, 118, 124, 137, 138, 187, 188, 191, 208
therapeutic approaches, 196
therapeutic interventions, 153
therapeutic targets, 157, 164
therapeutics, viii, 105, 188, 190, 192, 194
therapy, 41, 54, 96, 109, 111, 117, 122, 159, 164, 170, 172, 193, 224
thinking, 264
thioredoxin, 136
threat, 34
threshold, 27, 176, 227
thyroid, 247
tight junction, 65
time, 13, 15, 17, 24, 25, 34, 57, 70, 77, 78, 90, 95, 114, 122, 126, 138, 163, 165, 171, 174, 201, 205, 219, 221, 222, 223, 225, 229, 233, 251, 264, 266, 267, 268, 270, 272, 274, 276
TIMP, 56
tissue, 48, 49, 56, 60, 61, 64, 77, 98, 100, 141, 163, 164, 165, 167, 171, 174, 175, 178, 180, 195, 201, 215
tissue plasminogen activator, 56, 61
TLE, 77
TLR2, 178
TNF, 165, 172, 173, 193, 195
Togo, 165, 183
tolerance, 95
Toll-like, 164
toxic, 68, 85, 92, 93, 97, 98, 99, 110, 119, 120, 138, 152, 185, 186, 187, 189, 190, 191, 192, 202, 203, 217
toxicity, 58, 93, 95, 101, 103, 114, 115, 118, 119, 120, 121, 122, 124, 138, 145, 181, 202, 205, 208, 210, 214, 216
toxin, 71, 72, 86, 96, 97, 108
toxins, 176, 203
traffic, 81, 248
training, 232, 238
trajectory, 11, 263, 266, 267
trans, 82, 146
transcranial direct current stimulation, 232, 235
transcription, 121, 146, 159, 167, 170, 172, 176, 248

transcription factor, 121, 167, 170, 172, 248
transcription factors, 167, 170, 172, 248
transcripts, 173, 181
transfer, 61, 63, 92, 125, 135, 195, 205
transforming growth factor, 41, 193
transgene, 39, 199, 206, 212
transgenic mice, 39, 40, 44, 47, 49, 54, 55, 58, 59, 61, 63, 64, 69, 70, 74, 80, 81, 85, 87, 88, 90, 91, 94, 95, 97, 98, 103, 107, 108, 109, 110, 111, 112, 114, 117, 119, 124, 138, 141, 142, 147, 150, 151, 152, 155, 159, 163, 166, 167, 169, 173, 175, 178, 179, 181, 184, 205, 206, 209, 215
transgenic mouse, vii, 39, 51, 85, 87, 89, 91, 95, 100, 105, 112, 114, 117, 118, 119, 120, 121, 122, 123, 124, 142, 170, 174, 177, 181, 199, 203, 205, 206, 208, 209, 210, 211, 212
translation, 126, 137, 142
translocation, 151
transmembrane, 43, 115, 126, 137, 171, 187, 202, 216, 217
transmembrane region, 187
transmission, 67, 69, 71, 72, 74, 76, 78, 79, 232
transplant, 52, 147
transplantation, 41, 53, 156
transport, vii, 37, 38, 50, 51, 52, 55, 57, 65, 69, 82, 104, 145, 146, 147, 152, 153, 157, 169, 177, 188, 197, 244, 247, 248
trauma, 149
traumatic brain injury, 76, 149, 150, 155, 156
tremor, 246
trial, 85, 89, 90, 92, 94, 99, 102, 105, 106, 119, 120, 121, 122, 123, 139, 140, 142, 143, 152, 153, 167, 175, 272
trial and error, 272
trichostatin, 200, 207
trichostatin A, 200, 207
trifluoroacetic acid, 127, 128, 129
triggers, 191
triglycerides, 147
TSA, 200, 207
tuberculosis, 163
tumor, 47, 52, 56, 62, 117, 139, 165, 171, 201
tumor cells, 52, 139
tumor necrosis factor, 47, 56, 165, 171
tumors, 117
tumour, 50, 55
turnover, 187
two-dimensional, 159
type 2 diabetes, 152

U

ubiquitin, 243, 244, 247, 248, 249, 250, 252, 253, 254, 259
Ubiquitin, 245
Ubiquitin-proteasome system, 245
UK, 245, 258, 259, 260, 266
umbilical cord, 52, 53, 62
umbilical cord blood, 53, 62
unfolded, 14
United Kingdom, 89
United States, 113, 121, 155, 157, 158, 162
updating, 238
urea, 127, 128, 129
urinary, 123
urinary tract, 123
urinary tract infection, 123
urokinase, 48

V

vaccination, 52, 55, 58, 62, 87, 88, 90, 94, 95, 96, 99, 100, 103, 105, 106, 108, 109, 110, 140, 141, 170, 172, 178, 180, 183
Vaccination, 87, 89, 94, 102, 112, 214
vaccine, 85, 88, 92, 93, 94, 95, 96, 97, 99, 102, 104, 105, 107, 108, 109, 112, 118, 119, 120, 142, 161, 164, 167, 172
valence, 13, 14, 16, 17, 22, 23, 26, 28, 29, 30, 32, 33
valenced information, 15
validation, 92, 142, 171
validity, 15, 89, 221, 222, 223
values, 76, 174, 228, 257
variability, 23, 225, 243, 245, 246, 247, 250, 251, 260
variables, 222, 229
variation, 58, 156, 269
vascular cell adhesion molecule, 172
vascular dementia, 168, 238
vascular disease, 122
vascular inflammation, 169
vascular system, 163
vasculature, 48, 49, 57
vasoconstriction, 101
vasopressin, 136
VCAM, 172
vector, 54, 62, 95, 96, 97, 105, 106, 108, 112
velocity, 135
verbal fluency, 277

versatility, 99
vesicle, 68, 71, 72, 73, 74, 75, 76, 78, 81, 82, 189, 217, 248
vessels, 51, 65, 169
veterans, 150
video clips, 16, 22
Vietnam, 150
virus, 86, 96, 105, 146, 164
viscosity, 254
visible, 40
visual area, 223
visual attention, 31
visual memory, 32, 222, 223, 231, 279
visual processing, 35, 269
visual stimulus, 233
visuospatial, 220, 231, 232, 253, 272, 273
VLDL, 146, 147
voxel-based morphometry, 219, 225, 227, 228, 235, 237, 240

W

walking, 248
water, 86, 87, 91, 93, 107
water maze, 86, 87, 91, 93, 107
water-soluble, 86
weakness, 248, 254
web, 121, 123
western blot, 128
white blood cells, 168
white matter, 11, 35, 40, 135, 221, 225, 227, 256, 258
wild type, 42, 44, 46, 94, 151, 166, 173, 201, 206
windows, 35
wine, 123
Wisconsin, 270, 272, 276, 278
withdrawal, 253
women, 122, 140, 143
Women's Health Initiative, 122, 143
workers, 97, 98, 100, 117, 131, 136
working memory, 9, 17, 21, 23, 31, 219, 221, 224, 232, 234, 235, 236, 237, 238, 239, 240, 270, 272, 273
workspace, 272
wound repair, 247

X

xenobiotics, 126

Y

yang, 57
yeast, 125, 140, 213
yes/no, 9, 21
yield, 27, 28, 29, 120
yin, 57
young adults, 11, 13, 14, 15, 264

Z

zinc, 46, 47, 48, 49, 50, 64
Zn, 203, 215